NARRATIVE THERAPIES
WITH CHILDREN AND ADOLESCENTS

Narrative Therapies with Children and Adolescents

Edited by

CRAIG SMITH
DAVID NYLUND

Foreword by Melissa Elliott Griffith

THE GUILFORD PRESS
New York   London

© 1997 The Guilford Press
A Division of Guilford Publications, Inc.
72 Spring Street, New York, NY 10012
www.guilford.com

Printed in the United States of America

This book is printed on acid-free paper.

Last digit is print number: 9   8   7   6   5   4   3   2

Library of Congress Cataloging-in-Publication Data

Narrative therapies with children and adolescents / edited by Craig
Smith, David Nylund; foreword by Melissa Elliott Griffith.
    p.   cm.
Includes bibliographical references and index.
ISBN 1-57230-253-4
1. Child psychotherapy.   2. Storytelling—Therapeutic use.
3. Family psychotherapy.   I. Smith, Craig R., 1954–   .
II. Nylund, David.
RJ505.575.N37   1997
618.92'8914—dc21
                                                97-35905
                                                  CIP

I play it cool
And dig all jive.
That's the reason
I stay alive.

My motto,
As I live and learn,
is
Dig and Be Dug
In Return.

—Langston Hughes

After all, what is reality anyway? Nothin' but a
collective hunch. My space chums think reality was once a
primitive method of crowd control that got out of hand.

—Jane Wagner

The world's most renowned, expert computer scientists spent 10 years
programming the most sophisticated computer on the face of
the earth. The computer had more memory capacity than any other
ever made and could respond with lightning-quick speed. They
programmed every bit and byte, every iota of information from
every conceivable discipline since the dawn of civilization. After this
exhaustive effort was complete, the computer was finally ready to
respond to any of the scientists' questions! They thought long and
hard for a suitable question. Finally, one typed in the query, "Will
computers ever replace human beings?" Within a micro-second, the
computer flashed, "That reminds me of a story. . . ."

—Anonymous

Calvin and Hobbes

by Bill Watterson

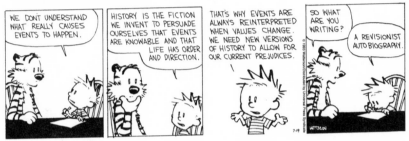

Contributors

Janet Adams-Westcott, PhD, Laureate Psychiatric Clinic and Hospital, Tulsa, Oklahoma

Tom Andersen, MD, PhD, Institute of Community Medicine, University of Tromsø, Norway

Harlene Anderson, PhD, Houston Galveston Institute; Taos Institute, Houston, Texas

Pam Barragar-Dunne, PhD, RDT-BC, Department of Theatre Arts and Dance, California State University at Los Angeles, Los Angeles, California; Drama Therapy Institute of Los Angeles, Los Angeles, California; private practice, Los Angeles, California

Lisa Berndt, MSW, Project Respect, San Francisco, California

Katherine Ceske, PhD, Kaiser Permanente, Mental Health Department, Stockton, California

Gene Combs, MD, Evanston Family Therapy Center, Evanston, Illinois; Chicago Center for Family Health, Chicago, Illinois

Victoria C. Dickerson, PhD, Bay Area Family Therapy Training Associates, Cupertino, California; Mental Research Institute, Palo Alto, California

Cheryl Dobbins, MA, Caring Parents and Safe Step Programs, Children's Counseling Center, Santa Rosa, California

David Epston, MA, CQSW, The Family Therapy Centre, Auckland, New Zealand

Jennifer C. Freeman, MA, Graduate School of Professional Psychology, John F. Kennedy University, Orinda, California; private practice, Berkeley, California

Jill H. Freedman, MSW, LCSW, Evanston Family Therapy Center, Evanston, Illinois; Chicago Center for Family Health, Chicago, Illinois

Lorraine Grieves, Vancouver Anti-Anorexia League, Vancouver, British Columbia, Canada

Tom Hicks, MSW, PsyD, Solana Beach Counseling Center, San Diego, California; Marriage, Family, Child Counseling Program in Counseling and School Psychology Department, San Diego State University, San Diego, California

Ian Law, Family therapist and training provider, British Columbia, Canada

Sue Levin, PhD, Houston Galveston Institute, Houston, Texas

Dean H. Lobovits, MA, Graduate School of Professional Psychology, John F. Kennedy University, Orinda, California; private practice, Berkeley, California

Stephen Madigan, MSW, PhD, Yaletown Family Therapy, Vancouver, British Columbia, Canada

David Nylund, MSW, LCSW, Kaiser Permanente, Mental Health Department, Stockton, California; Midtown Family Therapy, Sacramento, California; Professional School of Psychology, Sacramento, California

Colin Sanders, MA, The Pacific Youth and Family Services Society, Peak House, Vancouver, British Columbia, Canada; Yaletown Family Therapy, Vancouver, British Columbia, Canada

Peggy Sax, MA, MEd, Stone Mill Associates, Middlebury, Vermont

Craig Smith, PhD, MFCC, Solana Beach Counseling Center, San Diego, California; Marriage, Family, Child Counseling Program in Counseling and School Psychology Department, San Diego State University, San Diego, California

Kathleen Stacey, MA, Southern Child and Adolescent Mental Health Service, Adelaide, South Australia, Australia; Department of Public Health, Flinders University, Adelaide, South Australia, Australia

Kathy Weingarten, PhD, Family Institute of Cambridge, Watertown, Massachusetts; Harvard Medical School, Boston, Massachusetts

Jeffrey L. Zimmerman, PhD, Bay Area Family Therapy Training Associates, Cupertino, California; Mental Research Institute, Palo Alto, California

Acknowledgments

FROM BOTH OF US:

We want to thank Seymour Weingarten, Editor-in-Chief at The Guilford Press, for having the courage to take a risk with us. Jeannie Tang, Production Editor at Guilford, deserves special kudos for her tireless, behind-the-scenes coordination of our book. We also are both indebted to Michael Hoyt for his ongoing consultation and support throughout the editing process.

FROM DAVID NYLUND:

First and foremost, I want to express my gratitude to the contributors to this book, with a particular thanks to my co-editor, Craig Smith. He has become like a brother to me. This book came about only because of our enduring friendship.

My special gratitude goes to my partner, Liz Colt, for her reassurance, passion, and wisdom. I also thank her for her significant contribution at both the editing and proofreading stages.

Michael White, David Epston, and Karl Tomm have been a constant source of inspiration and influence on my work. Victoria Dickerson and Jeff Zimmerman have shaped my way of working. I also thank them for bringing other narrative therapists throughout the world to Northern California. I appreciate our growing friendship and Jeff's introducing me to the Grateful Dead! Stephen Madigan has encouraged me to write and supported my ideas. I also appreciate his tireless efforts in organizing the annual Narrative Ideas and Therapeutic Practices Conference.

I also want to recognize a growing California narrative community that shares ideas and gets together annually at a California participant's conference. This group includes David Marsten, Roxanne Rankin, Larry Zucker, Tom Hicks, Rick Maisel, Hasana Fletcher, Sandy Braff, Jim Walt, Sandy Walt, Linda Crawford, Pam Barragar-Dunne, Craig Smith, Kevin Fitzsimmons, Holly Jones, Charley Lang, Stephanie Gregory, Peggy Simpson, Debora Brooks, and Irene Williams.

I especially want to give thanks to José Rivera and Jack Gilliland at Kaiser Permanente, Stockton, for their innovative leadership and continuing support of diversity and a narrative practice. I also thank my colleagues in the mental health department at Kaiser—Victor Corsiglia, Paula Tucker, Robert Fernbach, Tom Elmore, Katherine Ceske, Todd Fetherston, Edwina Serventi, Curtis Chun, Alison Kemps, Sharon Hodges, Gean McFadden, Mike McFadden, Pat Wong, Linda Liem, Larry Meade, Beth Wilson, David Richwerger, Shiela Fergusson, Jan Moore, Suzanne Fraga, Juliana Petrosh, John Traylor, Michael Duveneck, and Robin Fennel—with whom I have worked over the past 7 years. Their support of narrative therapy and their participation in reflecting teams have enriched me. Another Kaiser colleague to whom I am indebted for her very special contribution to the book is Laura Padron.

I very much value my friendship and colleagueship with John Thomas, who has been a catalyst in the development of Midtown Family Therapy.

I am grateful to my parents, Gerald and Anita, my grandmother, Billie, and my brothers, Brett and Eric, for their support, encouragement, and love. I know this postmodern stuff is confusing (hazy?), but I think they'll be proud of this project!

Finally, I thank my son, Drake, for his love and friendship and for showing me the wonder of life and his mother, Dorene, who makes it possible for me to work on this book and shows that a postmodern family can work.

FROM CRAIG SMITH:

I want to thank all the unnamed friends and colleagues who have shared their enthusiasm and support. I also want to acknowledge the members of my extended family and my family, especially my parents. In addition to all of their terrific, invaluable support through the years, my parents have encouraged me not to accept conventional institutional authorities, such as the medical establishment, on blind faith.

I also want to express my gratitude toward Linda Terry for her eagerness to include cutting-edge ideas in San Diego State University's Marriage, Family, Child Counseling Program, and for her enthusiastic support of Tom Hicks and myself over several years. Special thanks also to Jennifer Andrews and David Clark at Phillips Graduate Institute. In addition to their personal support, they have made an enormous contribution by building an oasis where students can learn social constructionist and collaborative ideas in Southern California. They have sprouted seeds and carefully watered them, and I have been delighted to witness the growing awareness that has occurred as a result of their tireless efforts. In addition, they have brought many of the contributors in this book to Los Angeles for workshops, and have created helpful videotapes through Master'sWork Productions that have been very useful for my professional growth and for narrative therapy training. Through these opportunities, I have gotten to know many of the contributors in this book personally, which has been a wonderful experience.

I also wish to share my appreciation for my clients over the last 15 years. They have given me the privilege of hearing some of the most poignant and touching aspects of their lives. Also, their feedback on what I've done that has helped and hindered our work together has been invaluable. I feel blessed to be able to do work that I love. In addition, I have benefited tremendously from supervisees' and trainees' well-considered questions and concerns. I continue to learn, grow, and be inspired by all of these conversations, and look forward to more in the future!

I would like to thank Bill O'Hanlon, Bob Schwarz, Stephen Madigan, and Linda Crawford for the tremendous work they have all done in creating exciting, valuable, cutting-edge social constructionist therapy conferences. Pioneers of narratively oriented therapies also deserve special mention for creating numerous possibilities for the rest of us. These inspiring trailblazers include Harlene Anderson, Michael White, David Epston, Harry Goolishian, and Tom Andersen. I also want to express my heartfelt warmth and appreciation for Karl Tomm and Tom Andersen; both Karl and Tom have had an enormous impact on me personally and professionally. Like stalwart friends, their gentle and respectful voices continue to guide me and I feel tremendous gratitude for all they have done for our profession.

I'd also like to recognize all the inspirational and thoughtful people (including some from this book) who post messages on the largely postmodern therapy, computer bulletin board called MFTC-L. They have helped me reflect on many important therapy issues and refine my thinking. Thanks to Ken Stewart for his former "crowd-control" e-mail tagline and to Jeff Chang for his generous solution-oriented resources.

Special thanks to Melissa Elliott Griffith for graciously agreeing to do the Foreword for our book. Her delightful, homespun warmth and wisdom are like a breath of fresh air for our too often stodgy profession.

I'm indebted to the stellar cast of characters who collectively forged this book. I thank them for all their creative and thoughtful chapters. I sincerely hope that through e-mail, computer bulletin boards/World Wide Web sites, future articles, innovative workshops, and so on, we can develop and broaden the conversations that we started here with interested others!

I'd also like to extend my sincere appreciation to the following people who patiently plodded through my early, dense, and bloated drafts of my chapter for this book. I can honestly say this chapter has been "co-constructed" with their apt suggestions! The voices woven into the choir my chapter represents include David Pare; Kathy Weingarten; Peggy Sax; Kathleen Stacey; Erin Galloway; David Nylund; Liz Colt; participants in the Houston Galveston Institute theoretical seminar, including Leonard Bohannon, Sue Levin, Jamie Raser, Diana Carleton, Solomon Yusim, Lorianne Reeves, and Judy Elmquist; Tom Hicks; Larry Laveman; and Wendy West.

The last two people mentioned deserve extra-special kudos. These two wonderful "alliterative" friends (both having the same first and last initials!) provided "double duty" in reading my laborious drafts twice and providing excellent suggestions. Larry was a fantastic supervisor for me many years ago. In his warm, insightful, humorous way, he consistently encouraged me to develop my own, young therapist voice. But he was always there to provide structure or advice when I fell flat on my face. He has continued to support me personally and professionally, and I am very grateful to him. Wendy "Hank" West is a dear cyber-pal whom I met on MFTC-L about 3 years ago. She has been a continual source of camaraderie, integrity, learning, warmth, respect, and inspiration, and has taught me a lot about enduring, at-a-distance friendship. Thanks so much for being you, Wendy!

This montage of appreciation would definitely not be complete without mentioning my sidekick, co-trainer, co-supervisor, and dear friend of 10 years, Tom Hicks. Tom introduced me to narrative therapies. His continually evolving ideas about therapy and social constructionism has inspired and broadened me. He is passionately devoted to his craft, to growing, and to being a genuine "dialogic" participant with me and with others. I am very grateful for how he has helped me stretch in personal and professional ways, even when he had to drag me kicking and screaming! His relaxed humor and ability not to take himself too seriously have been gifts of lightness. As much as I have benefited from my travels to stellar workshops and conferences, like Dorothy after "OZ," I've begun to realize "There's no place like home!" Tom, thanks so very much.

Finally, there's my co-editor and good friend, David "Trams" Nylund. Combining the dependability and sure-handedness of baseball star Alan Trammell with the breezy, irreverent wit of Groucho Marx, he was a joy to work with throughout this project. He was reliably always a quick phone call or e-mail away for coordinating myriad details, and his delightful humor helped me keep things in perspective. He also is one of the most positive and supportive people I know, and I treasure our friendship along with our professional ties.

Foreword

I once saw an advertisement in a fancy gardening catalogue for the most wonderful gift: for a not-so-small fee, a pot of luscious, blooming houseplants would be delivered to the recipient's doorstep at the beginning of every month for one year. I wanted to give this gift to someone who would really appreciate it—me! What a delight it would be to grow flowers in the kitchen in February, to receive a surprise in September. Best of all, I could surely keep anything alive for a month, and then, just as the wilting would begin, the next pot would arrive!

I never indulged this wish to give myself this year of flowers, but in writing the Foreword for this book I have received an even better gift. For months, chapters have arrived on my doorstep from Craig and David, and I have eagerly studied them and incorporated them into my practice. I have given my partner and my coworkers sneak previews so that we could consider the ideas together. Unable to wait for the publication of this book, I shared the drafts with persons I work with in supervision and in therapy. Not only have the ideas from these chapters blossomed, but I can keep them alive for much more than a month. Not all parts of every chapter have been right for flourishing in the climate of my practice, but neither have there been any weeds. Indeed, everything I adopt becomes a hybrid, first with my own thinking, then with the experiences of the persons I talk with in therapy.

There is a great variety to be found in this collection. Some authors conduct their therapeutic conversations with words, and others more with art. Some work with the family in the room, some with only the children in the room, and others mostly with the parents. Some authors call themselves "narrative therapists" and some say their work is "narratively informed," but others never use the word "narrative" as a descriptor for their work. As a collection, then, what is the common thread? All these authors employ a mutualistic approach to therapy. All work within a social constructionist or postmodern perspective where no one view of reality is objectified as the correct view. Common to these chapters is the spirit of hope, wonder, and curiosity that can be felt in the relationships between these therapists/authors and the persons who come to them as clients. Each therapist genuinely seems to be learning from the client. Rarely, if ever, will the reader find the words, "As I expected . . . ," because these therapists do not already know, nor even desire to predict, the thoughts and actions of the clients. They delight in the creativity of the persons with whom they work. Their delight is contagious to us, the readers, and surely to the children and parents with whom they consult.

Still, within this common thread, two strands are distinguished. Some therapists employ a "reauthoring" approach where, together, client and therapist reconstruct a new narrative, less limiting and more freeing than that which existed before. Other therapists employ a "dialogic" or "hermeneutic" approach which focuses on multiple narratives and provides a space for clients to consider their many voices as a way to enter more liberating dialogues.

This is a distinction that has received little attention in the literature, yet it is often a central discussion in conference hallways and in internet chats. I find this distinction informative, as I consider different choice points in a therapy. However, for me, it is not about choosing an approach that will have absolute rule over my work, but about making choices which will influence me at the minute-to-minute level, within a session. Both the narrative and the hermeneutic epistemologists have enriched and anchored my work; indeed, too much would be lost if I were to relate to them in either/or ways.

Over and above these distinctions is the commitment shared by each author in this volume to democracy in therapy. If these practitioners claim foreknowledge about the persons they see in therapy, it is that these persons know as much and more about how their lives are and should be than do therapists. Inspired by them, I have tried to catch myself when I think I "know best" or am seduced by a sense of superior foresight. I want to be on the side of democracy and equality. A simple test can keep me in check on this. It is to ask the question, "Would I speak my thoughts aloud to my consultees?" Even more relevant to this book, "Could I wholeheartedly offer clients my communications to other professionals about their lives?"

To the latter question, the authors and editors of *Narrative Thera-*

pies with Children and Adolescents would give a resounding "Yes." I would be equally comfortable offering this book to persons doing therapy and persons in therapy, including those whose lives were opened to us in these chapters. I would offer it to them with confidence that they would experience honor and hope. Undoubtedly, they would bring back some revisions. But the test of our integrity as therapists is not that we get the final vision right, but that we work and speak and write in a way that is always open, open to receiving the revisions of those with whom we work.

MELISSA ELLIOTT GRIFFITH
Clinical Assistant Professor in Psychiatry
The George Washington University Medical Center

Preface

This book started as an offhand conversation about 3 or 4 years ago during a casual moment at a narrative therapy conference in Vancouver. We had become good friends and were talking about a variety of things. We were struck by how many excellent narrative therapists working with children and adolescents were at this conference. Along with many other tangential conversations, we innocently mused how neat it would be if someday a book could include these and other folks so more people could experience their work.

We both forgot about this conversation. Then, about 2 years later, Dave recalled it and suggested we bring this idea to life. After dialogue back and forth, we decided to contact others to see whether they would be interested in contributing. To our delight, they were. The Guilford Press was very supportive of this book as well, and voilà!

Both of us really enjoy being around children and adolescents and working with them in therapy. We are also passionately committed to helping young clients have a substantial impact on shaping therapy interactions, whether in private practice, school, residential, or other institutional settings. This passion extends to supporting a collaborative, mutual posture with all clients, young and old. Since we each enjoy different ways of practicing narrative therapy, we have chosen to focus on a variety of ways of doing narratively oriented work in this book.

This book is attempting to fill a much-needed gap in the family/systemic therapy literature. Much of conventional family therapy focuses on working with parents. Children's voices often seem to be minimized or not taken seriously as offering distinct and valid perspectives. *Narra-*

tive Therapies with Children and Adolescents attempts to honor their experiential and narrative worlds in systemic therapy. We hope this book will encourage systemic therapists to enter into young persons' experiences of the world and to bring forth creative solutions to problems.

One reason we became attracted to narrative and collaborative ideas was because of their respectful, inclusive, and nonpathologizing posture toward clients. We wish to embody this spirit with our various readers, no matter what theoretical orientation they may prefer. At the same time, we hope this book will provide readers with relevant differences that distinguish these relatively new narrative approaches from other useful and more familiar ways of working with children and teens. At various points in this book, contributors constructively critique traditional ways of working with clients as they highlight these differences.

The various contributors in this book all share postmodern assumptions, such as viewing clients as legitimate co-participants in determining therapeutic directions. However, as the plural title *Narrative Therapies* suggests, there are a number of stylistic and theoretical differences among contributors. For example, some authors feel that therapy is inherently a political act and that therapists should use this awareness in determining their actions. This could include addressing issues of power by such means as helping marginalized voices (e.g., children's voices) become more empowered relative to more dominant voices. This could also involve deconstructing sociocultural stories the therapist feels are oppressive, and minimizing opportunities to collude with narratives the therapist feels are oppressive.

There are other contributors using a narrative metaphor who focus on generating a multiplicity of narratives or voices so that dialogue can occur and so that clients can sort out which of these perspectives seem most fitting in different contexts. These authors attempt to create a therapeutic environment where clients can "say the unsaid"—say things they and others have never heard themselves say before. As this occurs, a spirit of self-reflexivity and dialogue can begin to overshadow previously limiting and adversarial monologues. New narratives about oneself and about others are generated as a result of this process.

We acknowledge that these represent significant theoretical differences. However, we prefer to think of these differences as multicolored threads in a rich tapestry of ideas, rather than as an invitation for pledging of allegiances and for wholesale rejection of differing perspectives. Likewise, we hope that you, our readers, will see this book as an opportunity to sample a large buffet. You may like a couple of aspects of one chapter, a few things from another, and so forth. Perhaps you will be stimulated to pursue a particular author's other writings as part of this ever-evolving meal! Above all, we hope that you will be inspired to develop and refine your own creative responses to these ideas, rather than feeling obliged to conform to any specific way of doing this sort of work.

The two of us embody these theoretical differences, along with this attitude of mutual respect. Dave currently tends to focus more on deconstructing oppressive stories, while Craig presently tends to emphasize creating a dialogue of inner and outer voices (perspectives). However, there are *many* shades of gray here: Dave has been inspired by a number of dialogic, collaborative language systems ideas, and Craig has also been very influenced by sociocultural practices from a re-authoring approach. We hope the different ways of thinking about narrative work that this book represents will stimulate exploratory and respectful discussions among others who also wish to include these different approaches in their ever-expanding narrative horizons.

After Craig's introductory chapter, the book begins with chapters on working with younger children, and concludes with chapters focusing on adolescents. We were both inspired by the "follow-up questions" format in *The New Language of Change* (edited by Steven Friedman; New York: Guilford Press, 1993). As in this book, we hope that our questions at the end of each contributor's chapter ask the sorts of questions you, our readers, might have asked, and that they create more of an intimate atmosphere. Whether or not Dave (DN) or Craig (CS) asks the follow-up questions you see depends on a variety of factors, including our time and the availability of the creative muse!

CRAIG SMITH
DAVID NYLUND

Contents

1

Introduction

COMPARING TRADITIONAL THERAPIES WITH NARRATIVE APPROACHES[1]

CRAIG SMITH

It is both exciting and formidable to offer an introduction for this book. I hope to provide a helpful way of understanding some of the unique narrative assumptions that the contributors to this book utilize. Since their chapters are focused on clinical transcripts, they don't have the opportunity to go into these assumptions in any great depth.

This collection doesn't include another important and increasingly popular postmodern approach to working with children: solution-oriented therapies. Many of the comparisons with traditional therapies mentioned in this introduction also apply to solution-oriented therapies. There are also a number of excellent books and articles available for

---

[1]Narratively oriented therapies are one of several types of postmodern therapeutic approaches. The reader may also wish to explore others, such as Ericksonian and solution-oriented therapies (in regard to the latter, see Footnote 2). Postmodernism is said to have many life-giving roots. These include feminist ideas; the ideas of philosophers and cultural historians, such as Foucault, Derrida, Nietzsche, Heidegger, Gadamer, Wittgenstein, Bakhtin, and Rorty; anthropological and sociological sources; literary criticism; personal construct theory; and humanistic and client-centered influences.

pursuing this innovative approach with children or teens.[2] The present collection focuses on a variety of approaches using a narrative metaphor.[3]

In addition, I want to highlight one particular point. One of the aspects of postmodernism[4] that is especially dear to me is the idea that no one person or approach has the "definitive answer." Although I prefer to orient myself with postmodern assumptions and utilize a narrative metaphor to describe my work, I want to emphasize that traditional therapies can be quite effective. I sincerely hope that readers will *not* infer from this book that narrative, postmodern approaches to working with children are the only effective ones. Many traditional play therapy approaches, family therapy interventions, and so forth have proven helpful and workable for a variety of youth.[5] Also, my therapeutic work has benefited from exposure to many different traditional child therapies and parenting approaches.

Thus, I am not suggesting that all traditional ways of working with and empowering children should be abandoned. Indeed, some of the contributors to this book find that clients like the therapist to occasionally bring in ideas from traditional clinical literature and research for discussion with the clients. This literature has enriched our appreciation for such things as the limitations of verbal therapy with young children; possible temperamental differences between youth; "red flags" that may signal trauma, sexual abuse, physical abuse, or neglect; and differing developmental and maturational capacities in children.

I am writing this chapter in order to introduce some assumptions

[2]See Chang (1996), Durrant (1989, 1990, 1993, 1995), Kowalski (1990), Kral (1986, 1989, 1994), LaFountain, Garner, and Boldosser (1995), Metcalf (1994), Murphy (1994), Pluznick and Rafael (to be published), and Selekman (1993), among others.

[3]Some contributors to this book, such as Tom Andersen, Harlene Anderson, and Sue Levin, don't label themselves "narrative therapists" but do think of therapy as helping clients' stories or meanings about themselves and others to expand or broaden. They also share many of the postmodern assumptions listed here. See the next-to-last section of this chapter for more discussion on this. Because of space limitations, we were not able to include other interesting uses of a narrative metaphor in therapy and developmental psychology. Spence (1982), Schafer (1992), and Stern (1990) offer a psychoanalytic application of narratives. Shawver (1996) offers a postmodern view of psychoanalysis. Eron and Lund (1996) provide an integration of strategic therapy and narrative therapy.

[4]Roger Lowe (1991) offers a succinct definition of postmodernism: "In general terms, Postmodernism represents a radical questioning of the *foundationalism and absolutism* of modern conceptions of knowledge" (p. 43; italics in original).

[5]I use the term "children" or "youth" to refer to both children and adolescents, for space considerations.

that distinguish narrative therapies from traditional ("modernist") approaches, and to clarify how two narratively oriented approaches differ from each other.[6] I hope this will provide a useful context for understanding why therapists in this book emphasize some aspects in their work with youth and de-emphasize others. Most of the assumptions discussed apply to work with both adults and children, but the section on assessment is focused more exclusively on children. Although I have attempted over the last 10 years to immerse myself in various postmodern articles, books, and workshops, my comments in this introduction reflect my *own* understanding of social constructionism and narrative therapies. Thus, different contributors to this book may have other ways of describing their work and their guiding assumptions.

As I shall explore in this chapter, narrative therapists assume that knowledge is socially constructed and that there are many valid, diverse ways of understanding ourselves and others. These ideas are seen as culturally informed and situated in ever-changing local contexts and relationships. Professional, social science ideas about human behavior are viewed as potentially useful ways (among many others) of thinking about clients' concerns, rather than as objective, empirically verified truths. Social constructionism, with its emphasis on partial, perspectival knowing, shifts conventional therapy's emphasis on objectivity and therapeutic certainty to an emphasis on intersubjectivity and therapeutic curiosity.

Traditional individual and systemic therapies generally assume that therapists' objectivity provides the foundation for their being experts in defining clients' problems and solutions.[7] I discuss examples from conventional psychoanalytic, cognitive, behavioral, humanistic, and family systems models to illustrate how traditional therapies assume that therapists are objective observers who discover what is "really" occurring with clients. Therapeutic use of suggestions, homework assignments, psychoeducation, interpretations, and confrontations can be helpful for clients. However, if therapists become convinced that their ideas are "true" and clients happen to find these particular ideas unsuitable, clients' voices can be inadvertently diminished, and other unwanted side

---

[6]I use "modernism" interchangeably with "traditional," "conventional," or "objectivist" therapies.

[7]I recognize that the term "traditional approaches" encompasses a very broad sweep of diverse therapeutic modalities. Some of the contrasts made between "postmodern" and "traditional" may be less distinct or relevant for a given form of traditional individual or family therapy. I hope that as a whole, however, many of the contrasting philosophical assumptions provide a useful way of thinking about narrative therapies.

effects for the clients can also occur. This scenario can limit therapists' creativity and effectiveness as well.

Rather than taking an authoritative stance with clients, narrative therapists attempt to adopt a curious, "puzzling-together" posture.[8] They help elicit clients' own meanings and experiences to assist them in generating more useful and empowering life stories. In some situations, this can involve becoming more familiar with the persons clients have talked to so far about their pressing concerns, and what their reactions have been to these external voices. Narrative ways of working can also involve helping clients separate from totalizing, pathological descriptions, or inviting them to explore potentially empowering alternative voices and stories previously de-emphasized in their lives. Thus, narratively oriented therapists see their contribution as facilitating a safe, exploratory therapeutic environment where diverse, nonpathological, alternative perspectives and stories can be entertained, rather than as expertly providing clients with authoritative, complete, or definitive responses.

Traditionally, comprehensive developmental assessments and histories are routinely used to help converge upon professionally defined meanings and causes for children's symptoms. Narrative therapists assume that there are many valid ways of explaining children's behaviors, in addition to professional or scientific methods. Thus, they like to include clients' and relevant others' perspectives along with therapists' professional and personal viewpoints in co-constructing this assessment information. In addition, they generally prefer to ask about developmental information as a specific response to particular family concerns, rather than conducting routine, comprehensive assessments. Furthermore, sociocultural and contextual factors are emphasized, as compared with more conventional intrapsychic emphases.

Finally, I compare and contrast two different ways authors in this book employ narrative metaphors, in order to provide a context for appreciating these distinctions. Although all the authors in this book embrace social constructionist assumptions, there are some differences in how these assumptions are utilized.[9]

---

[8]Narrative therapists prefer terms like "co-authoring" and "co-constructing" to underscore the quality of mutuality in work with clients (Hoffman, 1991, p. 12).

[9]If space permitted, it might also be useful to explore further comparisons between (a) traditional and (b) narrative approaches, such as (a) having one core, essential self versus (b) having multiple stories, voices, or selves; (a) privileging information about clients' pathology, diagnoses, and deficits versus (b) privileging clients' own experiences of their problems and their resources; and (a) therapeutic secrecy versus (b) therapeutic transparency.

SOCIAL CONSTRUCTION OF REALITY
AND PERSPECTIVAL KNOWING

In contrast to traditional systemic or individual therapies, narrative therapies share "postmodern"[10] assumptions. These assumptions contend that knowledge is socially or consensually constructed. That is, when we say that something is "true" or "factual," we can understand this as saying that a sufficient community currently accepts this information as "true" or "real."[11] For instance, those of us who are U.S. residents would probably agree that a dollar bill made out of paper is not *inherently and objectively* worth more than a quarter made out of nickel or silver. However, we quite routinely and matter-of-factly carry out financial transactions with the *pragmatic, socially constructed understanding* or agreement that paper bills are worth more than metallic coins. This constructed understanding is quite useful in the vast majority of our daily lives. But if we were to believe that this economic system reflects the "true or only way," this belief could restrain us from interacting with people who believe in a bartering economy or in another system of exchanging tokens.

This isn't meant to suggest that postmodernism implies "anything goes"—that whatever one person or community considers "fact" or "truth" is just as valid and acceptable as another person's or group's definition (Shotter, 1993, p. 13). Just as a bank won't accept Monopoly money for cash, assumptions about what is "real" can be very difficult to challenge. The fabric of our social world is often tightly woven; it determines what behaviors are considered acceptable and unacceptable, as well as which ideas and people are deemed relevant and worth following and which ones are "on the fringe."[12] This fabric is shaped by those with power to determine such things and is not easily unraveled (Monk,

---

[10]For general introductory purposes here, I loosely use the term "postmodern" interchangeably with "social constructionist" or "alternative" models. For additional definitions of what "social constructionism/postmodernism" entails for psychotherapy, see Cushman (1995, pp. 17–20), W. T. Anderson (1990), Gergen (1991), Berger and Luckman (1967), Neimeyer and Mahoney (1995), Sarbin and Kitsuse (1994), Shotter (1993), Parry and Doan (1994), Parker, Georgaca, Harper, McLaughlin, and Stowell-Smith (1995).

[11]Alan Parry (1991b) offers the idea that "any definition of the Real is but an old story that is no longer questioned" (p. 13).

[12]Some traditions may perpetuate power relations that silence certain voices (people of color, women, gays and lesbians, etc.). Rather than entering a "debate" to establish which tradition or perspective is "true," some therapists are courageously facilitating public conversations (on abortion, etc.) where opposing voices can learn from each other through respectful dialogues (Roth, Chasin, Chasin, Becker, & Herzig, 1992).

Winslade, Crocket & Epston, 1997, p. 35). Thus to say something is "socially constructed" doesn't mean it is easy to modify or disregard. As Stacey (1996) indicates, "Some people have more meaning-making power than others."

There are additional factors related to social or institutional power that determine the persuasiveness of one's truth claims in prevailing Western, industrial/technological cultures. These factors are pragmatic, time-tested, value-laden, and socially constructed criteria for deciding the credibility of different stories or descriptions within these cultures.[13] These criteria for plausibility include such things as the following: How coherent, consistent, or well-connected are the events being described? Do these accounts draw from commonly accepted cultural narratives, or do they seem unusual and odd (e.g., stories about extraterrestrial visitors)? Are events described sequentially so that there is a sense of movement through time, or are things mentioned more fluidly and haphazardly? Do narratives describe relevant features (who, what, where, when, etc.) in an explicit, economical, and selective way, or are they expressed in a vague, lengthy, roundabout fashion? (See Gergen & Gergen, 1986, pp. 25–26, 31; Robinson & Hawpe, 1986, pp. 113–116; Barry, 1991; Weingarten & Cobb, 1995.)

In our rapidly changing, commercial, busy, and complicated culture, it makes sense that for survival and efficiency, we often cling to these implicit guidelines as if they were anchors on a restless sea. However, these socially constructed criteria favor those who can present themselves in predictable, linear, "left-brain," consumer-efficient ways. If people in power rigidly use these signposts as objective, "true" evaluations of people's capabilities and worth, those who don't fit within the dominant culture (e.g., members of traditional native and indigenous tribes; artists; poetic, metaphoric, and nonlinear thinkers; children and adolescents; etc.) can easily be discounted, totalized, and pathologized (Tapping, 1993; Shotter, 1993, pp. 37–38; Stacey & Loptson, 1995).

Paul Dell (1982) suggests that rather than hiding behind the "objective" cloak of science, therapists might benefit from considering their diagnoses and determinations of "pathology" as reflecting their own particular biases and differing values about what healthy behavior is:

> Pathology exists in the domain of human intentions and values—not in the domain of science or in the domain of absolute reality. When we imply that a person is objectively and absolutely sick, we are confusing these two do-

---

[13]Utilizing a pragmatic worldview, John Amundson paraphrases William James's ideas when he suggests that "truth is the compliment we pay to ideas that earn their keep" (Amundson, 1996; personal communication, January, 1997).

mains and losing track of the value judgments which we are making. Similarly, and more importantly, when we then try to "fix" that person who (we imply) is objectively and absolutely malfunctioning, we are again confusing our values with absolute reality. In doing so, we may fool both ourselves and the "malfunctioning" other with regard to what we are doing: We are trying to implement our values without admitting, and, perhaps, without even knowing, that that is what we are doing. (p. 12)[14]

Postmodern therapies operate from the premise that all knowledge, including "scientific knowledge,"[15] is *perspectival,* rather than assuming that professionals have access to "objective truth" and that clients improve only when they concede to this knowledge. As seen through a narrative lens, therapists and their scientific theories of personality are immersed in predominant cultural influences and ideologies; thus, their knowledge and solutions for mental health are as biased and subjective as those of their clients.

Walter T. Anderson (1990) describes the difference between this perspectival knowing and objectivist/factual knowing by contrasting two different baseball umpires operating from these models.[16] Both offer their views on how to conceive of their role in calling balls and strikes. The objectivist umpire says, "There's balls and there's strikes and **I call 'em the way they are.**" The perspectival umpire says, "There's balls and there's strikes and **I call 'em the way I see 'em**" (p. 75; bold added for emphasis).[17]

---

[14]Similarly, John Shotter (1993) suggests that psychology be labeled a "moral" rather than a "natural" science (p. 23). Philip Cushman (1995) critiques traditional psychotherapy for assuming an insulated, "scientific," "philosophy-free," and "value-free" perch:

> Mental ills don't work that way; they are not universal, they are local. Every era has a particular configuration of self, illness, healer, technology; they are a kind of cultural package. They are interrelated, intertwined, interpenetrating. So when we study a particular illness, we are also studying the conditions that shape and defined that illness, and the sociopolitical impact of those who are responsible for healing it. (p. 7)

[15]Einstein pointed out, "It is quite wrong to try founding a theory on observable magnitudes [i.e., data] alone. . . . It is the theory which decides what we can observe" (quoted in Watzlawick, 1976, p. 58). See also Kuhn (1962) and Gergen (1991, p. 89).

[16]Giorgi (1970) suggests, "To say that all knowledge is in perspective essentially means that every stance that we take up with respect to the world opens up some possibilities and closes off others. . . . The establishment of the fact of perspectivity thus rules out any stance that can be all-knowing, and in effect, this rules out the possibility of an absolute stance . . ." (p. 162).

[17]Watzlawick (1976, p. 63) elaborates on some implications of this: "People remain consistently unaware of their discrepant views and naively assume that there is *one* reality and *one* right view of it (namely their own); therefore anyone who sees things differently must be either mad or bad" (italics in original).

In the illustration below, Ken Gergen (1991) offers another apt example of perspectival knowing; he suggests that people make conclusions and interpretations of situations based on "a particular community of interpretation" (p. 104). Perhaps as an alternative to the objectivist slogan "Seeing is believing," we might find it more useful to say, "Believing is seeing"!

> Consider for example, the line "Her boss approached her with steady gaze and ready smile." How is the reader to interpret the line? What is the author's intent? For a teenage sub-community obsessed with romance, the "steady gaze" and "ready smile" are the obvious signals of a budding love affair, so clearly the author intends to write about love. In contrast, a business executive might assume the author was describing a popular managerial style. If the reader were a feminist, however, the "steady gaze" and "ready smile" might reveal the nuances of sexual harassment. And for a Marxist, the author might be describing the seductive exploitation of the working class. In effect, each reader incorporates the author into his or her own perspective. (pp. 104–105).

Conventional therapies often refer to and identify their clients by their diagnostic category. Traditionally oriented therapists commonly ask, "What kind of intervention would you use with [diagnostic category] clients?" This type of question presupposes that a "scientific" diagnosis, which often reduces clients' complex lives to a few paragraphs, provides enough relevant information for determining generic interventions. Griffith and Griffith (1994) suggest that these diagnostic categories and subsequent interventions tend to honor only therapists' definitions of "reality" or "health"—and that clients are not welcome members in this club.

> [Traditional] approaches all employ [an] unseen "bureau of standards" that has the authority to declare what is real and what is not real about the problem. This "bureau of standards" which Francisco Varela (1979) refers to as the "community of standard observers," provides an authoritative reference for valid bodies of knowledge and methodologies that distinguish between reality and fantasy and objective and subjective truth. Therapeutic approaches judged worthy are those constructed from wisdom offered by the standard observers. However, the role of this community of standard observers is generally obscured, and their pronouncements are issued as objective facts. . . . none of these approaches includes the patient and his or her family members among the group of standard observers. They do not share the power accorded to the clinician and to the larger professional and scientific communities as experts able to define what is real and unreal. (pp. 21–22)

THE SCIENTIFIC COMMUNITY AS ONE SOURCE OF IDEAS: TRADITIONAL INDIVIDUAL AND FAMILY THERAPY APPROACHES

Thus far, I have explored how narrative therapists view reality as perspectival and negotiated in different social contexts and communities. Now I contrast this view with the modernist assumptions about "reality" which inform traditional therapies. Many of our long-held and unquestioned beliefs about ourselves and our world utilize modernist assumptions about what is "true" or "real." Thus, talking about these is a bit like trying to glance upward carefully to inspect one's own glasses while simultaneously wearing them! Like glasses at the end of one's nose that one is oblivious to, these ideas about reality have existed for so long and are so familiar in so many daily aspects that we take them for granted as simply "the way things are," and even reflecting on this topic can seem strange (Shotter, 1993, p. 4).

In an oversimplified way, modernism holds that we are capable of arriving at a universally true, objective reality that definitively separates "objective fact" from "subjective fiction."[18] Modernism privileges what it considers to be a steadily growing body of "objective knowledge" derived from scientific experimentation and anecdotal studies (Freedman & Combs, 1996, pp. 20–22). Some additional modernist assumptions include the following:

1. Theories and research about human behavior are comprehensively based on scientific methodology and anecdotal studies, and thus contain empirically verified "truth."

2. This "truth" is objective, unbiased, and universal.

3. Therapists, by virtue of their specialized schooling and training in human behavior, are the best authorities on the causes of clients' problems and on how to solve them. They are also able to distinguish "reality" from distortions/unreal projections, empirical statements from antiempirical statements, and so on.

4. Clients are much less familiar with the comprehensive body of scientific, objective knowledge. They also have various dysfunctions that distort, narrow, and bias their perceptions. Thus, whatever ideas clients have about their own lives and what to do about them are likely to be unreliable, biased, and suspect.[19]

---

[18]See Warnke (1987, pp. 2–3) for a fuller discussion.

[19]Like most things, there are exceptions in modernist therapy to this generalization. Certain humanistic theories, such as Rogerian therapy, privilege the client's voice a great deal.

5. Young therapy clients tend to be more impulsive and less "rational" than adult clients, and are also likely to be unreliable authorities on their own lives.

6. Thus, therapists' access to comprehensive, unbiased scientific research and objective psychological knowledge gives them superior ability to assess and solve clients' (especially young clients') problems. This makes therapists the best authorities on clients' lives, and they are best able to help clients adjust to "reality."

Individual Models

Each individual and systemic therapy school contributes to our ideas about issues clients are dealing with and ways to help them. Traditional, modernist approaches view psychotherapy as a social science similar to other scientific disciplines. Within the scientific paradigm, psychological ideas are often seen as "true" (empirically validated) rather than as one among many ways of making sense of our lives. Correspondingly, traditional therapists look through the lens of this "truth" (i.e., their particular theory of personality and psychopathology) to pinpoint the "real meaning" of their clients' behavior. Through a modernist lens, the therapist is an "objective observer" who merely takes in client impressions that are objectively there for trained eyes to see.[20] Melanie Klein, one of the pioneers among analytically oriented child therapists, provided one of many examples of therapists' unquestioned objectivity:

> For instance, little Peter . . . pointed out to me, when I interpreted his damaging a toy figure as representing attacks on his brother, that he would not do that to his *real* brother—he would only do that to his *toy* brother. **My interpretation of course made it clear to him that it was really his brother whom he wished to attack** . . . (Klein, 1964, p. 285; bold added for emphasis; italics in original)

Another child psychoanalyst, Adolf Woltmann (1964), described this objectivist capacity as "third-ear" and "third-eye" listening. He seemed

However, these arose as alternatives (exceptions) to the vast mainstream of traditional therapeutic approaches.

[20]Griffith and Griffith (1994) point out: "Heidegger (1962) recognized that the entire movement of Western philosophy and science since the Greek philosophers had been built on descriptions of the world made as if a human observer were in God's position, standing outside creation, not as part of it" (p. 29).

to indicate these as techniques for neutral or "objective" information gathering.[21]

> The psychoanalyst listens to the patient's free associations with the "third ear." The child therapist, whether he [*sic*] looks at a child's drawing, plastic creation, block or toy play, has to develop the 'third eye' in order to bring his understanding into proper focus. . . . Once the therapist has mastered the **real meaning** of the child's nonverbal language, he can then use it both diagnostically and therapeutically. (p. 325; bold added for emphasis) . . . Watching the child and his [*sic*] play activities, and trying to decipher the **real meaning** of his activities, is a sign of mature, professional responsibility. (p. 22; bold added)

It's significant that in the examples above, the words "really" and "real"[22] are used convergently to point to only *one* meaning—which is determined *exclusively* by the therapist and his/her theories about what counts as "meaning-full." The child's various comments and behaviors could lead the therapy in many different directions. Thus, thinking only in terms of one "real meaning" can drastically reduce the scope of therapy. This reduction has the advantage of providing a focus and singular direction for therapy. But it may prohibit more useful, alternative directions from being explored, and may inadvertently silence clients' divergent perspectives.

Although humanistic and child-centered approaches have significant differences from the analytic approaches referred to above, many share an underlying belief in one universally recognized, objective "reality" to which the therapist has superior access. Clark Moustakas (1964), one of the leading proponents of humanistic approaches with children, stipulated:

> The emotions of disturbed children and troubled children to a large degree, at the beginning of therapy, are diffuse and undifferentiated. . . . Children

---

[21]Psychoanalytically oriented child therapists are also encouraged to embrace the role of reality-based authorities to help children separate truth from fantasy (Frankl & Hellman, 1964, p. 231); Reisman (1973, p. 60).

[22]Conventional therapy's usage of the term "real" doesn't occur in a vacuum. Consider everyday, nontherapy experiences when people disagree with each other. How often do we hear urgings by one of the discontents for the other to "get real" or to "join the real world" (i.e., "see things my way")! From a young age, we are encouraged to believe that what *we* (or our families, etc.) firmly believe must be "real" or "true," and that *others* who just as passionately believe differently are "incorrect" and persuaded by "false" opinions rather than the "facts." Traditional ideas about truth can lead us to hit each other over the head with "reality," rather than genuinely trying to understand diverse perspectives and encouraging tolerance of this diversity.

have apparently lost contact with the people and the situations that originally aroused frustration, anger, fear, and guilt. Their emotions, in other
words, are no longer tied to **reality.** . . . The child now sees himself [*sic*] and
his relationships with people more as they **really are.** (pp. 417–418; bold
added for emphasis)

"Humanistic" or "relationship" theories are described as "nondirec-
tive" and do have significant differences from other traditional child
psychotherapies; however, they presume that the therapist can gain access to the child's "true feelings" by listening carefully and empathically:

> It is the therapist's role to listen empathically and extract from the child's
> play the child's **true feelings and desires.** This understanding is then reflect-
> ed back to the child in an accepting and understanding manner. The accep-
> tance and understanding confirm for the child that her or his feelings are
> valid and important and part of her or his self. (Brems, 1993, p. 266; bold
> added for emphasis)

Often humanistic therapists seem to talk as if the client's "true feelings
and desires" exist independently of the therapist's own values or biases
about what "true feelings" (or, conversely "false feelings") refer to. In
other words, from these descriptions, it seems as if the therapist simply
objectively mirrors or reflects back these "true" feelings from the child,
much as a glass mirror reflects the image of whoever walks in front of it.
From a postmodern perspective, the therapist's assessment of the
"truth" of these feelings is colored by his/her theories and values. For
example, many humanistic therapists see these "true feelings" through
the lens of such concepts as the "authentic self" or the "inner child,"
which contain many values about what a person can or should be in order to be fulfilled.

Behavioral approaches also exemplify a belief in objective knowledge. The therapist is seen as more "objective" because she/he is skilled
in the "scientific method." The therapist's skill lies in "neutral" empirical observation and asking questions to break behavior down to objectively observable antecedent and consequent units. These observables
are then used to systematically manipulate the conditions affecting the
problematic behavior, so that change can occur. The client's *impressions*
of improvement are seen as "subjective" and inferior to the therapist's
superior empiricism.

> By being explained in terms of the target behavior and what is manipulat-
> ed, and by collecting empirical data on the preceding and consequent
> events and the target behavior, one can draw conclusions of an **objective**

nature on what **actually occurred. Impressions** of improvement [i.e., from clients] are essentially devalued as having validity because of the focus on **objectivity,** i.e., the direct measurement of behavior. (Fine, 1984, p. 9; bold added for emphasis)

Ollendick and Cerny (1981) also discuss the "objective" foundations of behavior therapy:

> Behavior therapists choose to describe behavioral events in terms of stimuli and responses, not because they see the world of human behavior in terms of sequences of stimuli and responses but rather because thinking about behaviors in these terms allows explicit and **objective** definition of the behaviors.... since behavior therapists bring a scientific orientation to the clinical situation and since they attempt to incorporate empirical methodology into their routine clinical efforts, they come very close to the realization of the scientist–practitioner model endorsed by the APA Boulder Conference ... (p. 9; bold added for emphasis)

In addition, mainstream cognitive therapy approaches such as Ellis's rational–emotive therapy share the same positivistic (or "empiricist") beliefs that therapists have objective knowledge and can separate "rational" from "irrational" beliefs. Thus, these approaches strive to help children and adults become more "rational, objective" beings:

> The cognitive limitations of the early childhood period can often result in children's acquiring beliefs about themselves and their surrounding world that are **untrue** and **irrational** and that, if not corrected, can have an extremely deleterious effect on their future well-being. (Ellis & Bernard, 1983, p. 19; bold added for emphasis)

Family Therapy Models

Even though family therapy offers a interpersonal perspective rather than an intrapsychic or individual one, traditional family therapy models retain modernist assumptions, such as the therapist's being an expert on what constitutes healthy or dysfunctional behavior (McNamee, 1996, p. 129). Marvin Fine (1984) mistakenly assumes that *all* therapists share this premise: "Every therapeutic approach has, at least implicitly, a set of assumptions or generalizations about the characteristics of the well-functioning person, or, as we would put it, the well-functioning family system" (p. 137).

Fine goes on to share his specific assumptions, which include "clear subsystem boundaries" and "correct hierarchies," acknowledging that these represent structural and some strategic approaches.[23] In addition, he names major intervention techniques, including "reframing," "re-structuring tasks," "reinforcing tasks," "paradoxical interventions," and "metaphorical tasks" (pp. 146–150). Each of these interventions shares traditional assumptions that the therapist knows what clients should be doing differently—in other words, what "healthy" behavior is. For example, reframing often involves positive connotation in order to get clients to be more receptive to doing what the therapist thinks is needed. Thus, reframing can be used as a technique to get clients to do the tasks the *therapist* unilaterally decides will create helpful systemic change.

> We delivered the following interventions: 1) We told the family that Mark's low motivation to study was related to his worrying about his father. Mark's way of being loving and loyal to his father came by way of dys-functioning and thus allowing father to feel needed and useful. 2) we then suggested that every evening, Mark was to report to Sara and to make two choices: (a) which one-hour block he was to use for a task we would sug-gest, and (b) whether he was going to use that hour to study or to worry about his father. (Fine, 1984, p. 153)

Other traditional systemic approaches also share the belief that therapists have privileged, "objective" access to what constitutes "healthy" communication and appropriate systemic change. Reisman (1973) comments on Satir's and Ackerman's models:

> Satir . . . has described the role of the family therapist as that of an expert in communication and a model of clear, congruent message transmission. . . . The role of the family therapist, according to Ackerman, . . . is similar to that of the individual therapist. He [*sic*] communicates his empathic under-standing, tries to point out defensive operations and maneuvers, clarifies the conflicted feelings and beliefs within and between members of the fam-ily . . . (p. 239)

Thus, we have seen that both traditional individual and systemic models share certain foundational objectivist assumptions. From an individual

---

[23]Structural and some strategic approaches see systems as biological (or conventionally de-fined "family") entities with a healthy or dysfunctional "structure" and healthy or dys-functional "alliances" between family members. These approaches focus most heavily on notions of "hierarchy" and "power," and therapist–client interactions are often described in chess-like terms such as "moves" and "countermoves" and "challenging" the family structure (Minuchin & Fishman, 1981, p. 67). The therapist directs his/her attention to family structure because this is seen as driving the symptomatic behavior. The clients are in a less privileged position because of their ignorance of these dynamics (Haley, 1976, pp. 38–39).

perspective, the therapist has access to the "true" picture of the problem and to what is "really" happening or being felt inside the client (see also Brems, 1993, p. 265; Strean, 1970, p. 14; Mishne, 1983, p. 278; Reisman, 1973, p. 10; Fogel, 1993). Systemic models expand the observational field to include family members, but rely on similar assumptions that the therapist knows the most functional or correct way for family members to function and communicate with each other. Regardless of their philosophical assumptions, traditional systemic and individual therapies have helped many clients. This seems particularly evident when the client experiences the therapist as being warm, nonjudgmental (i.e., not evaluating the client on the basis of differing and opposing values), and empathic (Miller, Hubble, & Duncan, 1995; Duncan, Hubble, & Miller, 1997). In the next section, I explore what may occur when clients and therapists do indeed disagree about values or beliefs.

HOW THERAPISTS' ASSUMPTIONS OF "OBJECTIVITY" CAN LIMIT THEIR RECEPTIVITY TOWARD CLIENTS' PERSPECTIVES IN CLINICAL APPLICATIONS

I have discussed the conventional notion that therapists are trained to think of themselves as objective and comprehensive experts in human behavior. From this popular perspective, it follows that most of us have been taught that certain types of clients simply lack training in particular skills, and that our job is to empathically and efficiently provide them with these specific tools (Monk et al., 1997, pp. 83–84). Frequently this involves educating clients in how to be appropriately assertive, how to listen more empathically, or how to communicate more effectively by using tools such as "I" messages. Many clients have benefited from this instruction and have felt more empowered to deal with difficult situations in their lives.

From a narrative perspective, however, this educational posture may also have unwanted side effects in some situations. These could include such things as clients' having to turn to outside "experts" in the future when problems arise, feeling unable to pursue topics outside a therapist's structure when this feels less relevant to their pressing concerns, implicitly conceding to prevalent, oppressive cultural ways of interacting, or mistrusting *their* own unique solutions and perspectives (Shotter, 1993, p. 14; Nylund & Corsiglia, 1994; Zimmerman & Dickerson, 1996). Hence, our assumptions about a therapist's objectivity and a client's psychopathology or skill deficits may inadvertently privilege the therapist's voice and limit how much the client can influence the shape of therapy. Lowe (1991) points out that traditional therapies tend to assume fixed dichotomies between therapist and client while privileging the therapist's role in these dualities:

> The notion of therapy as an art of conversation—where the therapist is a co-participant *in* a conversation rather than an expert who *uses* conversation—can be seen as an attempt to displace dualities such as subject-object, rational-irrational, depth-surface, and form-content, where therapists are identified with the term on the left of the hyphen and clients with the term on the right. The subject-object duality encourages the positioning of families as objects of study, assessment, and intervention, while enabling therapists to abstract themselves from their social context and position themselves as objective observers and agents of change (i.e., subjects). (p. 46; italics in original)

If a therapist believes that she/he is inherently more objective than the client, she/he may inadvertently discredit the client's perceptions. For example, Stanley Greenspan, a well-known child psychiatrist whose books are often used in graduate schools and therapy settings, describes how to interview parents of children seen in therapy. In describing one particular case, his language suggests that he has access to "nondistorted" perceptions, in contrast to the child's perceptions. He also implies that he has a "truer" perspective on the father/husband than the wife/mother does:

> Of particular interest is to what degree these **distorted perceptions** of the child reflect displacements from problems that the parents are having with one another. . . . Here one can see that mother perceived her husband as cold (**he was actually much warmer than she thought**) in order to protect herself against her feelings. (Greenspan, 1981, p. 176; bold added for emphasis)

Greenspan (1981) urges therapists to use their "intuition" in evaluating children during the initial session and in general. He assumes that it's possible for a therapist to have direct, objective, and complete access to a child's inner experiences (including the child's moods, affects, capacity for relationships, etc.):

> The child's affects, thoughts, and interpersonal experience—to the extent that they are revealed in the interview—give you a detailed picture of the relative richness or poverty of the child's inner life, which you can then compare with the expected norm. **Moreover, they give you a sense of what it feels like inside the child's skin.** For example, a child may not have any overt problems, but the shallowness of his [*sic*] inner life is conveyed by the few primitive affects he manifests. You observe only some sadness, a little

envy, a little jealousy: you see **no capacity** for love, empathy, or sharing . . . you sense the child's inner emptiness. . . . In sum, even though there were no major symptoms in evidence—in fact, it was not even clear why the child was brought in—you have both observed and sensed that he has little depth . . . (p. 138; bold added for emphasis)

In the quote above, note Greenspan's usage of definitive, absolute language, which invites us to assume that his descriptions are objective and most certainly true. No mention is made of whether the child may agree or disagree with the therapist's perceptions. Indeed, the therapist's perspective seems to merge with the child's, and we may even forget that this isn't the child's account! Thus, the child's personal experience of his/her own reality is seemingly irrelevant.

Furthermore, a therapist's intuition and observations are largely focused on one criterion: How does this child compare with other children his/her age? Anything clients do in the intake that deviates from the therapist's developmental expectations is automatically suspect. Thus, therapists are encouraged to take a critical posture toward whatever deviates from "the norm," rather than to take a more open, curious, and appreciative stance toward this uniqueness.[24]

Let us see how assumptions about therapists' objectivity like those mentioned above can influence how therapists relate with children and other clients. The following transcript from Ellis and Bernard (1983) utilizes a cognitive model in illustrating their approach to an 8-year-old girl who was sent to therapy after her parents' separation. I include much of this verbatim exchange because I think it highlights many important distinctions between a traditional, authoritative stance and a more narrative, collaborative one.

> The following is a transcript of an interview conducted by the first author with an 8-year-old girl [who] was referred for therapy just after her parents' separation. She had become very hostile and had started to act out. Her concerns were highlighted when her parents started dating other people. During this first session, she was helped to understand what her beliefs were and how they were leading to her fears. . . .
>
> [Later in transcript:] T: What makes you so upset?
>
> C: I don't know.
>
> T: Well, think about it. Do you know anybody else whose parents got divorced?
>
> C: Yeah, my friend Emily. . . .

---

[24]"As you gain experience, you will get a sense of the initial types of behavior **acceptable** from a new patient, child or adult" (Greenspan, 1981, p. 21; bold added for emphasis).

T: How would Emily feel if her mother remarried?

C: I don't know

T: Huh?

C: I don't know.

T: You don't know what she wants. Do you think everybody would feel as upset as you if their mother remarried?

C: Probably.

T: Probably? Well, wait a second. Check that out. How do you know that?

C: I don't know.

T: That's right, you don't know. As a matter of fact, some kids are very happy when their mom remarries.

C: Happy?

T: Some of them are real happy about it.

C: They've got to be nuts.

T: No, they don't have to be nuts. Some of them like the idea, **so it really can't be the fact that your mom may remarry that makes you sad, could it?**

C: Yes. It does.

[Later:]

T: And you see what makes people upset—it's the way they think about things. If you thought differently about it, you wouldn't feel sad about it. Do you know that?

C: No.

T: Well, it's true. You think that it would be a pretty terrible thing, don't you?

C: No.

T: No? What do you think about it?

C: Well, I just think I wouldn't like it.

T: You just think you would not. But you don't know for sure, do you?

C: Right.

T: That's like if somebody says, 'Why don't you try these peas?' If you have never had peas before, and you say, 'No, I'm not going to try it—I don't think I'd like peas. I can tell by the way they look.' But you really don't know whether or not you like peas, do you?

C: I don't like them.

[Later, in talking about her reaction to her father's not coming home again:]

T: There are lots of things in the world that are bad that aren't terrible.

They're just a little bad. Or they may be a lot bad, but they're still not terrible. Do you think there's just one kind of bad and that's awful?

C: No, I don't.

T: What do you think?

C: I think it's—it's crummy.

T: It's crummy. that's right—**it's just crummy.** It's too bad that your father's not ever going to live at home again, isn't that unfortunate. And tough? But it certainly isn't terrible. It's not going to kill you if he doesn't come home, is it?

C: No.

T: You're not going to die?

C: No. I'll die of old age.

T: You'll die of old age, right. You're not going to turn into some kind of bad person because your father's not going to come home, are you?

C: No.

T: So it doesn't seem like such a catastrophe, if he . . .

C: It isn't.

[End of transcript]

[Ellis and Bernard conclude the transcript section by saying the following:] This example reveals the use of **empirical disputation to "check out" and correct the young girl's antiempirical assumptions concerning the consequences of her parents' divorce.** Persistent and directed questioning elicited a variety of beliefs and feelings [that] appeared to be responsible for the client's state of unhappiness and misbehavior. Even within the initial session, it can be seen that it was possible to identify and begin to challenge irrational concepts such as the "catastrophic" effects of possible remarriage. (pp. 78–87; bold added for emphasis)

The reader may well argue that this transcript illustrates an exaggerated and nonempathic confrontational style that many traditional therapists would not use. I think this is a very worthwhile point. It's also quite possible that this therapist spent time prior to this session building rapport and a supportive relationship. However, my hope is that these transcript "exaggerations" provide a heightened example of what is generally done with the best intentions in a much more supportive, gentler, and more subtle therapeutic style.[25]

---

[25]Various types of traditional play therapy from a variety of modalities are frequently used with young children. I will leave it to the reader to determine to what extent his/her theoretical preconceptions may allow for or preclude the following four concerns.

First, traditional therapists often implicitly reduce the scope of what can be talked about in therapy by focusing on particular content that interests the therapists and/or conforms to their theoretical lens. They do this with good intentions rather than maliciously; they are simply following the conventional wisdom that therapists are experts on the causes of and solutions to clients' problems. In the vignette above, we can probably safely imagine that this girl had a number of different reactions to and experiences about her parents' separation. From this entire range of experiences, the therapist reduced what could be discussed to one domain: arriving at the "empirical" or "real" meaning ("crummy," "unfortunate," etc.) of this separation between her parents. Anything that did not support this meaning was challenged, and any other topics not related to this domain that the girl might introduce were probably ignored.

Second, conventional therapists can inadvertently impose their preferred views of reality upon their clients in the name of empirical science, and this can have unfortunate side effects.[26] It would seem that this therapist assumed (1) that this girl's views of her parents' separation were distorted, and (2) that the therapist's job (as a representative of empirical thinking) was to help her "correct" these views. He disputed her "antiempirical assumptions." From the examples he gave, apparently what is empirically "terrible" is when someone "dies" or turns into a "bad person." According to this therapist, the "correct" empirical response to anything short of these conditions is to call the situation "tough" or "unfortunate."

Can we say that everybody, or everybody who is "rational," would agree what is empirical and what isn't? What if this child was raised in the Roman Catholic tradition, which holds that divorce or separation is not justified? Would it not then be understandable and "rational" if she felt this separation was "terrible"? Is there only one way of being rational (the therapist's or the dominant culture's way)? Or are there many "rationalities," depending on one's values and sociocultural beliefs? If we accept that different, viable "rationalities" or communities of interpretation exist, is it possible that this therapist's impositions could actually have added undue anxiety and self-doubt? Could the girl have begun to mistrust her own previously helpful perceptions about life, to become more dependent on others, and to lose her own voice?

---

[26]Lynn Hoffman suggests:

> For me, the most serious challenge to the field of mental health follows the postmodern argument that much "normal social science" . . . perpetuates a kind of colonial mentality in the minds of academics and practitioners. . . . therapists of all kinds must now investigate how relations of domination and submission are built into the very assumptions on which their practices are based. (1991, p. 9)

Third, when a therapist adopts a confrontational, expert posture, how is she/he able to determine that her/his disputations and confrontations are successful in shifting the client's perceptions? In the case above, how would this therapist have known the difference between a simple client concession to the more powerful therapist and a genuine shift in the client's cognitive appraisal?

All therapists can occasionally get carried away by their own enthusiasm about a particular idea or story and not be clear about where a client is. Because of the power differential, frequently clients don't feel free to share their disagreements or concerns with the therapist in a verbal manner.[27] Many therapists check in with clients at these times to emphasize their genuine concern for having the clients' reactions privileged.[28] If a therapist's ideas are not helpful, ideally the therapist can be responsive and let go of this particular inquiry, and the client can then orient the therapist toward more useful directions. Alternatively, the client and therapist can have a dialogue clarifying both of their positions to determine how they should proceed from here. With this mutual honesty and collaboration, simple concessions or attempts to please the therapist are less likely to be confused with legitimate changes.

Fourth, a traditional therapist may become particularly fixed on certain theoretically predetermined content. The therapist may be so convinced of the "empiricism" or "truth" of his/her theoretical frame that it becomes unquestionable and unavailable for discussion. Thus, he/she may be more likely to attribute pathology or "resistance" to the *client* and not to the *theoretical frame* if the client finds the therapist's ideas or direction unsuitable. For example, the therapist in the transcript above might well have attributed "fault" or "resistance" to this girl if she had continued to insist that she felt sad about her mom's remarrying or that this separation was "terrible."

If this happens, it can lead to a lessened ability to experience the client's legitimate disagreements and sense of disconnection with the therapist. If indeed the girl in the transcript felt alienated from the therapist, was there anything conceivable she could have said or done that would

---

[27]Tom Andersen (1991, p. 50; 1995, p. 15) and Griffith and Griffith (1994, p. 86) have provided a unique and extremely valuable contribution for therapists who sometimes privilege clients' spoken words and miss unspoken somatic expressions. These authors have emphasized how clients' discomfort with particular discussions in therapy is often expressed by a sigh, a glance, shallow breathing, or other bodily indications.

[28]Tom Andersen (1995) shares how he goes about trying to privilege the client's voice: " . . . I have to wait and see how the other responds to what I say or do before I say or do the next thing. . . . I have to go slowly enough to be able to see and hear how it is for the other to be in the conversation" (p. 15).

have successfully conveyed to him that he was not connecting with her felt experience or resonating with her most pressing concerns? Or would this therapist's firm objectivist belief in what is "real/empirical" have made it likely that her disagreements or sense of disconnection would be seen through the lens of the client's "antiempiricism" or her "resistance"?

Often therapists indirectly or directly offer supportive suggestions, interpretations, or confrontations that clients find helpful. Clients often enter therapy with expectations that therapists are supposed to do these things, and if a therapist and client have fairly similar values and perspectives, these suggestions can often be quite useful. But when clients *disagree* with therapists' underlying assumptions or values, sometimes the therapists' well-intended interventions can combine with client concessions to form a vicious, self-perpetuating cycle of therapist ignorance and client self-blame. If a client senses that a therapist is implicitly and indirectly steering him/her toward the therapist's preferred story or "reality," this may make it more difficult for the client to express disagreement openly. If the client doesn't express this genuine disagreement and keeps this hidden, this in turn can deprive the therapist of feedback that might help her/him reflect on the usefulness of this therapeutic direction. Furthermore, if adult or child clients doubt the legitimacy of their own uncomfortable reactions to the therapist's interventions, they may concede to the "expert's" perspective and blame themselves for experiencing discomfort with the therapist's agenda. On top of whatever presenting problems clients bring to therapy initially, this self-blame can feed feelings of despair and hopelessness.

Often the only client escape from this pathologizing cycle is conforming to *the therapist's idea* of healthy behavior. O'Hanlon and Weiner-Davis (1989) describe this sort of disturbing pattern as a therapist-driven or theoretical "self-fulfilling prophecy."[29] Hubble and O'Hanlon (1992) refer to this sort of process as "theory countertransference":

> Unfortunately, most therapists have what we call "delusions of certainty" or "hardening of the categories." They are convinced that the observations

---

[29]O'Hanlon and Weiner-Davis (1989) aptly comment:

> One of the problems we see with holding these ideas as unquestioned 'Truths' is that the beliefs therapists hold often influence the data and outcomes in therapy. We therapists sometimes unwittingly create self-fulfilling prophecies (or perhaps we should call them other-fulfilling prophecies, in this case). If we believe that there is a deep, underlying problem, we might prompt the creation of one in the course of therapy. If we believe clients are sick and incapable, they may begin more and more to fulfill our expectations. (pp. 31–32)

This subject of how therapists can affect what they in turn observe is described as "second-order" therapy (Hoffman, 1990, p. 5; Golann, 1988).

they make during the assessment process are "real" and objective. They are certain they have discovered *real* problems. . . . Lacking from the discussion of countertransference in the psychoanalytic literature has been much examination of the ways in which the therapist's "theory" influences the work. While it was widely accepted that the person of the psychoanalyst . . . could be facilitative or disruptive, less attention was paid to how the clinician's overall conception of the human condition and therapy would affect treatment outcomes. (pp. 25–27; italics in original)

AN ALTERNATIVE TO THERAPEUTIC "OBJECTIVITY" AND CERTAINTY: CURIOSITY, "THERAPEUTIC LOVING," AND OPENING SPACE

Jon Amundson and Kenneth Stewart (1993, p. 118) provide a convenient summary distinguishing traditional models ("a therapy of certainty") from postmodern models ("a therapy of curiosity") (see Table 1). Similarly, Karl Tomm (1991; see also Freedman & Combs, 1996, pp. 269–272) discusses these positions of certainty and curiosity as reflecting a wide continuum of closing space and opening space with clients.[30] He prefers whenever possible to open space for the client to consider *more* empowering distinctions and preferred behaviors, rather than to close space on the client's ability to continue *less* desirable behaviors. Tomm proposes two additional terms to describe these positions: He refers to the therapist's reducing options or closing space[31] as "therapeutic violence," and contrasts this with the therapist's increasing options and opening space, or "therapeutic loving." Tomm (1991) speaks of these positions as "ethical postures," and utilizes Maturana's definition of violence as "any imposition of one's will upon another" and of loving as "opening space for the existence of the other."[32]

---

[30]Different narrative therapists also often have differing ways of relating with clients in different contexts. Some tend to be more open and uncertain at times, and others can be more definitive at times.

[31]It's understandable why therapists are traditionally referred to as "shrinks."

[32]Tomm (1991) uses some narratively oriented approaches, but doesn't identify himself as a "narrative therapist." He gives the example of opening space regarding a suicidal client. Ethically, therapists need to do everything possible to prevent clients from actually attempting suicide. But there are different therapeutic postures therapists can adopt in this effort. From a curious, opening-space posture, he might separate a person's identity from habits or ways of being (externalized) and ask, "What habits or ways of being would have to die for you to consider wanting to live?" If the client didn't respond to these invitations and explorations, Tomm acknowledges that he would have to consider utilizing more traditional measures to close space on the client's ability to do harm to himself/herself (measures such as a suicide contract, hospitalization, etc.).

TABLE 1. A Therapy of Certainty and Curiosity

A therapy of certainty	A therapy of curiosity
Is uncomfortable with ambiguity; needs to have structure and clarity	Can tolerate confusion and ambiguity without moving to premature closure
Quickly insists on a diagnosis and adheres to descriptions from those diagnoses	Moves more slowly in defining the problem, taking time to consider the experience in the room
Relies on problem-saturated descriptions of client behavior	Takes care to discover exceptions to the problematic behavior
Clients who don't "get it" are seen as "resistant" and this resistance must be subverted, broken through, etc.	When it seems that clients don't "get it," it may be that we haven't asked the kind of questions that will move the therapy forward
Is concerned with asking and answering "why" questions	Asks circular questions and examines the effects of the problem
Closes space by narrowing observations to ones' constructions/predispositions	Opens space by considering observations from many system levels
Assumes that a symptom serves just as a function . . .	Does not assume symptoms to be doing anything in particular, and may fit many theoretical explanations
Operates from a first-order perspective and does not consider the therapist–client system	Operates from a second-order perspective, always considering the therapist–client system
Is concerned with teaching, explaining, disseminating "expert knowledge"	Asks questions, looks for the special indigenous knowledge of the client
Discounts or overlooks the resources of the client	Takes care to discover what strengths are present . . .

Note. From Amundson and Stewart (1993). Copyright 1993 by the American Association for Marriage and Family Therapy. Reprinted by permission.

If we wished to adopt a less certain and more open, exploratory posture with the girl in the transcript above who was concerned about her parents' separation, how might we do this? We could begin by asking her how she would like to spend this time in therapy together, or by asking her to express more fully what *she* was most concerned about in this difficult situation. We might ask whether she had spoken to anyone about her concerns, and, if so, what her reactions were to these others' ideas. If suggestions were offered by these people, had any proven helpful so far? (See Andersen, 1991, pp. 47, 61; Lax, 1991.)

A curious, opening-space conversation might also involve facilitating some dialogue between the girl and one or both parents (either in person or in her imagination). This dialogue could involve each person's having an opportunity to express her/his worries, appreciations, and so forth, and to genuinely hear the others' concerns and internal/external voices in a fresh way. For example, while seeing the girl alone, we might ask this girl to imagine what her mother or father might say (externally) if either were to overhear her express her biggest concerns. We also could inquire whether her mom and dad might be thinking or feeling something different inside themselves from what they expressed out loud. These distinctions could lead to more hypothetical conversations and implications, which might expand how this girl thought about and in turn reacted to her concerns (i.e., beyond "acting out") and to others (H. Anderson, 1993).

Similarly, we could invite this girl to speak from another's perspective (Tomm, 1992) to try to imaginatively generate other, yet unconsidered, ways of understanding and coping. For example, we could ask her whether it might be okay to talk to her "as if" she were her mother. If she was open to this, we could ask her "mother" things like why this separation was occurring, how her "daughter" was reacting to this separation, how she could help her "daughter" feel better about what was occurring, and so on. With this girl's permission, we might also use this information to discuss things with the parents or to involve them as a family unit in therapy.

Narrative therapists using a re-authoring approach might begin by inviting this girl to talk about things she enjoyed doing that had no direct connection to the presenting problem of acting out, and spend time simply joining with this girl as a unique human being with varied interests. Such an invitation can often help to reduce children's sense of blame and embarrassment. She might be asked whether she understood her parents concerns and knew why she was in therapy. Her parents' concerns (i.e., her "temper") might gradually be spoken of in an externalizing way—for example, "So it sounds like your parents are concerned about what happens when 'temper' is around?" (Epston & White, 1992; White, 1989; White & Epston, 1990). Externalizing conversations could thus be used to help separate her sense of her identity and personhood from the problem at hand ("temper") and to empower her in her relationship to this problem. She might be asked what effects "temper" had on her parents, on her, on how she was treated by her parents, and so on. The therapist could ask her whether it might be possible for her to be angry or sad without letting "temper" get the better of her, and, if so, how (Freedman & Combs, 1996).

Rather than continue a possible adversarial relationship, the parents might be invited to assist the girl in relation to this anger. Thus, they might be asked to watch for and record times when she was able to "out-trick temper." They also might be asked what these achievements told them about her particular qualities and abilities as a person. In addition, the girl might be interested in hearing from other kids (by letter, videotape, etc.) who had made some headway with her situation, or in helping children who were not as far along as she was, in order to increase the "audience" for her successes in dealing with this (Monk et al., 1997; Zimmerman & Dickerson, 1996).

The various collaborative, narrative interactions described above are ways to increase the chances that children's unique voices and preferences will be taken seriously and will significantly influence therapy. Narratively oriented therapists are very interested in listening quite carefully to how children describe their concerns. These descriptions are not used as a way to interpret what is "really" being said. Neither are they primarily used for normative comparison for later correction or challenge. But if the therapist doesn't use these traditional ways of relating to children in therapy, how does the therapist decide what to focus on?

Narratively oriented therapists continually invite all clients to share their ideas about what therapy should focus upon, rather than carrying this entire presumption and burden of therapeutic focus on their own shoulders. These therapists are oriented by attempting to grasp *what clients want for their lives and how this connects to what they want from therapy.* Examples of questions that can help co-construct this therapeutic focus include the following: Who initially had the idea for therapy, and who sees the behavior in question as a problem? Does the client agree or disagree with this perspective? Do others' or the client's own reactions to this "problem" interfere with her/his life or with how she/he would prefer to be? Who would the client hope could hear and understand her/his biggest concerns? What difference would this make if they could? (See H. Anderson, 1993; Andersen, 1991; Monk et al., 1997; Zimmerman & Dickerson, 1996.) Thus, rather than seeing themselves as encyclopedias of psychological wisdom, or as "nannies" who steer clients in more "healthy, functional" ways, narratively oriented therapists are more like "midwives" who help clients bring forth their often unclear, partially articulated concerns and their preferred ways of responding to these concerns.

Is there any difference in how narrative therapists think of children's expressions and adult expressions? Yes and no. As pioneers in the play therapy literature have indicated (Axline, 1947), young children often have difficulty verbalizing certain things and often prefer to express themselves in play activity. Narrative therapists also utilize creative and expressive play modalities (drawings, puppets, role play, etc.). However, rather than using these modalities to interpret children's "real" feelings or to determine what needs to be corrected, narrative therapists use these to help children express and expand upon preferences within their metaphoric worlds.

Another difference between children and adults for many narrative therapists is children's particular vulnerability to having their voices co-opted by adults who have more power in the world (Stacey & Loptson, 1995). Thus, narratively oriented therapists try to take special care to insure that children have the freedom in therapy to speak in their own voices.

Most narrative therapists would probably agree that aside from these differences, they don't react substantially differently to children's stories and adults' accounts. Whatever preconceptions they have about children's development are held just as flexibly as whatever ideas they have about adult behavior. With all ages, the focus in on helping clients express and enlarge their stories or voices about themselves and others.

TRADITIONAL AND NARRATIVE PERSPECTIVES ON ASSESSMENT

Objective, Therapist-Determined, Singular Assessments versus Intersubjective, Mutually Determined, Multiple Assessments

Many traditional texts about working with children and adolescents focus heavily on doing comprehensive developmental assessments and histories, and on using such instruments as the House–Tree–Person test, family drawings, the Children's Apperception Test, the Thematic Apperception Test, and a family genogram. The contributors to the present volume don't emphasize these aspects in their chapters. I hope that by the end of this section, the reader will understand why such assessments and testing aren't highlighted.[33]

---

[33]Griffith and Griffith (1994) offer their perspective on how clinicians might use such things as traditional psychological testing/assessments without privileging the assumed "certain" and "expert" status of these instruments, and while opening space for clients to have the last word on *their* experience:

> The patient's experience, not a scientific or societal standard, is the ultimate judge of the worth of the work between clinician and patient. Rather than stating, "It is great you are so much better. Your Hamilton Depression Scale shows that you are no longer depressed," one would ask instead, "How is the depression now compared to where we started? What things do you notice that tell you this? Your Hamilton Depression Scale Score is less than one-half of what it was when we started. Is this better or worse than your own assessment?" (pp. 74–75; bold added for emphasis)

We have seen earlier how therapists are traditionally encouraged to pinpoint and converge upon the "real meaning" of the client's behavior. Similarly, when families first come to therapy, most therapists assume that their job is to take all the varied, diverse complexities families are immersed in and place these within some universal, clearly defined assessment or diagnostic categories that simplify and make sense of these intricacies.

> Find out exactly when each problem began and what precipitated it—e.g., a family crisis, a certain event, the child's (or his [*sic*] family's) conflicts about his development. Your goal is to obtain a brief history and complete cross-sectional picture of the presenting illness. . . . A detailed knowledge of the child's functioning across the board requires great patience and systematic focusing. . . . It will, however, tell you about *all* the problem areas and their contexts. This sort of detailed history is crucial to your fully understanding not only the current problems, their likely precipitants, and their pervasiveness, but also the related strengths and vulnerabilities that the child possesses. (Greenspan, 1981, p. 178; italics in original)

Greenspan's language assumes that with a rigorous and detailed examination, the therapist can single-handedly sift through data to arrive at an objective determination of what the problem is and what caused it. Notice the words he uses that fit this objectivist world: "exactly," "complete . . . picture," "fully understanding," "*all* the problem areas and their contexts." This view suggests metaphorically that a singular problem is objectively "out there" waiting to be carefully unearthed and pieced together to form the "true picture," and to be compared with other clinical case descriptions that will confirm this picture. This traditional search for a singular problem or singular reality connects to psychotherapy's emphasis on objectively comparing and evaluating clients before intervening.[34]

These determinations assume an objective view of reality that all rational people agree on. But what if we begin questioning whether there is a singular, "true" problem to be found? What might happen if we thought in terms of *many* "problems," depending on the perspective

---

[34]Parry (1991a) describes how Freud and others in the modernist tradition assumed it was their professional responsibility to translate clients' symptoms and concerns into an exclusive, "professional," abstract theoretical realm where the "real" meaning of the symptoms existed:

> Psychotherapy was especially a child of modernism. Equipped with theories that explained problems in living on different levels than they were experienced by their sufferers, therapists became particularly prominent cultural exemplars of the modernist tendency to require an authority to pronounce on the underlying meaning of people's experiences. (p. 38)

sought (H. Anderson, 1993, p. 324)? Often, for example, a child's teacher, parents, siblings, grandparents, friends, coach, school counselor, and therapist have very different and yet equally credible ideas about what is really going on. Some therapists generally think of problems as defined by clients and by those persons clients are in relevant conversation with about these problems, which could include all of the people in this example.[35]

From a narrative perspective, no single individual, including the therapist, has omniscience. That is, no one can form a complete, panoramic, exhaustive view of reality or of the problems clients bring to therapy. Each person involved in the problem scenario would be seen as having a valid yet partial perceptual claim or explanation for what the problem is and what should be done about it. Thus, from a narrative standpoint, *the initial focus of therapy is on trying to grasp the local meanings and understandings of everyone involved, through creating a mutual, comfortable, and safe conversational environment.* This can involve respectfully exploring their ideas about such things as these: what therapy should focus on; how the problems arose; how the problems are affecting various people; what might help solve the problems; what sorts of solutions have already been considered or successfully utilized; and so forth.

Standard versus Contextual Use of Assessment[36]

Conventionally, many who work with children assume that in order to help children and families, an elaborate and exhaustive developmental/family history, beginning with infancy, must *always* be done.[37]

---

[35]Harlene Anderson and Harry Goolishian (1988) originated the idea of a conversational system as contrasted with conventional ideas about a "family system." This idea has been variously referred to as the "problem-determined system," the "problem-organizing/problem-dissolving system," and so on.

[36]Often therapists are required by their agencies or funding sources to complete a comprehensive psychosocial form that asks for children's developmental history in many domains. Narrative therapists separate this *institutional* requirement from a *theoretically necessary* one, and they are likely to be open with clients about this institutional constraint, while acknowledging that clients may or may not find these questions particularly relevant.

[37]Like Greenspan (1981) and other traditional child psychotherapists, Reisman (1973, pp. 20–25) sees children's psychological problems as explained by a universally applied developmental framework, including "retardations of development" (speech, language, motoric problems), "fixations/developmental arrests" (persistence of inappropriate behaviors or impulses), and/or "regressions" (temporary immature behavior after an environmental stressor). See also Mishne (1983), Ellis and Bernard (1983, p. 19), Shaefer and Millman (1977, p. 21), and Brems (1993).

Many traditional clinicians believe that in order to be a professional, competent therapist, the therapist must continually be assessing and evaluating how well or poorly each child client measures up to (the therapist's ideas about) age-appropriate development in a large variety of domains, no matter how far adrift this exploration departs from the family's pressing concerns.

Greenspan's (1981, pp. 186–187) routine assessment inquiry includes asking each family about the child's "early feeding and weaning," "early differentiating experiences," "birth of siblings," and "toilet training," along with many other aspects. From a traditional perspective, these sorts of comprehensive developmental inquiries are linked to "empirically verified findings" that provide definitive answers to why children with these characteristics behave in a problematic manner and what sorts of environmental and intrapsychic explanations are viable.

Narrative therapists have found some of these findings useful, but they also strive to privilege clients' unique sociocultural situations and clients' own understandings about their concerns. Many narrative therapists are quite familiar with the professional literature's ideas about developmental milestones and capacities. When at any particular moment families' concerns seem to relate to these developmental theories, they can draw from this resource to wonder aloud with families about possible connections and ask clarifying, detained historical questions pertaining to this specific issue.[38] For example, parents may be concerned that their 4-year-old isn't responding to their requests, and the narratively oriented therapist may begin wondering if this could be connected to the parents' use of complex, abstract language. The therapist may then tentatively offer developmental ideas from the scientific, professional discourse (developmental stages, expectations, etc.) or from his/her experiences with other clients or with his/her own family. The therapist can then ask whether the parents have considered these ideas before, or, if not, how well these fit with their particular family in this unique context. Thus, these developmental inquiries are specifically related to these particular parents' pressing concerns, rather than occurring in a more comprehensive and universally applied fashion.[39] The therapist also

---

[38]When I first began thinking of assessment in less global and more situationally defined ways, I worried that I might be missing something important that I could have gotten in a more comprehensive, standard developmental history. However, my experience has been that if I continue to stay connected to what clients are saying and to my own internal reactions, these important considerations seem to emerge in timely ways.

[39]In a number of educational or parenting contexts, it may be very important to consider how a child's motoric, visual, auditory, emotional, and/or general information processing compares with that of other children.

checks in with the parents to insure that this exploration has personal relevance for them. In this way of working, the therapist's professionally informed ideas about what is happening are not given special, unimpeachable status, and these ideas are not seen as "the truth" to which clients must concede in order to improve. This assumption requires therapists to be comfortable with ambiguity and to embrace multiple realities. In the example above, perhaps the therapist has overlooked other factors the parents are aware of, which could just as credibly account for the child's problematic behavior. A narrative therapists' expertise is in adopting a mutual, relational posture to help the conversation move forward in helpful, often unpredictable directions, not in unilaterally providing definitive assessments or conclusive therapeutic solutions.

Assessing Normative, Intrapsychic Capacities versus Listening for Contextualized, Sociocultural Understandings

Systemic thinking, feminist theories, and postmodern therapies have suggested that people's behavior cannot be understood apart from their *unique, systemic, sociocultural contexts* (Pare, 1995). For example, to label a housewife as having a "dependent personality disorder" isolates her from all the other women struggling with this issue in Western society, and obscures how these characteristics are fostered and encouraged by prevailing gender expectations of women (Hare-Mustin, 1987; Goldner, 1988; Weingarten, 1994, 1995).

Many therapists have recently become more aware of varied situational factors affecting clients, such as differences in culture, race/ethnicity, sexual orientation, gender, and family lifestyle. However, these ideas haven't yet significantly influenced how we conduct routine assessments of children. Traditional ideas such as Greenspan's (1981, pp. 16–43) seven "categories of observation" continue to be prevalent in many mental health agencies. These categories are used to determine how well or poorly a young client's reactions match up to his idea of universally applicable "age-appropriate expectations." One of Greenspan's categories is called "human relationship capacity," and this supposedly determines how well children can form interpersonal relationships in all situations.

I offer the following example from Greenspan (1981) to demonstrate how traditional approaches often give a clinician free license to interpret a child's behavior without regard to whether this particular child, family, or culture would agree with the clinician's understanding

[40]The clinician is constrained, however, by his/her therapeutic orientation and by whatever the dominant psychotherapy culture considers to be a "professional" or "reasonable" interpretation.

or not.[40] There is no or very little discussion of contextual, sociocultural factors influencing such a clinical evaluation. In fact, these are actively *discouraged* in favor of making universal and fixed developmental pronouncements about the child's intrapsychic world. In his example for evaluating a child's "human relationship capacity," Greenspan suggests:

> As you enter the waiting room and relax for a minute between patients, you want to observe both the interaction between the child and whoever brought him and between the child and others in the room. Is he being affectionate, or withdrawn and aloof? Is he making contact with others; how much distance does he maintain from them? Simply by watching for a half a minute or so, you get an impression of how the child has negotiated all the available human relationships in the waiting room. **Do not dismiss from consideration or excuse on situational grounds what the child has chosen to do.** (p. 19; bold added for emphasis)

From a narrative perspective, we can't separate our conclusions about such intrapsychic abilities from our culturally and historically informed preconceptions and theories about what "affectionate" behavior is or what "making contact" consists of. What one sociocultural tradition sees as respectful distance, another may see as aloof and withdrawn.[41]

Narrative therapists also assume that clients' shifting and contextualized meanings often play an extremely pivotal role in how they behave. For example, suppose that just before coming to the waiting room, the parent in Greenspan's example told the child, "You better behave or else the doctor will get very mad at you!" This child may typically be more spontaneous and outgoing, but *now* may in this context be very "withdrawn" in order not to risk offending the therapist. Rarely will parents spontaneously disclose to the therapist such contextual communications given to a child unless the therapist asks them in a supportive manner what the child's understanding is of this meeting.

In short, it is possible that allowing standardized developmental preconceptions to become the universal, unquestioned "norm" for evaluating children puts therapists in danger of forming reductionistic conclusions about their young clients. Such conclusions overlook a more nuanced, contextualized grasp of children's experience, and ultimately

---

[41]Feminist scholars have pointed out that most of our theories about human behavior have historically been based on male subjects and male theorists. Furthermore, men's ideas about such things as "closeness" or "distance" are often very different from how women often view these. See Belenky, Clinchy, Goldberger, and Tarue (1986, pp. 6–7), Gilligan (1982), and Jordan, Kaplan, Miller, Stiver, and Surrey (1991).

(though inadvertently) impose dominant cultural assumptions upon children. (See Freedman & Combs, 1996, p. 31.)[42]

Rather than thinking of children as being governed strictly by internally developed, universal psychological structures or character deficits, narrative therapists tend to see children's behavior in more sociocultural, reciprocal, and contextual terms (Shotter, 1993, p. 14). These factors relate to assumptions by narratively oriented therapists that people's actions are guided by culturally derived meanings and stories they continually construct about their worlds and about themselves. These meanings shift, depending on whom people are with and how these others react to them in a particular context. The reader can see that these contextual fluctuations don't make for quick, tidy, "one-size-fits-all" evaluations of intrapsychic experience! Many narrative therapists view the professional literature's age-specific assessment categories or developmental stages as tentative guidelines for clinicians and families to use, modify, or discard as they find suitable.

Assessment as a Discrete Stage for Neutral Information Gathering versus Continual Assessment and Influential Questions

Traditionally, assessment is thought of as the first discrete stage in the overall therapy process, leading to subsequent treatment plan and intervention stages. Narratively oriented therapists tend to think of assessment, or the gathering of relevant information, as occurring *continually* throughout therapy.[43] They think of the therapist as always "on the way to understanding" what is being said, but never fully arriving (H. Anderson and Goolishian, 1992, pp. 32–33).

In addition, "assessments" can be more than simply neutral information gathering. Even though the therapist is only asking questions and not making statements, these questions steer the clients' responses in some directions and not others. Clients develop ideas about what

---

[42]Alan Parry (1991a) suggests:

> If family therapy were to embrace a fully narrative paradigm and identify itself as a kind of literature rather than as an applied science, it could not only work with people at the level at which they describe their experiences, but it could also move beyond the disposition to categorize and reduce a person's story according to the degree to which it exemplified a particular discrepancy from a norm described by a theory. (p. 40)

[43]Some narratively oriented therapists may choose not to use the term "assessment" to describe *any* of their work, because this term is typically identified with ideas of comparing and diagnosing clients, and this is not a primary focus.

types of information the therapist thinks is relevant and are likely to omit unrequested information from other aspects of their lives. Some questions can also have a therapeutic effect or a harmful effect (Andersen, 1991, pp. 50–57; Tomm, 1988, 1992). Many narratively oriented therapists using re-authoring ideas often intentionally ask questions to legitimize previously overlooked aspects of children's lives (resources, abilities, strengths, etc.) and to begin co-constructing more preferred stories about their lives (White, 1989; White & Epston, 1990; Zimmerman & Dickerson, 1994).[44]

SOME DIFFERENCES BETWEEN CONTRIBUTORS TO THIS BOOK: RE-AUTHORING AND HERMENEUTIC EMPHASES[45]

Although the therapists represented in this book share many assumptions and ways of working, there are significant differences among them as well. Many therapists in this book have been strongly influenced by Michael White and David Epston's re-authoring approach to narrative therapy. After exploring this narrative tradition, I discuss the hermeneutic and dialogic approach espoused by Harry Goolishian, Harlene Anderson, and Tom Andersen, which some therapists in this volume utilize.[46]

---

[44]If the reader would like to explore nontraditional developmental approaches, Brett Steenbarger (1991) draws some cogent contrasts between traditional "stage-based theories of human development," (which he asserts "pathologize developmental diversity" (p. 288), and socially constructed, "contextualist" developmental models. John Morss (1996) and Erica Burman (1994) also critique traditional developmental models from a variety of perspectives. In addition, Alan Fogel (1993) has written an excellent book that takes a relational, contextual, and flexible view of child development. See also Hoffman (1991) and Cushman (1995).
 A reader who is specifically interested in further writings on child development using a narrative metaphor might pursue research in sociolinguistics and narrative language development, such as Dennie Wolf's (1990, 1993). Wolf provides a scholarly and detailed look at how children develop and acquire different "voices" or ways of speaking, depending on the context and on the people they are relating with.

[45]I have chosen these terms to honor the contributors' *own* ways of describing their work, and I don't intend to suggest that these terms are inherently mutually exclusive. I also sometimes substitute the word "dialogic" for "hermeneutic."

[46]I have given a lot of consideration to the idea of specifying which authors use which of these two approaches in this book. However, many of the authors in this volume use both approaches in differing degrees. In addition, I would feel uncomfortable speaking in behalf of different contributors on this issue, since they know the nuances of their work much better than I do. I hope that the reader can gain some cues by taking the conceptual distinctions outlined in this section and noting which guiding assumptions various authors appear to emphasize in their chapters.

Re-Authoring Approaches to Narrative Therapy

White and Epston have made a very significant contribution by illustrating how clients internalize social discourses that totalize and pathologize them. For example, a youth may come to therapy with a temper or attention problem. Our dominant culture often speaks as if the *child* is the problem (i.e., "This is an angry child" or "This is a conduct-disordered child"), rather than talking in terms of the child facing or dealing with a particular problem. White and Epston originated the idea of having "externalizing conversations" with a client so that the person's identity is separate from the problem. They see this as a helpful way of politically resisting a potentially harmful cultural tradition. In addition, this way of speaking often frees clients to take more responsibility for coping successfully with these problems, since their very personhood is not being challenged. (See White, 1989; White & Epston, 1990; Roth & Epston, 1996; Foucault, 1977; Monk et al., 1997, pp. 99–102; Freeman, Epstein, & Lobovits, 1997.)

Furthermore, many clients find that talking about their problems as separate from their personhood gives them greater hope for change and decreases their self-blame. It also allows the clients to examine and deconstruct the particular socially constructed messages and ways of thinking that feed the problem. Often a therapist asks about the effects of an "externalized" problem on a client and on others. The therapist may also ask about the sorts of promises, threats, or other tactics the (personified) problem uses to try to keep the person in its grip. As the problem story is co-constructed in these sorts of externalized ways, the client often feels freer to let go of chronic, habitual, and disempowering ways of thinking and being. In turn, progressively separating himself/herself from this problematic lifestyle allows the client to consider more empowering self-narratives that have been lying dormant in the background, unnoticed and neglected. (See White, 1989; White & Epston, 1990; Freedman & Combs, 1996, pp. 58–63; Monk et al., 1997, pp. 102–106; Zimmerman & Dickerson, 1996.)

With families and couples, problem patterns can be externalized. In some situations, each participant in a problem pattern can be invited to take responsibility for how she/he has inadvertently contributed to this pattern. Thus, in a "pursuer–withdrawal" pattern, both people can begin to notice how one's (externalized) "withdrawal" habit contributes to the other's (externalized) "pursuing" habit and vice versa. In other situations, all participants can be invited to pool their resources to collectively overcome (externalized) relationship restraints such as "bickering" or the "rift" (Zimmerman & Dickerson, 1996, p. 52).

After clients' problems have been externalized and their problem stories have been explored, clients are invited to explore aspects of their lives that don't fit the "problem-saturated" or "old" stories. For example, children who are predominantly anxious will have some moments, no matter how small or fleeting, in which they are a little less anxious. Therapists become curious about these aspects ("unique outcomes"). Re-authoring therapists may ask anxious children questions such as these: "How were you able to be less anxious at that moment? What did you do or say to yourself that may have helped you have more influence on the 'anxiety'? Have there been other moments like these? What do these moments say about your hopes and personal qualities?" (See White, 1989; White & Epston, 1990; Freedman & Combs, 1996, pp. 67–68, 89–91; Monk et al., 1997, pp. 106–112; Zimmerman & Dickerson, 1996, pp. 79–86).

Previously, clients have often trivialized and dismissed these "unique outcomes" as lucky or insignificant. But as therapists express curiosity about these, life is breathed into these moments, and collectively these previously isolated moments can form the building blocks for "new" or "alternative" stories. Thus, *instead of a client's being totalized as the problem* ("I'm just an anxious person"), *the client can be seen as immersed in two contrasting stories or life directions* ("I'm a person who has been in the grip of 'anxiety'" [old story]; "I'm a person who is able to have some influence on 'anxiety'" [new story]).

Next, therapists using this approach will often ask clients which life directions they prefer. If clients indicate that they prefer the new, alternative stories of themselves, they can be asked to describe what they like about these directions. This helps insure that clients are heading in ways *they* prefer, rather than simply trying to please their therapists. If clients prefer these alternative ways of being, therapists can then help them find ways of making these stories endure in the face of invitations to return to their old stories. For example, a therapist can invite a client to wonder who might encourage and support a developing story about influencing "anxiety," or who might have anticipated that the client has this capacity to keep "anxiety" in its place. The client can then be asked what the next preferred step might be. The more the therapist expresses curiosity and explores implications of this emerging story, the more "real" or concrete it becomes. This concreteness in turn helps this alternative account survive. Various innovative re-authoring therapists have used very creative ways of helping the preferred story grow and endure. Many invite clients to consider consulting with previous or current clients who have dealt with similar concerns (via letter writing, videotape sharing, leagues, etc.). In addition, many re-authoring therapists write letters to clients between sessions or have celebratory certificates or parties to help highlight their blossoming alternative stories and help them endure. (See White, 1989; White & Epston, 1990; Freedman &

Combs, 1996, pp. 237–263; Monk et al., 1997, pp. 110–116; Nylund & Thomas, 1994; Lobovits, Maisel, & Freeman, 1995; Madigan & Epston, 1995.)

Therapists who utilize these deconstructive, externalizing, re-authoring ways of working are often particularly attuned to helping clients re-examine sociocultural messages to discover which ideas genuinely fit them and which don't. For example, many mothers have had to deal with years of "mother blame" for such things as incest, battering, and so on. Even though men perpetrate these injuries, predominant sociocultural ideas have suggested that women are implicitly to blame for what happened (e.g., by not being satisfying sexual partners for the husbands/incest perpetrators) and have tended to excuse men from being held accountable.[47] Thus, women clients in this situation can be invited to separate themselves from this (externalized) "mother blame" in order to re-evaluate these cultural assumptions. Depending on a client's particular concerns and contexts, additional sociocultural dimensions for exploration could include themes of oppression based on race/ethnicity, sexual preference, age, gender, or class (White, 1995; Freedman & Combs, 1996; Tamasese & Waldegrave, 1993; Zimmerman & Dickerson, 1996, pp. 61–76).

Hermeneutic/Dialogic Approaches

Re-authoring approaches have proven helpful for many clients in many different contexts. Let us now turn our attention to another helpful approach that has some different emphases. The hermeneutic emphasis described here is based on the work of Harry Goolishian, Harlene Anderson and Tom Andersen (Andersen, 1991, 1993; H. Anderson & Goolishian, 1988, 1992; H. Anderson, 1997). In contrast to the re-authoring focus on helping clients free themselves from oppressive stories, hermeneutic or dialogic approaches assist clients in moving from stuck monologues to more liberating dialogues. Hermeneutic methods don't intentionally try to use externalizing conversations, or try to invite clients to take a different position toward (externalized) problems by examining their tricks, exploring how they have managed to overcome these problems, or the like. Furthermore, they don't attempt to consolidate a client's unique outcomes into a durable, alternative story. Instead, they attempt to facilitate clients' dialogue with many different internal and external narratives (or voices) "in a state of coexistence," without necessarily inviting clients to step more fully into any particular narra-

---

[47]Two excellent resources for dealing with survivors of abuse and with perpetrators of abuse are Durrant and White (1990) and Jenkins (1990), respectively.

tive (Penn & Frankfurt, 1994, pp. 219–222). The premise here is that many different "selves" or voices are called forth in different relationships and situations. Dialogic therapists provide a safe haven for exploring and sorting through these voices, so that clients can respond in more flexible and satisfying ways. (See Anderson, 1996; Penn & Frankfurt, 1994, pp. 219–222; Seikkula, Aaltonen, et al., 1995, pp. 65–69; Gergen & Kaye, 1992, pp. 179–181.)

We have seen how re-authoring therapists successfully co-construct coherent old and new story lines that invite clients to have a different relationship with their presenting problems. Hermeneutic approaches extend the familiar conversations about clients' presenting concerns into new, uncharted territory, so that misunderstandings or limited understandings preventing successful coordination with others can be dissolved. Their goal is to create a safe environment where a free flow of previously unsaid stories and new realizations can occur (H. Anderson & Goolishian, 1988; Griffith & Griffith, 1994, pp. 65–93; Schnitzer, 1993, pp. 446–447). I realize that this may sound vague. In order to give a clearer idea of what this process entails, let me try to share how I understand problems arising from a hermeneutic perspective.

Because our interaction with ourselves and with others is so complicated, we often construct abbreviated stories that simplify things and allow us to proceed quickly with life. We make snap judgments and assume things about others' expectations, motivations, and so on. We see what we expect to see as we move through our regular, patterned lives, and we don't notice many other potentially helpful nuances (Andersen, 1992b). If we are able to navigate successfully through life and coordinate satisfactorily with others with these "make-do" narratives, we generally feel content. However, sometimes our assumptions don't work so well, and problems develop: Others change and don't do what we anticipated; we are mistreated by others and we don't have an adequate reply; the stories we always silently hoped for in our lives suddenly don't seem possible.

Frequently we respond adequately to these challenges by such things as negotiating compromises with the others, finding authentic voices that successfully convey how we feel mistreated, or dialoguing with ourselves about how to move on in spite of our revised hopes. However, when these sorts of internal and/or external conversations resolving these disconnections, misunderstandings, and hurts are currently beyond our grasp, *we often feel stuck*. From a hermeneutic framework, this is when clients often pursue therapy (Griffith & Griffith, 1992, p. 9).

An example may help illustrate how clients become stuck in competing monologues that prevent a satisfying resolution of their pressing concerns. Suppose a father becomes irritated with his son, telling himself and perhaps saying out loud, "The problem is, he is lazy!" Since this is the only voice he presently hears (within himself), he continues to treat the boy as if this were the "true" story. He may decide he has to increase his demands on this child to "show him how to be responsible." Meanwhile, the child has formed assumptions or stories about the father as well ("He is mean! He likes to boss me around!"). Operating with this equally limited, stuck, monologic perspective, the child then rebels against the "mean" parent by doing even less responsible things than before, further confirming the father's monologue that the child is truly lazy.

As these "dueling" monologues (H. Anderson, 1993, p. 332) continue, and as this problematic cycle escalates, other people may become involved. The child's teacher may be alarmed by his defiance and talk with the school counselor, who in turn meets with the boy and father. The parents may consult their minister to seek his/her advice. As the father discusses his "laziness" concern with others, he may be exposed to new, possibly contradictory explanations. In addition to "laziness," the father may also start wondering about the minister's mention of the child's "needing more spiritual guidance." In addition, he also may be pondering the school counselor's suggestion to "spend more time" with his son.

As in this example, when clients finally wind up on therapists' doorsteps, they often have had a variety of internal and external conversations about their pressing concerns (what is causing them, what the best solutions are, etc.). However, clients are often confused and generally haven't had an adequate opportunity to reflect on their various reactions to these voices and how best to proceed. Clients frequently don't voluntarily share these confusions (or their doubts whether therapy should even be pursued at all) with therapists they have just met. If a therapist doesn't ask about internal and external conversations related to a client's coming to therapy, the therapist and the client may begin to feel out of sync with each other.

In order to connect with clients' unspoken doubts, their experiential worlds, and with how they presently make sense of their pressing concerns, dialogic therapists often begin therapy by becoming curious about what sorts of discussions or thoughts led up to this meeting. They may ask questions such as these: "What is the history of the idea behind this meeting? Who is involved with this situation [or who is worrying about this situation besides yourself]? Who had that idea [for therapy] first? What were your own reactions to this idea about coming to therapy?"[48]

---

[48]See the earlier reference in this chapter to conversational, "problem-determined systems" as described by H. Anderson and Goolishian (1988); see also Andersen (1991, p. 61) and Lax (1991, pp. 130–131).

The therapists then follow their curiosity about unspoken aspects in clients' subsequent responses.

For instance, in the earlier example, the father may indicate that the school counselor first had the idea for family therapy. Thus, the therapist may try to get a clearer sense of whether this family understands more specifically what the school counselor had in mind for counseling. The father may say he isn't really sure, but it seems that the counselor wants the parents to give their child more attention. The therapist can then explore what others' reactions to this idea are. The child may agree, but Dad may disagree with the school counselor's "needing more attention" idea. If so, the therapist can ask each of them in turn to *elaborate* on why they agree or disagree. The father may also respond by mentioning the minister's "spiritual guidance" theory, and this idea can be explored as an additional resource for consideration, along with the school counselor's hypothesis.

Like a musician patiently tuning an instrument before playing with others, the therapist asks these sorts of questions in order to get "up to speed" and provide very relevant background information on how clients are likely to filter and understand what the therapist says. In addition, these questions help establish a comfortable, compatible working relationship. For example, before introducing a wild animal into a new habitat, zoologists carefully explore this habitat's ecology to insure that there is a good fit. Similarly, therapists working this way like to explore clients' particular, local "ecology of ideas" (Bogdan, 1984) before introducing new perspectives, so that the therapist's contributions aren't experienced as either "too familiar" or "too unusual" (Andersen, 1991, p. 46).

As the son and father elaborate on their reactions to the school counselor's "attention" idea, they are helping the therapist get oriented to how they experience themselves and each other (Tomm, 1991), as discussed above. At the same time, these spontaneous elaborations may express nuances that neither one has ever heard the other say before. If so, *change subtly occurs as clients' familiar assumptions about themselves begin to shift and expand.* (See Andersen, 1995, p. 33, 1992a, 1994; H. Anderson, 1993, pp. 325, 328; Seikkula et al., 1995, p. 73; Swim, 1995, p. 108; Smith, 1995.) For example, the son may say that he agrees with the school counselor's suggestion, because his dad never does anything fun with him—he's always "yelling at me about something." Following the spontaneity and curiosity of the moment, the therapist may ask about the son's reaction (internal conversation) when his dad does this. The son may say that he feels his dad doesn't love him— that he fears he loves his older brother more.

While Dad listens to these new elaborations, his previous monologue about his son's laziness may begin to loosen and dissolve. He may begin to reflect back on their previous confrontations, and may now suddenly remember the look of sadness in his son's eyes when he tried to get the boy to be more disciplined by sternly insisting he take out the trash. Since the therapist has created a safe, exploratory environment to "say the unsaid," the father is now more open to his son's perspective (Schnitzer, 1993, pp. 446–447). He may now be eager to begin a dialogue with his son and learn more about how long he has felt this way, what things the father has inadvertently done that makes him think "Dad likes my older brother better," and so on.

Similarly, if the therapist turns to the father and asks him to share his internal reactions as he was listening to his son, the son may also be able to see and hear his father in new ways that help to dissolve his previous notion that his father doesn't care for him. Ideally, this spirit of curiosity, self-reflexivity, and dialogue will transfer to future misunderstandings and support a mutually respectful relationship (H. Anderson, 1993, p. 332; Swim, 1995, p. 111).[49]

Tom Andersen (1996) indicates that he is primarily focused on *how* stories get told (i.e., from which perspective/voice), rather than emphasizing the content of any particular story.[50] He is concerned about this question: "Who can talk to whom about which issue here and now?" This orientation generates wonderings about things such as these: "Who prefers to talk about this topic? Who would prefer not to talk about this right now? Who might prefer to be silent and listen? How would you like me to participate here with you? Would someone prefer to watch and listen behind a one-way mirror? Are there others that we should be including in these talks?" (Andersen, 1991, p. 46).

These sorts of process-oriented questions also help therapists to be mindful of various speaking and listening formats that might maximize opportunities for self-reflection and for understanding others in new

---

[49]Hans-Georg Gadamer has discussed some inspiring and respectful ways of understanding genuine dialogue. Georgia Warnke (1987) describes Gadamer's thinking about this:

> Genuine conversation is based upon a recognition of our own fallibility, on a recognition that we are finite and historical creatures and thus we do not have absolute knowledge. . . . each participant in a genuine conversation must be concerned with discovering the real strength of every other participant's position . . . as someone who despite heritage, quirks of expression or the like is equally capable of illuminating the subject matter. (p. 100)

[50]Peggy Penn and Marilyn Frankfurt (1994) have written an excellent article that describes some helpful ways of "creating a dialogic space" (p. 222) and uses the idea of "narrative multiplicity" to accommodate many different selves or stories for different contexts.

ways. For example, clients may be so accusatory and defensive that they may be freer to express their own voices and to consider the others' perspectives if each person meets separately with the therapist or if one is in a listening position while another one talks exclusively with the therapist. In addition, there may be others in the "problem-determined system" (friends, extended relatives, social workers, etc.) who can be invited to help support clients' voices or to offer new perspectives, enabling dialogue to occur.

Andersen originated the idea of "reflecting processes," in which clients can shift back and forth from a "talking position" (outer conversation) to a "listening position" (inner conversation). Reflecting processes can occur in different ways—with a reflecting team,[51] or just with the therapist's speaking to one person while others "listen in." In the example above, where the therapist speaks with the son while the father "eavesdrops," it's possible that the father listens more fully and less defensively when he doesn't have to prepare for an immediate reply. In addition, clients can have imaginary, hypothetical conversations with important others who cannot be present. They can be asked how one of these other important voices might react to their concern, and in turn how they might reply to this external voice.[52]

Dialogic/hermeneutic therapists assume that in between sessions, clients may have had whatever internal or external conversations were needed for last week's problem to dissolve, and may no longer need to discuss that particular issue in therapy. Thus, these therapists don't assume that previous themes or stories will still be relevant (H. Anderson, 1994; Swim, 1995, p. 110). If they are, the client will probably mention these, or the therapist can ask if what they are talking about today connects with previously developed narratives. Tom Andersen's method for allowing a client maximum freedom to determine each therapy's agenda is to ask the client at the beginning of *each session,* "How would you like to use this meeting?" This allows the client to talk about cutting-

---

[51]Reflecting teams can be used in a variety of ways. However, in general they provide a format where clients and the therapist can silently "listen in" while previously silent, observing team members have the opportunity to share their observations and to engage in dialogue with each other. This team may talk for about 10 minutes or so. Afterward, the clients and therapist talk about what conversations stood our during the team's discussions. Clients and therapists often experience this process as a very helpful opportunity to consider many different perspectives on their concerns (Andersen, 1991; Andrews & Frantz, 1995).

[52]From my perspective, Karl Tomm's (1992) "internalized-other interviewing" is a very creative, empowering method to bring others' voices within the client to life and to play with ways to expand these voices.

edge concerns, solutions, or whatever else has immediate relevance at each new meeting (Andersen, 1991, p. 47).[53]

Anderson and Goolishian's idea of "not knowing" expresses a central feature permeating this dialogic way of working (H. Anderson, 1993, p. 330). They have indicated that this does *not* mean that the therapist pretends to have no prior knowledge or biases, or never shares ideas with the client (H. Anderson & Goolishian, 1992, pp. 29–30; Seikkula et al., 1995, p. 67). Rather, they describe this as setting aside whatever preconceptions the therapist might have about what the client is saying, in order to privilege the client's descriptions.

Personally, I often find it easier to embrace a "not-knowing" stance when I am more quiet and still as the client is speaking. Before responding, I try to ask myself whether I've really listened to what the client has just said, or whether I'm busy thinking of my next question. I find it tempting to become immersed in my own assumptions about what the client means, and I often experience a sense of urgency to "make" things happen. To cope with these temptations, I continually attempt to attune myself to the client. I try to notice changes in the client's tone of voice, emphasis, physical posture, and the like as guides for discerning what the client seems *most moved by* in each utterance. I often find that these utterances depart from our previous themes or narratives.

Like an exuberant dog galloping to and fro with abandon, generative dialogue has a life of its own, with unpredictable twists and turns. All participants, including the therapist, risk changing in this fluid process. The therapeutic conversation may unpredictably trigger a sudden burst of energy as a client recalls an important memory or pressing concern, or has a new realization that diverges from our previous conversations. I try to stay with and ask the client to elaborate on these sudden, significant departures. Thus, I don't want either to ignore these emergent moments or to prematurely rush in and impose previous connections or themes for my own sense of security and certainty (H. Anderson, 1993, p. 341). I frequently fall short of my goal to adopt a "not-knowing" stance, but when I'm able to come from this place, I feel much more connected on a moment-by-moment basis with my clients. Sometimes I'm able to catch myself coming from a more certain, "knowing" place. If I have any doubts that I may have inadvertently diminished a client's pressing concerns or voice, I attempt to

---

[53]Some clients may not know at the beginning of a session what they wish to focus on. Thus, an alternative way to allow clients to determine the agenda is to ask, "Do you know how you would like to use today's time or would you like to just talk out-loud for a while and see where things go?" (Hicks, personal communication, September, 1996)

check in immediately to see how the client has experienced what I just said.

The re-authoring and hermeneutic approaches utilized in this book have each helped many different clients. Many narratively oriented collaborative therapists feel more comfortable or familiar with one of these two approaches. However, as more therapists continue to be exposed to these and other postmodern and modern approaches, some creative combinations have emerged (Smith, 1995). Some therapists in this compilation have drawn from both the re-authoring tradition and the hermeneutic or dialogic traditions in unique ways. To give one of many possible examples, this blending can include things such as facilitating dialogues between externalized voices (e.g., "temper") and relevant others in the conversational system (e.g., the client's sister).[54] The problem's voice can respond to the sister's "inner" and "outer" voices, and the client can then reflect on the processes of this dialogue. Thus, the client can be asked something like this: "What does 'temper' tell you to do with your sister? What does your sister say to you when the 'temper' gets in between the two of you and gets you to swear at her? After she says this, what do you think she says *to herself* about what she just did? What does 'temper's' voice whisper in your ear then? What would 'temper' think if it could hear what your sister was thinking inside instead of what she actually says? As we're talking about this [external conversation], would you be willing to say what you are saying to yourself now [internal conversation]?" Each client reflection can yield a new perspective or voice, which can in turn be included in the ever-evolving dialogue with others and within the client.

This relatively open inquiry can yield a lot of unexpected new perspectives on the client's pressing concerns, and allows the therapist to stay connected moment by moment to wherever the client's reactions happen to diverge. Furthermore, when a client talks about enacting a new solution, there is another option besides focusing on the content of the client's story (i.e., how the client was able to accomplish this, developing unique outcomes, etc.). Clients can be asked to process what it is like (internally) to hear themselves say what they have just said (externally) (Hicks, personal communication, January, 1996). This allows clients freedom to respond from a variety of perspectives, rather than simply responding from the perspective of the new story or comparing their reaction with the old

---

[54]In addition to the examples above, a great many re-authoring therapists use a variation of Andersen's reflecting team or reflecting processes as a regular part of their therapy. For example, see the Section "The Community as Audience: Reauthoring Stories," in Friedman (1995).

story. There are a number of other ways to combine an externalizing, sociocultural approach with a dialogic approach that invites clients to sort out various internal and external voices.[55]

CONCLUSION

This introductory chapter has provided some comparisons between traditional and narrative therapy approaches with youth. It has explored objectivist ideas privileging therapists as the best authorities on clients problems and lives. We have seen that therapists espousing a variety of individual and systemic approaches can use their privileged, expert status to focus narrowly on what they consider to be significant. These approaches can be quite effective if clients agree with their therapists' direction. Indeed, the professional, scientific literature can be used as a potentially helpful resource rather than as a universal, normative, and definitive standard. However, if clients don't experience these professional findings as helpful, their voices may be inadvertently disregarded, or they may be blamed and pathologized. In addition, therapists who insist on their "truth" can find their *own* sense of creativity, wonder, excitement, and receptivity progressively diminished—to the point of eventual burnout. Focusing exclusively on professionally derived, interpretive schemas can provide familiarity, but this can also restrain therapists from successfully hearing and utilizing clients' idiosyncratic expressions. Utilizing rather than challenging clients' own descriptions can help therapists to join with them in meaningful ways, and these descriptions can be used as organic springboards toward alternative perspectives and resolutions.[56]

The traditional orientation differs from narrative approaches, which have been strongly influenced by such social constructionist ideas as perspectival knowing. These approaches attempt to collaborate with clients in determining what gets discussed and what ideas are most useful. Rather than adopting an "expert" posture and focusing on theoreti-

---

[55]I currently prefer to identify myself as a "dialogic narrative therapist," since I find it helpful to externalize problematic voices and cultural aspects supporting these, along with a primary focus on facilitating a criss-crossing or dialogue between inner and outer perspectives.

[56]Milton Erickson was a creative pioneer in advocating a principle of "utilization" (Erickson & Rossi, 1981). See also Miller et al. (1995) for their research on effective therapy; they conclude that clients often experience therapists as empathic when the therapists speak in the clients' "language and worldview . . . rather than in the terminology of their own treatment model" (p. 58).

cally predetermined meanings, therapists attempt to open space for clients' different voices or stories to be co-constructed. These new, mutually generated considerations can often be very different from what the therapists *or* the clients might have exclusively generated or even imagined. These collaboratively generated discussions can lead to previously unconsidered distinctions and possibilities for restoried lives with more satisfying resolutions.

This chapter has also compared traditional approaches to assessing childhood development with alternative approaches. The former emphasize universally applied, comprehensive, and intrapsychic features, whereas the latter see development in more situational, specific, and contextual terms. Therapists who are especially focused on comprehensive, age-appropriate "norms" may find it more difficult to listen more openly to youth and understand what most concerns *them* as unique individuals in their particular contexts. Finally, the chapter has discussed some distinctions between narratively oriented therapists who emphasize re-authoring aspects, and those who focus more on dialogic conversations and on how clients' stories are being told.

I hope that this introduction helps orient you, our readers, in some useful ways as you explore this book. Many of us growing up in mid- to late-20th-century Western culture have benefited from very well-intentioned traditional ideas about children and therapy. I hope this book will encourage those of you who are excited about cutting-edge, collaborative possibilities with youth to consider the diverse, creative ideas in this book as a springboard for following your own hearts and for finding your mutual pathways with clients!

REFERENCES

Amundson, J. (1996). Why pragmatics is probably enough for now. *Family Process, 3*(4), 473–486.

Amundson, J., & Stewart, K. (1993). Temptations of power and certainty. *Journal of Marital and Family Therapy, 19*(2), 111–123.

Andersen, T. (1991). Guidelines for practice. In T. Andersen (Ed.), *The reflecting team: Dialogues and dialogues about the dialogues.* New York: Norton.

Andersen, T. (1992a). *Reflecting processes: Dialogues about dialogues* [Videotape]. Los Angeles: Master's Work Productions.

Andersen, T. (1992b). Reflections on reflecting with families. In S. McNamee & K. J. Gergen (Eds.), *Therapy as social construction.* Newbury Park, CA: Sage.

Andersen, T. (1993). See and hear, and be seen and heard. In S. Friedman (Ed.), *The new language of change: Constructive collaboration in psychotherapy.* New York: Guilford Press.

Andersen, T. (1994). Workshop presented at the California Family Studies Center/Phillips Graduate Institute, Los Angeles.

Andersen, T. (1995). Reflecting processes; acts of informing and forming: You can borrow my eyes, but you must not take tham away from me! In S. Friedman (Ed.), *The reflecting team in action: Collaborative practice in family therapy*. New York: Guilford Press.

Andersen, T. (1996). Workshop presented at the California Family Studies Center/Phillips Graduate Institute, Los Angeles.

Anderson, H. (1993). On a roller coaster: A collaborative language systems approach to therapy. In S. Friedman (Ed.), *The new language of change: Constructive collaboration in psychotherapy*. New York: Guilford Press.

Anderson, H. (1994). *Collaborative therapy: The co-construction of newness*. Workshop presented at the meeting of the American Association for Marriage and Family Therapy, Chicago.

Anderson, H. (1996). Workshop presented at the California Family Studies Center/Phillips Graduate Institute, Los Angeles.

Anderson, H. (1997). *Conversation, language, and possibilities—A postmodern approach to psychotherapy*. NY: Basic Books.

Anderson, H., & Goolishian, H. (1988). Human systems as linguistic systems: Preliminary and evolving ideas about the implications for clinical theory. *Family Process, 27*, 371–393.

Anderson, H., & Goolishian, H. (1992). The client is the expert: A not-knowing approach to therapy. In S. McNamee & K. J. Gergen (Eds.), *Therapy as social construction*. Newbury Park, CA: Sage.

Anderson, W. T. (1990). *Reality isn't what it used to be*. San Francisco: Harper & Row.

Andrews, J., & Frantz, T. (1995). Reflecting teams in case consultation and training: Two for the price of one. *Journal of Collaborative Therapies, 3*(3), 14–20.

Axline, V. (1947). *Play therapy*. Boston: Houghton Mifflin.

Barry, A. K. (1991). Narrative style and witness testimony. *Journal of Narrative and Life History, 1*(4), 281–294.

Belenky, M. F., Clinchy, B. M., Goldberger, N. R., & Tarlile, J. M. (1986). *Women's ways of knowing: The development of self, voice, and mind*. New York: Basic Books.

Berger, P. L., & Luckman, T. (1967). *The social construction of reality*. Garden City, NY: Doubleday.

Bogdan, J. (1984). Family organization as an ecology of ideas: An alternative to the reification of family systems. *Family Process, 23*(3), 375–388.

Brems, C. (1993). *A comprehensive guide to child psychotherapy*. Needham Heights, MA: Allyn & Bacon.

Burman, E. (1994). *Deconstructing developmental psychology*. New York: Routledge.

Chang, J. (1996, June). *Solution-oriented therapy with children and their families*. Workshop presented at Therapeutic Conversations 3, Denver, CO.

Cushman, P. (1995). *Constructing the self, constructing America*. Reading, MA: Addison-Wesley.

Dell, P. (1982). *Pathology: The original sin.* Paper presented at the First International Conference on Epistemology, Psychotherapy, and Psychopathology, Houston, TX.

Duncan, B., Hubble, M., & Miller, S. (1997). Stepping off the throne. *Family Therapy Networker, 21*(4), 22–33.

Durrant, M. (1989). Scaling fears: Making exceptions to problem behavior meaningful. *Family Therapy Case Studies, 4*(2), 15–31.

Durrant, M. (1990). Saying "boo" to Mr. Scarey: Writing a book provides a solution. *Family Therapy Case Studies, 5*(1), 39–44.

Durrant, M. (1993). *Residential treatment: A coopertive, competency-based approach to therapy and program design.* New York: Norton.

Durrant, M. (1995). *Creative strategies for school problems: Solutions for psychologists and teachers.* New York: Norton.

Durrant, M., & White, C. (Eds.). (1990). *Ideas for therapy with sexual abuse.* Adelaide, South Australia: Dulwich Centre Publications.

Ellis, A., & Bernard, M. (1983). *Rational–emotive approaches to the problems of childhood.* New York: Plenum Press.

Epston, D., & White, M. (1992). *Experience, contradiction, narrative and imagination: Selected papers of David Epston and Michael White, 1989–1991.* Adelaide, South Australia: Dulwich Centre Publications.

Erickson, M. H., & Rossi, E. L. (1981). *Experiencing hypnosis: Therapeutic approaches to altered states.* New York: Irvington.

Eron, J., & Lund, T. (1996). *Narrative solutions in brief therapy.* New York: Guilford Press.

Fine, M. (1984). *Systematic intervention with disturbed children.* New York: SP Medical and Scientific Books.

Fogel, A. (1993). *Developing through relationships: Origins of communication, self, and culture.* Chicago: University of Chicago Press.

Foucault, M. (1977). *Discipline and punish: The birth of the prison.* London: Allen Lane.

Frankl, L., & Hellman, I. (1964). The ego's participation in the therapeutic alliance. In M. Haworth (Ed.), *Child psychotherapy.* New York: Basic Books.

Freedman, J., & Combs, G. (1996). *Narrative therapy: The social construction of preferred realities.* New York: Norton.

Freeman, J., Epston, D., & Lobovits, D. (1997). *Playful approaches to serious problems: Narrative therapy with children and their families.* New York: Norton.

Friedman, S. (Ed.). (1995). *The reflecting team in action: Collaborative practice in family therapy.* New York: Guilford Press.

Gergen, K. J. (1991). *The saturated self: Dilemmas of identity in contemporary life.* New York: Basic Books.

Gergen, K. J., & Gergen, M. (1986). Narrative form and the construction of psychological science. In T. Sarbin (Ed.), *Narrative psychology: The storied nature of human conduct.* New York: Praeger.

Gergen, K. J., & Kaye, J. (1992). Beyond narrative in the negotiation of therapeutic meaning. In S. McNamee & K. J. Gergen (Eds.), *Therapy as social construction.* Newbury Park, CA: Sage.

Gilligan, C. (1982). *In a different voice: Psychological theory and women's development.* Cambridge, MA: Harvard University Press.

Giorgi, A. (1970). *Psychology as a human science: A phenomenologically based approach.* New York: Harper & Row.

Golann, S. (1988). On second-order family therapy. *Family Process, 27,* 51–64.

Goldner, V. (1988). Generation and gender: Normative and covert hierarchies. *Family Process, 27*(1), 17–31.

Greenspan, S. (1981). *The clinical interview of the child.* New York: McGraw-Hill.

Griffith, J. L., & Griffith, M. E. (1992). Owning one's epistemological stance in therapy. *Dulwich Centre Newsletter, No. 1,* 5–11.

Griffith, J. L., & Griffith, M. E. (1994). *The body speaks: Therapeutic dialogues for mind–body problems.* New York: Basic Books.

Haley, J. (1976). *Problem-solving therapy.* New York: Harper & Row.

Hare-Mustin, R. (1987). The problem of gender in family therapy theory. *Family Process, 26,* 15–28.

Heidegger, M. (1962). *Being and time.* New York: Harper & Row.

Hoffman, L. (1990). Constructing realities: An art of lenses. *Family Process, 29,* 1–12.

Hoffman, L. (1991). A reflexive stance for family therapy. *Journal of Strategic and Systemic Therapies, 10*(3–4), 4–17.

Hubble, M., & O'Hanlon, W. H. (1992). Theory countertransference. *Dulwich Centre Newsletter, No. 1,* 25–30.

Jenkins, A. (1990). *Invitations to responsibility: The therapeutic engagement of men who are violent and abusive.* Adelaide, South Australia: Dulwich Centre Publications.

Jordan, J. V., Kaplan, A. G., Miller, J. B., Stiver, I. P., & Surrey, J. L. (1991). *Women's growth in connection: Writings from the Stone Center.* New York: Guilford Press.

Klein, M. (1964). The psychoanalytic play technique. In M. Haworth (Ed.), *Child psychotherapy.* New York: Basic Books.

Kowalski, K. (1990). The little girl with the know-how: Finding solutions to a school problem. *Family Therapy Case Studies, 5*(1), 3–14.

Kral, R. (1986). Indirect therapy in the schools. In S. de Shazer & R. Kral (Eds.), *Indirect approaches in therapy.* Rockville, MD: Aspen.

Kral, R. (1989). The Q.I.K. (Quick Interview for Kids): Psychodiagnostics for teens and children—brief therapy style. *Family Therapy Case Studies, 4*(2), 61–65.

Kral, R. (1994). *Strategies that work: Solutions in the schools* (2nd ed.). Milwaukee, WI: Brief Family Therapy Center Press.

Kuhn, T. (1962). *The structure of scientific revolutions.* Chicago: University of Chicago Press.

LaFountain, R., Garner, N., & Boldosser, S. (1995). Solution-focused counseling groups for children and adolescents. *Journal of Systemic Therapies, 14*(4), 39–51.

Lax, W. (1991). The reflecting team and the initial consult. In T. Andersen (Ed.),

The reflecting team: Dialogues and dialogues about the dialogues. New York: Norton.

Lobovits, D., Maisel, R., & Freeman, J. (1995). Public practices: An ethic of circulation. In S. Friedman (Ed.), *The reflecting team in action: Collaborative practice in family therapy.* New York: Guilford Press.

Lowe, R. (1991). Postmodern themes and therapeutic practices: Notes towards the definition of 'family therapy.' *Dulwich Centre Newsletter, No. 3,* 41–52.

Madigan, S., & Epston, D. (1995). From "spy-chiatric gaze" to communities of concern. In S. Friedman (Ed.), *The reflecting team in action: Collaborative practice in family therapy.* New York: Guilford Press.

McNamee, S. (1996). Psychotherapy as a social construction. In H. Rosen & K. Kuehlwein (Eds.), *Constructing realities: Meaning-making perspectives for psychotherapists.* San Francisco: Jossey-Bass.

Metcalf, L. (1994). *Counseling toward solutions: A practical solution-focused program for working with students, teachers, and parents.* Needham Heights, MA: Allyn & Bacon.

Miller, S., Hubble, M., & Duncan, B. (1995). No more bells and whistles: Effective therapy doesn't have much to do with either theory or technique. *Family Therapy Networker, 19*(2), 53–63.

Minuchin, S., & Fishman, H. C. (1981). *Family therapy techniques.* Cambridge, MA: Harvard University Press.

Mishne, J. (1983). *Clinical work with children.* New York: Free Press.

Monk, G., Winslade, J., Crocket, K., & Epston, D. (Eds.). (1997). *Narrative therapy in practice: The archaeology of hope.* San Francisco: Jossey-Bass.

Morss, J. (1996). *Growing critical: Alternatives to developmental psychology.* New York: Routledge.

Moustakas, C. (1964). The therapeutic process. In M. Haworth (Ed.), *Child psychotherapy.* New York: Basic Books.

Murphy, J. J. (1994). Brief therapy for school problems. *School Psychology International, 15,* 115–131.

Neimeyer, R., & Mahoney, M. (Eds.). (1995). *Constructivism in psychotherapy.* Washington, DC: American Psychological Association.

Nylund, D., & Corsiglia, V. (1994). Attention to the deficits in attention-deficit disorder: Deconstructing the diagnosis and bringing forth children's special abilities. *Journal of Collaborative Therapies, 2*(2), 7–17.

Nylund, D., & Thomas, J. (1994). The economics of narrative. *Family Therapy Networker, 18*(6), 38–39.

O'Hanlon, W. H., & Weiner-Davis, M. (1989). *In search of solutions: A new direction in psychotherapy.* New York: Norton.

Ollendick, T., & Cerny, J. (1981). *Clinical behavior therapy with children.* New York: Plenum Press.

Pare, D. (1995). Of families and other cultures: The shifting paradigm of family therapy. *Family Process, 34*(1), 1–20.

Parker, I., Georgaca, E., Harper, D., McLaughlin, T., & Stowell-Smith, M. (1995). *Deconstructing psychopathology.* Thousand Oaks, CA: Sage.

Parry, A. (1991a). A universe of stories. *Family Process, 30,* 37–54.

Parry, A. (1991b). If the doors of perception were cleansed. *The Calgary Participator, 1*(2), 9–13.

Parry, A., & Doan, R. (1994). *Story-re-visions: Narrative therapy in the post-modern world.* New York: Guilford Press.

Penn, P., & Frankfurt, M. (1994). Creating a participant text: Writing, multiple voices, narrative multiplicity. *Family Process, 33,* 217–231.

Pluznick, R., & Rafael, R. (1994). *An alternative story for child welfare: Building safety in therapeutic relationships.* To be published.

Reisman, J. (1973). *Principles of psychotherapy with children.* New York: Wiley.

Robinson, J., & Hawpe, L. (1986). Narrative thinking as a heuristic process. In T. Sarbin (Eds.), *Narrative psychology: The storied nature of human conduct.* New York: Praeger.

Roth, S., Chasin, L., Chasin, R., Becker, S., & Herzig, M. (1992). From debate to dialogue: A facilitating role for family therapists in the public forum. *Dulwich Centre Newsletter, No. 2,* 41–48.

Roth, S., & Epston, D. (1996). Developing externalizing conversations: An exercise. *Journal of Systemic Therapies, 15,* 5–12.

Sarbin, T., & Kitsuse, J. (Eds.). (1994). *Constructing the social.* Thousand Oaks, CA: Sage.

Schaefer, C., & Millman, H. (1977). *Therapies for children: A handbook of effective treatments for problem behaviors.* San Francisco: Jossey-Bass.

Schafer, R. (1992). *Retelling a life: Narration and dialogue in psychoanalysis.* New York: Basic Books.

Schnitzer, P. (1993). Tales of the absent father: Applying the 'story' metaphor in family therapy. *Family Process, 32*(4), 441–458.

Seikkula, J., Aaltonen, J., Alakare, B., Haarakangas, K., Keranen, J., & Sutela, M. (1995). Treating psychosis by means of open dialogue. In S. Friedman (Ed.), *The reflecting team in action: Collaborative practice in family therapy.* New York: Guilford Press.

Selekman, M. (1993). *Pathways to change: Brief therapy solutions with difficult adolescents.* New York: Guilford Press.

Shawver, L. (1996). What postmodernism can do for psychoanalysis: A guide to the postmodern vision. *American Journal of Psychoanalysis, 56*(4), 371–394.

Shotter, J. (1993). *Conversational realities: Constructing life through language.* Thousand Oaks, CA: Sage.

Smith, C. (1995). *One way of incorporating two different narrative therapy approaches: "Collaborative language systems and "decnstructive-externalizing."* Paper presented at Narrative Ideas and Therapeutic Practice: The 3rd Annual International Conference, Vancouver, B.C., Canada.

Spence, D. P. (1982). *Narrative truth and historical truth.* New York: Norton.

Stacey, K. (1996). Workshop presented at San Diego State University.

Stacey, K., & Loptson, C. (1995). Children should be seen and not heard?: Questioning the unquestioned. *Journal of Systemic Therapies, 14*(4), 16–32.

Steenbarger, B. (1991). All the world is *not* a stage: Emerging contextualist themes in counseling and development. *Journal of Counseling and Development, 70*(2), 288–295.

Stern, D. (1990). *Diary of a baby.* New York: Basic Books.

Strean, H. (Ed.). (1970). *New approaches in child guidance.* Metuchen, NJ: Scarecrow Press.

Swim, S. (1995). Reflective and collaborative voices in the school. In S. Friedman (Ed.), *The reflecting team in action: Collaborative practice in family therapy*. New York: Guilford Press.

Tamasese, K., & Waldegrave, C. (1993). Cultural and gender accountability in the "just therapy" approach. *Journal of Feminist Family Therapy, 5*(2), 29–45.

Tapping, C. (1993). Other wisdoms, other worlds: Colonization and family therapy. *Dulwich Centre Newsletter, No. 1,* 3–4.

Tomm, K. (1988). Interventive interviewing: Part 3. Intending to ask circular, strategic, or reflexive questions? *Family Process, 27*(1), 1–16.

Tomm, K. (1989). Externalizing the problem and internalizing personal agency. *Journal of Strategic and Systemic Therapy, 8*(1), 54–59.

Tomm, K. (1991). 2-week externship in systemic therapy through the Univ. of Calgary, Alberta, Canada.

Tomm, K. (1992). *Interviewing the internalized other.* Workshop presented at the annual meeting of the American Association for Marriage and Family Therapy, Miami, FL.

Varela, F. J. (1979). *Principles of biological autonomy.* New York: Elsevier N. Holland.

Warnke, G. (1987). *Gadamer: Hermeneutics, tradition, and reason.* Stanford, CA: Stanford University Press.

Watzlawick, P. (1976). *How real is real?* New York: Random House.

Weingarten, K. (1994). *The mother's voice—Strengthening intimacy in families.* New York: Harcourt Brace.

Weingarten, K. (Ed.). (1995). *Cultural resistance—Challenging beliefs about men, women, and therapy.* New York: Haworth Press.

Weingarten, K., & Cobb, S. (1995). Timing disclosure sessions: Adding a narrative perspective to clinical work with adult survivors of childhood sexual abuse. *Family Process, 34*(3), 257–270.

White, M. (1989). *Selected papers.* Adelaide, South Australia: Dulwich Centre Publications.

White, M. (1995). *Re-authoring lives: Interviews and essays.* Adelaide, South Australia: Dulwich Centre Publications.

White, M., & Epston, D. (1990). *Narrative means to therapeutic ends.* New York: Norton.

Wolf, D. (1990). Being of several minds: Voices and versions of the self in early childhood. In D. Cicchetti & M. Beeghly (Eds.), *The self in transition: Infancy to childhood.* Chicago: University of Chicago Press.

Wolf, D. (1993). There and then, intangible and internal: Narratives in early childhood. In B. Spodek (Ed.), *Handbook of research on the education of young children.* New York: Macmillan.

Woltmann, A. (1964). Concepts of play therapy techniques. In M. Haworth (Ed.), *Child psychotherapy.* New York: Basic Books.

Zimmerman, J., & Dickerson, V. (1994). Using a narrative metaphor: Implications for theory and clinical practice. *Family Process, 33,* 233–246.

Zimmerman, J., & Dickerson, V. (1996). *If problems talked: Narrative therapy in action.* New York: Guilford Press.

2

"I Am a Bear"

DISCOVERING DISCOVERIES

DAVID EPSTON

I was introduced to Bjorn, aged 7, by his mother, Gerde. By chance I had very recently returned from Stockholm, where I had been teaching and visiting friends and their two children, Emilie and Bjorn. Visiting the Stockholm Zoo, I took delight in watching two native bears playing in water and noted that "Bjorn" meant "bear." So I must have looked confused or seemed not to hear as Gerde repeated herself. "Bjorn," she said, "like in Bjorn Borg!"

I broke free of my memories of Stockholm and replied with some excitement: "Yes, yes . . . I know. Matter of fact, I know what your name means. Do you?" Neither Gerde nor Bjorn knew. I informed them that "Bjorn" means "bear," and felt pleased to make this known to them. Bjorn seemed not to know what to make of this association, so I asked him: "Are you bear-like?" He was still lost, but grinned.

We entered my office and Gerde took over. She informed me that Bjorn had been referred by a pediatric specialist, whom they attended in the first instance on account of a kidney infection. The major symptom

Except for the "Editorial Question," this chapter is reprinted (with very minor revisions) from Epston (1992). Copyright 1992 by Dulwich Centre Publications.

of this had been urinary frequency. However, antibiotics had been prescribed and the infection was arrested.

Despite this both immediate and happy outcome, Bjorn felt the need to attend toilets more and more. They returned and were given the opinion that this would resolve itself in time, and an appointment was made to review this in 3 months. Bjorn increasingly felt required to attend toilets—so much so, in fact, that it was interfering with his schooling, as he continually had to absent himself and he found it difficult to sleep at night due to his frequent toileting. In fact, on the way to our meeting, they had to call into three petrol stations for the selfsame purpose. The pediatrician advised the family to consult me.

Gerde informed me that Bjorn feared that he would wet his pants and that this had become an overwhelming concern of his. I inquired whether she felt that this "problem" had been investigated medically to her satisfaction. She assured me it had, but she and Bjorn's father were of the opinion that this had now become "a habit." "Do you think this habit has started to have a life of its own?" She lamented that this was certainly the case. Their answers to my "relative-influence questions" (White, 1986) developed a compassion we all shared for the plight of this young boy. There seemed little in his life that had been spared by the problem's humiliating prospect of wetting his pants.

As chance would have it, Bjorn, in an aside, mentioned that the day before our meeting, he had gone from "morning tea to big play" without having to go to the toilet. I seized upon this with alacrity and requested permission to record our conversation, because I suspected this could very well be "bad news" for his problem. This both dramatized what was to follow and positioned Bjorn as its protagonist.

DAVID: Now Bjorn, you remember yesterday, the 31st day of October ... it could be a really important day in your life, couldn't it? ... because on that day, for some reason or other ... I don't know yet but we'll find out ... you—*you*—did something really, really important. You won over your habit. Before, you couldn't hold on to your peepee,[1] but yesterday you got some strength, some bearlike strength inside of you to do this. And I asked you because I think it's very interesting how it was that you were able to be so strong all day yesterday. Your strength ... how long did it last?

BJORN: It lasted between morning tea and big play.

DAVID: Between morning tea and big play.

---

[1] "Peepee" was the word contributed by Bjorn's mother, Gerde.

BJORN: Yes, between them.

DAVID: So on a day when you were feeling weak and your habit was strong, how many times would you have gone between morning tea and big play?

BJORN: Maybe about two.

My introduction positions me as commentator, as eyewitness to events that are about to unfold before me. Subjunctivizing is introduced by the suggestion of "it could be a really important day in your life, couldn't it?"

Jerome Bruner makes a case for what he refers to as "subjunctivizing" as a means to contribute to the creation of new possibilities and new realities. I am aware that this term is somewhat awkward, but I remain faithful to it in order to acknowledge my source:

> I have tried to make the case that the function of literature as art is to open us to dilemmas, to the hypothetical, to the range of possible worlds that a text can refer to. I have used the term 'to subjunctivize,' to render the world less fixed, less banal, more susceptible to recreation. Literature subjunctivizes, makes strange, renders the obvious less so, the unknowable less so as well, matters of value more open to reason and intuition. (1986, p. 159)

Mystery and intrigue are brought about by the proposition that "on that day, for some reason or other . . . I don't know yet but we'll find out . . . you—*you*—did something really, really important." The frame of inquiry into what "knowledge" made from "morning tea to big play" possible is set by the temporal distinction "Before . . . but yesterday . . ." The putative solution is externalized by the allegation that "you got some strength, some bear-like strength inside of you," connecting it to bear-likeness and objectifying it so that it can be matched up to the externalized problem—the "habit/problem," so called. Gerde had already conveniently separated the problem from the medical discourse through which it had very appropriately been interpreted and "treated." This double externalization allows the problem and the solution/alternative knowledge of self to "face" each other. Instead of the problem speaking of the identity of the person, the person is now positioned to speak of and to the problem. This permits alternative discursive practices, many of which I have come to associate with unconsidered possibilities and previously unheard-of discoveries.

DAVID: Yesterday, the 31st day of October, was a pretty good day for you. And you were telling me that you felt pretty proud of yourself for winning and not losing. Are you curious . . . do you know what "curious" means? Are you wondering how it was on Wednesday you were able to be so strong? Are you wondering? I know I am wondering. I am very curious. Are you very curious?

BJORN: Yes.

By expressing my curiosity and wonderment rather than employing conventional evaluative/assessment/classificatory formats, I indicate the potential location of "knowledge" in the other's experience.

DAVID: Can you think of anything you did differently that you don't really want to forget? . . . Did you have a dream or anything that told you what to do? Did your teddy bear tell you something . . . did it give you some special ideas? Did your mum or dad give you some special strength food? What made you so strong?

BJORN: I don't actually know what it was.

DAVID: Have you got any guesses?

BJORN: It just came up.

I start by asking an open-ended question that I don't necessarily expect to be replied to; my purpose is more a matter of orientation to the doing of difference. I then expect, as is the case here, to propose any number of possibilities for the young person to examine and consider. Often young persons will quickly associate with one of them or be encouraged either to generate or discover one of their own. When working with young children, we probably need quite an array of these at our disposal, and I zealously add any novel sources to my stock. My intended purpose in proposing dreams, magic, and so forth is to recruit the young persons' imagination into the world of children, a realm I hope they will allow me into. A reading of children's stories can equip you with your own collection, which should indicate to young persons that you are willing to enter their life-world rather than their being required to explicate themselves according to the adult world.

DAVID: Your strength just came up. Really! Can you think of any other times your strength just came up like that? . . . Maybe not just to do with your habit, but when you are running, cycling, or playing . . . or swimming when your strength just came up in a hurry like that . . . and lasted for a fair while?

BJORN: It does it sometimes at swimming . . . sometimes.

DAVID: So sometimes at swimming you feel very strong.

BJORN: I feel I've got power and can go a bit faster.

DAVID: Really! Is that right? When does that happen?

BJORN: It sometimes happens at backstroke or lying on my back and kicking.

DAVID: And all of a sudden you don't feel tired . . . you feel powerful?

BJORN: It just comes up.

DAVID: Is it a good feeling?

BJORN: Yep!

This series of questions attempts to locate further examples of "strength coming up" and, once again, I am careful to suggest some likely sites: running, cycling, playing, or swimming. Bjorn acknowledges possessing at times the externalized power/strength, but relates it to himself in a random way ("It just comes up").

DAVID: Do you think you are growing up? And do you think your power has anything to do with that?

BJORN: Yep . . . 'cause I've got bigger . . .

DAVID: Taller and more muscle?

BJORN: Taller.

GERDE: He has grown 5 centimeters in the last few months. We just measured him.

DAVID: Do you think you will grow out of this problem . . . this habit? Do you think your strength will take you away from it?

BJORN: I don't really know if it is.

DAVID: Do you think you are growing up and getting stronger, and, of course, your habit stays the same but you are getting stronger? . . . Look, where is this power coming from? I know you have a powerful name. Do you think your teddy bear is giving you power? Do you think he is starting to worry about you . . . after all, that's what teddy bears are for—to look after kids? What do you think teddy bears are for?

BJORN: Make you sleep.

GERDE: Actually, he has something else to give him strength . . . a cow, Micky. She always travels along with us.

DAVID: A power cow . . . I've never heard of those before.

BJORN: When I cuddle her, it makes the power come.

DAVID: How long does it take?

BJORN: Twelve minutes.

DAVID: Is that all?

BJORN: The power comes out.

The first questions potentially link "power/strength" to the notion of growing up, an idea particularly appealing to young people. Also, given his age, it is very likely that either Bjorn or his mother will report favorably on his growing up. And I then go on to speculate as to the source of his power, and I do so because I am alternatively using "teddy bear"/"teddy bjorn." Much to my surprise, his primary cuddly toy is a cow. Bjorn discovers from his experience a means to "make the power come." By doing so, he purports to be the agent of the externalized "power/strength/solution."

DAVID: How do you do that?

BJORN: I think the power comes because it was fun playing with her . . . giving them food and milk.

DAVID: So do you figure it has something to do with having a good time? Is that why you get power?

BJORN: I get power sometimes when I ride my bike . . .

DAVID: I can understand that. So look you've got a lot of sources of your power. One, bike riding. Two, backstroke.

BJORN: And lying on my back and kicking.

DAVID: Lying your back and kicking strong. You've got a power cow. And you've got your power teddy bjorn. You've got a lot going for you, haven't you?

BJORN: Yah!

The sources of power are reiterated and summed up. They derive from his own experience and his relationships to his fantasy familiars.

DAVID: Can I suggest something and you tell me if I am right or wrong? Maybe you didn't know until we got talking here today that you had all this power and for that reason, your habit was winning over you? You didn't know you had such power . . . you didn't put it together? . . . You had power here and here but didn't put it against your habit, right? You used your power for your cycling, for your getting to sleep at night, used your power for having a good time, for swimming fast and kicking hard. But you didn't know that you could use your power against your habit . . . you didn't know that. What do you think?

BJORN: Dunno.

This series of questions theorizes about this habit's current status. The suggestion that "not knowing" both the existence and extent of his powers is his weakness obviates the "not knowing." The "not known" becomes known.

DAVID: Well, first of all, did you know you had so much power?

BJORN: I didn't really know that I had it.

DAVID: Is it good to know that you are no such weakling? Is it good to know that you are powerful?

BJORN: Yep!

DAVID: This is no surprise to me. You know why? Two reasons—first, because I knew what your name meant. Number two, you look rather powerful. (*Turning toward Gerde*) He looks healthy and strong. You know how you can tell a sick-looking person, and they certainly don't look like him. Can I just feel your muscles?

In "knowing" that he has so much power, Bjorn is redescribing himself in terms of powerful attributes, rather than "weakness"/"growing down"/"wetting your pants."

I ceremonially invite him to remove his coat and flex his biceps. His parents are in the health food business, and not surprisingly, he is a picture of good health. Gerde looks on with pleasure in Bjorn's self-delight at impressing me with his physical strength, which augments the sources of power he can draw upon. Gerde provides another example, and that is her pride in how high he can climb trees.

DAVID: What do you think would happen if you gathered up all your power? . . . You've got a lot of power and a lot of helpers. If you got it all together and put it against your habit, what do you think would happen? Who would win, your habit or you?

BJORN: Me!

DAVID: Good! I think so too. (*To Gerde*) If I understand your pediatrician, Bjorn has had something of a setback and lost some of his strength, and more importantly his confidence . . . no kid would want to wet their pants . . .

GERDE: That's his main concern, actually; he's always saying he's afraid of wetting his pants. That's what actually bothers him. I really think he has enough power because all through these times, he's never wet his pants.

DAVID: I didn't know that. You're stronger than what you think you are? Do you think you are stronger than what you think you are? Do you think your problem is trying to trick you into thinking you are a bit of a weakling when in fact you are quite a strong and powerful person?

BJORN: It tries to say that . . .

DAVID: What does it say to you?

BJORN: It just says . . . it thinks that I'm a weakling but I'm not.

DAVID: Good. What if you talked back to it?

BJORN: I try to do it.

DAVID: What do you say back?

BJORN: I say . . .

DAVID: I just wonder if we got together and worked out some power talk for you. Do you think this would really scare your habit? . . . teach your habit a lesson? Would you like to teach your habit a lesson? Teach your habit that it doesn't really know how strong you are? You can't be tricked into thinking you are a weakling? What do you think about that? Would you like to do that?

BJORN: I always say at night . . .

DAVID: Yah, what do you say?

BJORN: When I've gone to the toilet maybe 12, 11, or 10 times I say: "That's the last time." If I have to go again I'll say: "No, that's the last time and that's it."

DAVID: What do you think would happen if you tried that after 7 times? If you said: "Look, I'm sick of 11 times, I think I'll get powerful after 7?" What do you think would happen? Do you think you could do it if you used your strength like you are using it?

BJORN: I think I could have done it because I've done it one night. I had to go toilet . . . one night, then I held it. I held it the whole night until the next morning.

DAVID: You didn't?

BJORN: It was only one night it happened.

DAVID: That was a good night to remember, wasn't it?

Finding out some information about this fear of wetting his pants, along with the fact that he never has, allows me to inquire: "Do you think you are stronger than what you think you are?" This is followed by the personification of the problem as a trickster, tricking Bjorn "into thinking you are a bit of a weakling when in fact you are quite a strong and powerful person?" This provides two self-descriptions, one based on the mischief or malevolence of his problem, and the other more in accordance with his mother and myself. Such a question has the effect of deconstructing the "truth" of his problem's version of himself. This leads Bjorn to recollect having talked back to his problem and having asserted an alternative version of himself, one consistent with this version that has been both resurrected and generated by this conversation. The question revising down his self-assertion from 11 times to 7 times is important for allowing action to be taken at will rather than being contingent.

DAVID: Look, you sound ready. You are old enough, strong enough, and smart enough to go against this habit. Do you think you are? We might come up with some ideas to help you. Do you want to wait until you are older?

BJORN: I'll do it.

DAVID: (*To Gerde*) Would you be pleased for him to do it?

GERDE: Of course.

DAVID: I've got the impression from what you have been telling me that you have got all the power you need. But it's all over the place. It's not there when you need it. It's almost as if you've got a car, and you know petrol gives cars power. And you have got petrol in this tin over here, and this tin over here . . . but the car still doesn't go. You've got lots of petrol but you just haven't put it into the tank. Do you know what I mean by "petrol tank"? I think we've got to get the power into you. Okay? And then you can use it for whatever you want to use it for. You can use it to break this habit . . . or you could also use it to swim faster or enjoy your life more. You ready for this?

BJORN: Yep!

With problems of this nature that require young people to take responsibility for the resolution of the problem, I often use "readiness questions" (White, 1986). In the exchange above, I restate the "double externalization," habit versus strength/power, by way of a rather elaborate metaphorical description. Bjorn consents to bring his power/strength to bear on his problem, and I consent to the requirement on our part "to get the power into you." That is the contribution others can make.

I suggested at the end of the session that Gerde drop in at her neighborhood library on the way home and get some books on bears, as I observed that, despite Bjorn's being bear-like, I didn't think he fully appreciated the parallels. She was only too happy to bring his bear-likeness to his attention. I, in turn, promised to make a cassette tape for him and forward it to him by post. For working with young people, I have substituted recorded tapes for letters as my medium of preference and necessity.

> White and I have written at some length detailing 'letters as narrative': Letters constitute a medium rather than a particular genre and as such can be employed for any number of purposes, several of which are demonstrated in this text. In a storied therapy, the letters are used primarily for the purpose of rendering lived experience into a narrative or 'story,' one that makes sense according to the criteria of coherence and lifelikeness. Accordingly, they are at variance to a considerable degree to those conventions that prescribe both the rhetoric and stylistics of professional letter-writing. By 'professional' letters, I am referring to those communications between professionals about persons and their problems. Typically, the persons who are subjects of these letters are excluded from any access to this record, even though their futures may be shaped by it. In a storied therapy, the letters are a version of that co-constructed reality called therapy and become the shared property of all the parties to it. (White & Epston, 1989, pp. 125–126)

Much to my dismay, I became very busy and wasn't able to find time to make a tape. About a week later, I rang Gerde to see if it was necessary and, if so, to make amends. Gerde was glad to hear from me, as for four successive nights, Bjorn had slept through the night without requiring to go to the toilet. Since then, he had remitted, and she urged me to send him a tape. I did so immediately and booked another appointment.

The following is a transcript copy of that taped "story":

> "Hello, Bjorn, David speaking . . . I decided against sending you this tape right away because I guessed you might need it a little bit later . . . and now is a very good time to start listening to this tape. It might be the very best time to listen to just before you go to bed . . . when it is dark or coming on dark . . . or if there was a time you felt you needed more strength.
>
> "Your problem has weakened your bladder, and I am sorry

about that . . . but little did your bladder and little did your problem know that your name was Bjorn . . . now it probably doesn't speak Swedish . . . it's probably an English-speaking problem so it doesn't know yet, but it will learn that your name means "bear." Now everyone knows that bears are very nice animals, but when they get angry they can be very strong and vicious. And when I met you recently I had a sense that you had a bear-like strength inside of you. And I wasn't surprised when you told me that on October 31st you had beaten your habit and proved to it how bear-like you were, because you went from morning tea time to the big break time without having to go to the toilet. You kept your strength. Usually if your habit was strong and it had weakened you, you would have had to go to the toilet twice.

"You told me you felt proud of yourself for winning, and when you told me that, I could see the pride all over your face. And then when I asked how was it that you got so strong all of a sudden, you said that your strength just came up in a hurry and lasted for a fair while. Now, Bjorn, that's not the only place or the only time your strength comes up. And there were some other places that it did. And you told me that when you are swimming, especially doing the backstroke or lying on your back and kicking, you said: "It just comes up!" It just comes up! Bjorn, do you think if you got angry you could make it come up? I don't know, but it's possible if you are as bear-like as your name tells me. And I wondered if your power had anything to do with your growing up. And your mum said that you were getting taller and more muscley. And that you had grown 5 centimeters since February. This made we wonder if in the very near future you're just going to grow away from your problem and grow out of it. You also told me that you felt powerful climbing trees. And isn't it interesting that bears are famous for their ability to climb trees?

"You have a powerful name, a powerful mind, a powerful body, and just one bit of you has been a bit weakened by your illness. Also you have some power friends . . . you told me that you had a teddy bear, a teddy bjorn. And when I asked if it would look after you, you said: "It makes me sleep. It makes me brave at night." You also have Mickey, the power cow. And when you cuddle her it makes the power come. Riding your bike also makes you feel powerful. So when I started thinking about it, Bjorn, there were many sources of your power. Your name, your bear-like name . . . your physical strength . . . your growing up . . . your ability to call up and call upon your power when you need it— swimming doing the backstroke or lying or your back kicking . . .

when you are cycling . . . climbing trees. These are all your sources of power. And you didn't know you had so much power. And you didn't know you could use your power against your habit. Your habit had better watch out if you put your power against it. It is a weak habit . . . a habit that usually affects young people, and it couldn't stand up to either your growing up or putting your power against it. So, Bjorn, all you have to do is call up your power instead of just letting it come. Now it just comes up when you need it. Do you think you need your strength and your power against your problem to weaken it and strengthen yourself?

"You said it was good to know you were so powerful. But I knew it, Bjorn, and your mum knew it. You have a powerful name, you look powerful, healthy, and strong . . . and when I felt your muscles they told me that inside of your body there was a lot of strength. There's just one little bit of you that has been weakened by your sickness. But you're no weakling. Bjorn, you could if you wanted to when you need to . . . gather all your power together . . . you've also got helpers in your teddy bjorn, and your teddy cow. And when I asked you who would win, your habit or you, it was pretty clear that your habit was a weak habit. And that you could win. But it has made you lose your muscle tone and your confidence, and made you afraid of wetting your pants. But remember you never have wet your pants.

"So, Bjorn, you are stronger than what you think you are. And your habit is trying to trick you into thinking you are a weakling. It is not so! Bjorn, this is not so! So, look, you are a powerful young person, but your problem is weakening you and making you miserable, making you not sleep at night. It is time to get angry with it, Bjorn, to strengthen yourself and not just let your power come up, but call it up.

"Bjorn, there is a secret formula for this, and I'm going to tell you what it is. What you have to do, if you want to weaken your habit and strengthen you, is to say this when you need it, and only when you need it. So listen very, very carefully . . . to what I'm going to say now.

"Are you ready, Bjorn? Really, really listen. And say after me when you need to . . . you don't need to say everything but just what you like of my words. These are magic power words. Very, very powerful. Ready?

> Problem, I am getting sick and tired of how you are making me think I have to go to the toilet all the time and making me believe I am going to wet my pants. Well, let me tell you, problem, I have **never** wet my pants and I **never** will. So I don't believe you **any**

more. Problem, my name is Bjorn. I am bear-like. Like a bear, I am a very nice and cuddly person, but when I get angry, **watch out!** I have more strength than you think. Until I met David, I just thought my power came up when I needed it, like when I am swimming backstroke, riding my bike, or climbing trees. Now I know I can call it up when I want to . . . when I am **angry. Problem, I need to teach you a lesson you will never forget.** I am going to make you **wait and wait** until you are sick of bothering me. I have all the power I need to do this. And if I feel weak, I have a teddy bjorn and teddy cow to give me courage and strength. And I have strong parents. So, problem, **you've had it!** You thought I was a weakling, a little pussy cat—**I am a bear!** (**Bold** types indicates vocal stressing.)"

I am now making it part of my regular practice to provide young persons with "taped stories." Doing so allows us as therapists to re-enter the world of children, a world many of us have forsaken. Tapes allow for direct access and can be employed by young persons at particularly strategic times, especially for those problems/habits that are most troublesome at night, like nightmares, night rocking, early morning asthma attacks, night fears, bedwetting, and so on. These tapes are constructed with reference to the narratives familiar to children. So, when I am ready, I approach my dictaphone, place it on the floor, and sit cross-legged in front of it and merely tell it a story.

I compose the "story" in much the same way as I might write a "letter as narrative" from my notes taken during the session. I read them over several times until a story line emerges in my imagination. In Bjorn's story, my hope was to convert the randomness of his power/strength "just coming up," to "calling it up" at those times he either required or desired it. I devised the "magic power words" as my vehicle for this transition from chance to volition. I also added "bladder retention training" but removed it from the frame of a "program," and located it in the narrative as a form of revenge. Such a frame is only possible in an externalizing discourse, in which a young person can relate to the problem in some way or other. It also made it likely for this young person to bear the discomfort of making his problem "wait and wait until you are sick of bothering me." The notion of "trick" admitted of another version, another "reading" of Bjorn's experience of his bladder and the urgency he felt.

Gerde canceled the next appointment 3 weeks later. She concluded it wasn't necessary, as the problem had vanished and she felt that attending the appointment would be a waste of time for me as well as for Bjorn. I contacted Gerde by phone several times up until a recent 6-month follow-up. She observed that Bjorn's only concern now was his unwillingness to travel on trans-Pacific flights, and that they didn't feel there was any cause for concern right now.

SUMMARY

I have been exploring for some time now the capability of young people to produce their own knowledge in relation to their concerns. Accordingly, my task is to assist them to produce their knowledge and, moreover, to know their knowledgeableness. For those adults committed to the view that children's problems are best resolved by the transfer of adult "expert" knowledge, the notion that young people can generate their own solutions often seems strange. I advance two propositions: (1) Taking young people seriously is hard for adults who expect young people to take them seriously, and (2) hypnotic phenomena are children's play.

With Bjorn, the alternative story contained both a re-presentation of the alternative knowledge to its inventor and suggestions of how this knowledge might be applied at his will. "Readiness questions" had reassured me that he was willing.

I refer to this approach to young persons' problems as "discovering discoveries," and my step-by-step summary follows:

1. Grasp the problem-saturated story.
2. Externalize the problem.
3. Personify the problem.
4. Make a discovery of a "unique outcome," a discovery that contradicts the person's or family's "storying" of events in his/her/their lives.
5. Speculate as to how this "unique outcome" might constitute a part-solution to the problem.
6. Invite the person/family to acknowledge this part-solution as an accomplishment.
7. Elaborate the particulars to the discovered solution practices, and invite the person/family to endow these practices with some significance in relationship to the problem, his/her/their self-descriptions, or his/her/their relationships.
8. Invite the attribution of heroic or virtuous properties for discovering these inventions; with young people, I suggest the domains of magic, wizardry, "mental karate," or the like (Epston, 1989, pp. 45–46).
9. Draw distinctions between these knowledge-based practices and those practices that have organized the person/family around the problem and contributed to his/her/their becoming problem-bound.
10. Promote the person/family from person/family-with-a-problem (or a problem-person/family) to a person/family-with-a-solu-

tion (or a solution-person/family, power-person/family, veteran[s] of the problem, consultant[s] to other victims of the problems, etc.) (Epston & White, 1990).

EDITORIAL QUESTIONS

Q: *(DN) When I first read this chapter, I was very intrigued with the practice of sending Bjorn a recorded tape of your voice as opposed to a written letter. I have incorporated it into my work with children, and it has been well received. What is your rationale behind this? What impacts has this practice had on the children you have worked with?*

A: Over the years, I have regularly replaced letters with oral stories told with young persons as their intended audience. My reasons are pretty obvious for doing so. First, such "storytellings" are closer to their experience of stories read or told to them by reading/telling adults. The young people are not required to have reading abilities, which would have been questionable for children of Bjorn's age or younger.

Second, the audiotaped "storytelling" can easily become the property of these young persons, and it is very likely that they can have ready access to it and call upon it at their bidding. I recall inquiring and learning that Bjorn could operate a cassette recorder/player without adult supervision.

Third, the tone and atmosphere of the reading of the story are in the style of bedtime stories, a time when most young people are more than willing to give their full attention for quite long periods of time. I try my best to "tell" these stories rather than read them off the page. I might rehearse them once or twice with a trial reading or two until I sense that I am ready to "tell" it rather than read it. For some reason or other, I have found it best to sit on the floor imagining that I am at a young person's bedside. I have, with parents' consent and them joining me, on occasion done the first "telling" *in situ* (e.g., the child's bedroom at bedtime in an instance of extreme and debilitating night terrors). This practice, on review, has invariably had a greater impact than I would have expected from a written text, such as a letter.

Q: *(DN) I am very much captivated by your work with children, as you attempt to enter their "worlds" and discover their special abilities and knowledges. Your work with Bjorn is a superb example of this. To enter into the worlds of children may be a challenging practice for therapists who have been trained to impart their expert knowledge to children. Any advice for therapists on how to identify the special abilities of children so that they can generate their own solutions?*

A: I suppose one of my purposes in co-authoring *Playful Approaches to Serious Problems: Narrative Therapy with Children and Their Families* (Freeman, Epston, & Lobovits, 1997) with Jenny Freeman and Dean Lobovits was to provide any number of means to do so. I don't want to review the book here, but I would like to excerpt one exercise I have found helpful in having therapists themselves rehabilitate their own "special abilities" from their childhoods. I developed this when I considered the history of my own rehabilitation. To cut a long story short, it happened in the months of preparation for a plenary address I was asked to deliver at the 1983 Australian Family Therapy Conference, held that year in Brisbane. The topic I was requested to address was "What are the main influences in your work?" This really perplexed me, and I recall the pains I went to in reviewing virtually every book, videotape, workshop, or colleagueship I had ever had in my family therapy "life." I was getting nowhere fast when to my amazement, my father, better known as Benny the Peanut Man, came to mind (see Epston, in press).

This discovery and what was to flow from it led me both to acknowledge and to re-embrace those "special abilities" that almost all my formal trainings had ignored and suppressed. In my workshops on the "Special Abilities and Knowledges of Young Persons and Adolescents," after a "warm-up" of transcripts of young people of various ages disclosing their "special" and at times marvelous abilities, I invite those in attendance to interview each other according to the following format of questions. For a more detailed account, see Freeman et al. (1997).

1. What "special" and now seemingly weird or childish abilities did you possess as a 4-, 5-, 6-, 7-, 8-, 9-, 10-, 11-, or 12-year-old?

2. What delights and satisfactions did these abilities afford you?

3. Can you recall any adult—a parent, an uncle/aunt, grandparent, schoolteacher, coach, or even the person who sold you candies at the neighborhood store—who you *knew* fully appreciated your special abilities?

4. (If your interviewed person cannot recall anyone, ask this question in place of 5:) If you had been available to your ——-year-old self as the person you are now, how might you have shown your appreciation of those special abilities? How might you have acted toward your ——year-old self so that your appreciation was in no doubt?

5. (Follows from 3:) In what ways did that adult person indicate to you that he/she knew you were "weirdly abled" but did not think your abilities were weirdness? Was it the way the person spoke to you? Was it the twinkle in his/her eyes? Or *what?*

6. Do you recall surrendering or suppressing these abilities—say, between the ages of 10 and 13? Was it in response to critical or belittling comments from a friend or teacher? Or did it have to do with the misunderstandings and subsequent fears of parents or other important adults in your life? Or did you conclude that these abilities were childish and should be left behind now? *Or what?*

7. When you came home to yourself as an adult person, did you think to acknowledge or rehabilitate any of your seemingly weird abilities? Under what circumstances?

8. Do any of these special abilities of yours now feature in your work with children? Or even with adults?

I then seek consent to interview those who enjoyed recalling such adult persons from their childhood reminiscences. I interview them about these people's "practices" of acknowledgment of young people's special abilities. And then I ask them this question: "You were quite young at the time, but despite that, do you recall what questions X used to ask you? And if not, can you just guess what questions you think X would have asked you, say if she/he came upon you while you were playing in the sand on the beach or were lying down looking up at the sky or whatever?"

I have found that such an exercise really assists people to respect such "practices," and, I hope, to consider incorporating into their work and to revalue in general the "worlds and wisdoms" of young persons.

REFERENCES

Bruner, J. (1986). *Actual minds, possible worlds.* Cambridge, MA: Harvard University Press.

Epston, D. (1989). Are you a candidate for mental karate training? In D. Epston, *Collected papers.* Adelaide, South Australia: Dulwich Centre Publications.

Epston, D. (1992). "I am a bear": Discovering discoveries. *Family Therapy Case Studies,* 6(1). (Reprinted in M. White & D. Epston, *Experience, contradiction, narrative and imagination: Selected papers of David Epston and David White, 1989–1991.* Adelaide, South Australia: Dulwich Centre Publications, 1992.)

Epston, D. (in press). Benny the Peanut Man. In D. Epston, *On catching up with David Epston: Published papers (1991–1995).* Adelaide, South Australia: Dulwich Centre Publications.

Epston, D., & White, M. (1990). Consulting your consultants: The documentation of alternative knowledges. *Dulwich Centre Newsletter, No. 4,* 25–35.

Freeman, J., Epston, D., & Lobovits, D. (1997). *Playful approaches to serious* problems: Narrative therapy with children and their families. New York: Norton.

White, M. (1986). Negative explanation, restraint and double description: A template for family therapy. *Family Process, 25*(2), 169–184.

White, M., & Epston, D. (1989). *Literate means to therapeutic ends.* Adelaide, South Australia: Dulwich Centre Publications. (Republished as *Narrative means to therapeutic ends.* New York: Norton, 1990.)

3

"Catch the Little Fish"

THERAPY UTILIZING NARRATIVE, DRAMA, AND DRAMATIC PLAY WITH YOUNG CHILDREN

PAM BARRAGAR-DUNNE

> Entertaining new and novel ideas requires room for
> the familiar.
> —ANDERSON (1993, p. 328; acknowledging an idea
>   originally attributed to Gregory Bateson)

Drama allows persons to embrace their creativity, spontaneity, and uniqueness. Role playing of the familiar provides the foundation for exploring the unfamiliar. Role playing, or observing the playing of different roles, creates the conditions for new possibilities and perspectives to come forth. By taking different roles, persons experience the world, others, and themselves through new lenses. Creative exploration releases alternative knowledges and opens space for new possibilities and change.

PLAN OF THE CHAPTER

This chapter focuses on the use of drama and narrative with young children. The chapter text consists of two main sections ("Theoretical Discussion" and "Clinical Examples"). The latter includes four cases, each spanning a period of 6 months to 1 year.

The first section invites the reader to discover ways that drama complements and integrates with narrative therapies through opening additional options and possibilities, utilizing collaborative processes, and inviting alternative stories. I attempt to deconstruct different types of play and creative therapy components to help the reader understand how this occurs. This section concludes with specific ways of using drama and narrative therapies (Barragar-Dunne, 1992a) based on concepts and techniques from 15 years of working with young children (Barragar-Dunne, 1988, 1992b, 1993a, 1993b).

Again, the second section explores four case studies; all involve children in a group home setting, ages 5 to 10. Selected sessions and portions of sessions illustrate specific drama and narrative techniques outlined in the first section—namely, the *Wonder Space, Transformational Circle, Consultant Corner,* and *Action Rituals* (Barragar-Dunne & Barragar, 1997).

THEORETICAL DISCUSSION

Drama and Narrative

Narrative therapies are rooted in collaborative, respectful, and relational processes. These can be enriched by utilizing drama processes, which invite additional avenues for creativity and spontaneity to come forth. Drama and narrative together can open and expand therapeutic space and possibilities for alternative stories, self-descriptions, and change.

In opening therapeutic space for children, drama and narrative offer opportunities to play out familiar stories as well as alternative or hypothetical stories. Playing and role taking—natural abilities for most children—open possibilities for expansion, exploration, and growth. Many young children have difficulty verbalizing experiences because of underdeveloped verbal and conceptual skills. When young children do talk, it happens most naturally as they talk through their actions, and these actions inform their experiences. Drama and narrative offer invitations for both child and therapist to interact and experience life in different ways. Robert Landy (1986, 1993, 1996) emphasizes in his writings that implicit in dramatic playing is the sense of the player as creative. Even if the roles are to a large degree predetermined (i.e., familiar), children still choose those roles that have meaning for them currently. Roles may be played for different reasons, such as to survive, to express a feeling, to meet a need, or to explore something new. Each act of role taking and role playing invites a child's creativity and sense of play, and opens space for a story to be told in different ways. Tom Andersen (1996) talks about how he orients himself toward broadening the client's repertoire for how the story gets told. Playing varied roles helps stories be told from various perspectives. Using drama therapy, a young child may take on the roles of mother, father, sibling, and many, many others. Each act of role reversal offers the possibility of understanding and playing the story differently.

I often have children begin by role-playing a situation in which they are pushed around by the problem (problem-saturated story; White & Epston, 1990). This role may be more familiar because it gets repeated over and over again. Drama then offers the opportunity to branch out and play a larger repertoire of roles.

The collaborative and narrative concepts central to the drama therapy enactments I describe include relational and bodily knowledge; collaboration/co-regulation and a nonexpert position; opening of therapeutic space; alternative stories; and externalization.

Relational and Bodily Knowledge

In keeping with collaborative and drama therapy concepts, a spontaneous, moment-to-moment interchange between child and therapist, usually felt on the nonverbal level, is a powerful way to show respect for the child. Tom Andersen (1996) speaks of four kinds of knowledge: "rational," "technical," "relational," and "bodily." Rational knowledge refers to theoretical, abstract ways of knowing. Technical knowledge describes practical, "how-to" knowing. Relational knowledge centers on how to be with a particular person at a particular moment. In this context, bodily knowledge refers to turning in to the client's and therapist's sensory or nonverbal expressions. With children, relational knowledge assumes particular importance. Relational knowledge allows the therapist to be sensitive at each moment to where the child is in her/his play activities, and not to intrude or become the expert. By tuning in to the child and responding with bodily knowing, the therapist assists in creating the conditions for an exchange of ideas (even nonverbal ones). To illustrate this point in work with children, imagine that a child performs an action (e.g., the child becomes a dinosaur puppet, roaring and scaring the townspeople). The child becomes moved by his/her own actions. In responding, the therapist is moved by what the child is moved by, not by some predetermined kind of response. This type of openness and spontaneity can foster a deeply felt mutual respect between therapist and child.

Collaboration/Co-Regulation and a Nonexpert Stance

The give and take inherent in drama lends itself to the narrative concept of "collaboration." For honest dramatic expression to happen, no lead players or "experts" exist, and players work collaboratively with each other. Collaboration and responding in the moment makes dramatic events come alive. By taking a nonexpert position, the therapist increases the chances of opening therapeutic possibilities and bringing forth the creativity of child clients.

Fogel (1993) refers to this kind of collaboration as "co-regulation," which occurs whenever individuals' joint actions blend together to achieve a unique and mutually created set of social actions. This co-regulation, a collaborative process characterized by spontaneity and creativity, becomes the fundamental source of developmental change. Co-regulation/collaboration allows the child to participate in the discovery of possibilities and alternatives.

Opening of Therapeutic Space

Many children benefit just by playing and using their dramatic imagination with a variety of materials and by adopting to different roles and perspectives. Sometimes a child will prefer particular kinds of materials to play with. When a therapist honors these preferences, the child experiences a therapy space that feels, safe, respectful, creative, and playful. All of these things help to open rather than to close or narrow the therapeutic space.

The form of drama (or way the story is told) allows a child to explore different kinds of experiences. A story may be told behind a puppet theatre, in an improvisation, as dialogue, as a ritual with masks, in a sandbox, with colored fabrics and music, and so forth. By playing different kinds of roles—from people to inanimate objects to animals—children also see life from different perspectives. Allowing all these options opens additional space. When many options and creative materials are available, participants experience an openness and freedom that become helpful for the therapeutic process. Children also show preferences at certain moments for different kinds of dramatic structures, which range from highly structured to loosely structured (e.g., free improvisational scene, structured role play, narrative story, etc.).

Expansion of Alternative Stories and Knowledges

Role playing allows a child to move backward and forward in time as a way of exploring the self in the past, present, and future. When playing a role, the child taking the role is *both* the role and *not* the role at the same time. For instance, a child playing a teacher is both the child (not teacher) and the teacher (not child) at the same time. This paradoxical relationship between a child and a role opens space for different kinds of experiences and options (i.e., observer, director, character, self) not previously experienced. This allows many perspectives to come forth. When these perspectives come forth, these lead to other perspectives that engender other alternative stories, and the process goes on.

Drama has many forms and roles, which lend themselves easily to the concept of expansion. The playing of actor, director, observer, and auxiliary (actor in another person's scene) each offers an expansion. An "alternative story" (a story that shows a child in a more preferred role or acting in ways that invite personal agency; White & Epston, 1990) receives further expansion through using different dramatic forms, such as story or narrative, dialogue, pantomime, or movement. One "unique outcome" (a scene that shows an alternative to the problem-saturated story; White, 1989) may invite the awareness of another unique outcome, which leads to another. Sometimes these scenes may be real-life scenes and at other times hypothetical or imaginary scenes.

Externalization

"Externalization" creates a separation between a person and a problem, and opens space to show preferred ways of relating to a problem (White & Epston, 1990). Externalization for children happens easily through the use of objects, puppets, life-size dolls, masks, and other creative materials (Barragar-Dunne, 1988, 1992a, 1992b). Inviting the exploration of the environment through objects becomes important for the child. These objects (which are varied in texture, shape, weight, and kind) become potential invitations for the child. Instruments, puppets, and dolls offer possibilities for exploring characters and stories. The child exercises her/his choice in which objects to explore. Objects help children to externalize and separate themselves from their problems and to become directors of their own stories. Externalization puts space between a child and a problem.

For example, a child who chooses a tarantula puppet to be "Mad Anger" may discover ways to develop a different relationship with anger. Another child who sets up "my world" in the sandbox externalizes his/her world as experienced. Because the child is the author of the world created, this opens possibilities for change and other options. When a world is viewed in miniature, it becomes visible in a different way than previously experienced.

In summary, drama integrates well with narrative by inviting additional avenues for creativity; expanding therapeutic space; and bringing forth possibilities for alternative stories, new self-descriptions, and change. In addition, drama and narrative can help the therapist to tune in to bodily and relational knowledge, to take a collaborative stance, and to utilize externalizing methods.

Kinds of Play

Ann Cattanach (1992, 1994), British play therapist and registered drama therapist, defines three kinds of play that offer different ways of expanding experience:

1. "Embodiment play" occurs when a child explores the world through the senses, using Play-Doh, Slime, clay, or other claylike substances, or other tactile materials. The senses invite exploration and a sense of knowing common to very young children, and provide them with the circumstances to enlarge their world.

2. "Progressive play" happens when children discover the world outside themselves through toys, dolls, or other objects. Through these objects, children can explore alternative stories. Objects such as toys, dolls, and puppets assist in externalization and help children to separate themselves from a problem and to expand their perspective.

3. "Role play" occurs when a child begins playing himself/herself in a familiar situation and then pretends to be someone else. The process of drama assists as an agent in the healing process, allowing transformation from everyday reality into dramatic reality. These transformational experiences create shifts in children, who experience these changes on a bodily, kinesthetic level.

"Dramatic play" (Barragar-Dunne, 1992b) is a more global, general term used to describe the play of young children as they take spontaneous roles on and off or engage in creative play. This play is often fragmented, short, totally involving, and spontaneous, and invites creativity. Dramatic play includes within it embodiment play, progressive play, and role playing as defined by Cattanach.

Therapy Space

An open therapy space with softness and a sense of flow can often create an invitation for exploration. Large soft pillows and a creative work space assist in fostering a sense of a therapeutic environment that becomes special and safe to children, much like preferred spaces from their natural environment (e.g., an attic, a closet, a tree house, or under a table) where they may enter their own world of make-believe. A therapy room that offers color, warmth, diversity, and a sense of openness and playfulness allows children to use these qualities to explore feelings, stories, ideas, and conflicts.

A therapy space will be enhanced by visible and audible invitations through simple musical instruments (a drum, triangle, bells, etc.). Other children may gravitate to a sandbox and toys, while still others may choose life-size dolls or puppets. Still others love to explore through art (paints, clay, Play-Doh, collage, etc.). A bag of fabrics of different colors, textures, and shapes; soft flexible balls of different sizes; stretch bags and stretch ropes; colored tissue paper; and various art supplies (see below) invite further participation and collaboration.

Narrative and Drama Therapy Concepts for Children

Narrative concepts coupled with drama therapy principles bring forth the development of the *Wonder Space, Transformational Circle, Consultant Corner,* and *Action Rituals* (Barragar-Dunne, 1997).

The *Wonder Space,* a special space designated by a fabric mat or some other special way, allows a child to focus on wondering. When a child enters the *Wonder Space,* she/he may draw, talk, or create a scene with small objects about something the child wonders about. At any time in the therapy session, a child or therapist may go to the *Wonder Space.* Variations of the *Wonder Space* may include a *Wonder Chair, Wonder Hat,* or *Wonder Box.* An older child may write down wondering questions in a creative journal (Barragar-Dunne, 1995).

The *Transformational Circle* is a special circle where change happens. This circle may be designated by a circle drawn in chalk or indicated by a large stretch rope or circular mat. To assist in communicating the understanding of transformation, the therapist may wish to use some of the following creative transformational games:

1. "Transformation of the Object." A pencil or other objects changes and becomes different things as it is passed in a circle.
2. "Ball Change." A Nerf ball, as it is passed in the circle, becomes a ball of different weights—a beach ball, a balloon, a bowling ball.
3. "Fabric Emotion." A piece of fabric is used to show one emotion and then used in a different way to show another emotion. For example, a child may use a piece of fabric to show sadness by drying his/her tears with a large handkerchief, and this fabric may then be transformed into a superhero's cape or a beautiful dress.

The child or therapist enters the *Transformational Circle* if either wants to change something or if either has experienced change. Those who enter draw, tell, or create with objects what has changed or what they would like to change.

The *Consultant Corner* is designed by a special table with art supplies. These include book-making and mural construction materials, white paper, colored marking pens, crayons, scissors, tape, large sheets of butcher paper, mask-making materials (i.e., paper plates, colored tissue paper, yarn), and stapler. The space also includes an audiotape recorder and blank audiotapes; musical instruments; a Polaroid camera; and a video camera, VCR, and blank videotapes. In the *Consultant Corner,* children share in whatever form they choose something they found helpful in therapy and would like to pass on to someone else. They may do any of the following:

- Write a letter.
- Draw a special picture.
- Make an audiotape recording.
- Write an ongoing book.
- Create a mural.
- Make a videotape.
- Recreate a special moment and photograph it.
- Make a picture book.
- Create a mask.
- Conduct an interview.
- Make up a song or piece of music.

Action Rituals assist children to make sense out of things, as well as sometimes serving as a friend to encounter a difficult obstacle. Repeating actions in a ritual often invites a sense of confidence and a safe place. Examples of specific *Action Rituals* illustrated in this chapter include the following:

- "Mother's Love"
- "Fabric Environment"
- "Dismantle and Fix"
- "Self-Talk"
- "Ringing the Bell"
- "Singing to Self"
- "Nurturance"
- "X'ing Out"
- "Catch the Little Fish"
- "Empty and Fill"
- "Going to a Special Place"
- "Drawing"

In summary, drama and narrative techniques for children assist the children by speaking their language and taking into account their preferences for movement, action, and experiential work.

CLINICAL EXAMPLES

Some young clients may come from situations in which they have experienced abuse. Such children have often been taken away from their families and are now in foster care or a group home setting. Often these children come to therapy with limited experiences in dramatic play or role playing. Although playing and taking roles are natural parts of the lives of many children, they sometimes appear diminished in children who have experienced abuse. Interacting with these children in a creative, collaborative therapy process requires sensitivity and openness.

Children in foster care or a group home situation often appear to be "insecurely attached." They have often been denied the essential reciprocal relationship with a fully committed adult. Often these children struggle against such things as low self-esteem, low trust, insecurity, vulnerability, depression, or hyperactive behavior. Assisting these children to uncover their strengths and to generate alternative stories and self-descriptions invites forward movement in their lives.

Background

To demonstrate my integration of narrative and drama therapy, four children (ages 5, 6, 7, and 10) are followed here over a therapeutic process spanning 6 months to 1 year.[1] Four to seven sessions are presented for each child. These sessions may be full sessions or portions of sessions, and are not necessarily in chronological order. All of the children come from a group home environment and have been removed by court order from their biological families because of parental substance abuse, child physical or sexual abuse, or other reasons. Thus, all of these children have been swept away in early childhood from those they have known and all that has been familiar. The children all live in their group home with caregivers who endeavor to provide a loving environment. In most cases these children will not return to their biological families, but will be placed in a more permanent foster care or adoption situation. They have all experienced abandonment, loss, anger, mistrust, and lack of security. They also share a desire to go forward and succeed.

---

[1]To protect confidentiality, names and circumstances have been changed to protect the identity of each client.

Inviting a capacity for self-nurturance, and respecting their individual histories, honor these children and invite the collaborative process to take place.

In this clinical section, I name various specific rituals (i.e., *Action Rituals*). These are names in quotation marks that describe what to me are relevant features of themes in a child's play. The particular child involved may view this ritual differently or have another name for it.

Ronald

1. "Mother's Love"

Ronald—a friendly, interactive 5-year-old, taken away from his mother when he was 2 years of age because of her drug abuse—enters the therapy space. Staff members describe Ronald as hyperactive and out of control, but appreciate his qualities of friendliness, curiosity, and eagerness. They raise concerns about Ronald's inability to control himself, and also indicate that he often shows strong anger or sadness, which they attribute to his abandonment as a child. It is their hope that in therapy, Ronald may honestly express his feelings and perhaps discover alternative ways of controlling and being in charge of his emotions.

Ronald continually asks questions as he plays with the toys, objects, art materials, and puppets throughout the therapy space. As he plays, I begin to feel his sadness. Ronald tells a story with the objects about a little boy who is taken away from his home. He says, "The mother loves the little boy, but she could not take care of him." As Ronald places the objects and continues the story, his sadness increases. Later he draws a picture and says, "This is a picture of my sad mother. My mother wants me to be with her and she is sad." I wonder to myself how Ronald might hold his mother's love in a special place. I also wonder how his mother's love might be a friend to Ronald. I try to imagine what his mother's love might say to Ronald in his present circumstances.

The story of sadness in Ronald's life reflects an undeniable part of his life in adjusting to the loss of his mother and the home he knew. He has not seen his mother since he was 2 years of age. The therapy environment provides a place for Ronald to tell the story of losing his mother. Throughout the therapy, the "Losing Mother" story repeats itself many times. I wonder whether repeating the story may help Ronald in trying to make sense of his experience, and I reflect to myself about the possibility of creating a ritual of "Mother's Love."

I enter the *Wonder Space* and wonder aloud with Ronald what he thinks about when he says the words "mother's love." "What color is mother's love . . . ? What shape is mother's love . . . ? How big is mother's love . . . ? What texture is mother's love . . . ?" Ronald talks about the largeness of his mother's love and says that his mother still loves him even though he is not with her. Ronald prefers to draw a picture of mother's love and asks me to draw with him. Ronald holds his mother's love in his heart. Ronald repeats the "Mother's Love" picture, which becomes a ritual throughout the therapy process.

2. Broken Houses and New Life

The room comes alive as Ronald runs in with boundless energy and begins setting up an intricate scene with little objects in the sand. This progressive play consists of constructing block-like buildings, lamp posts, cars, and people into a configuration of a city. Then an earthquake comes, and Ronald aggressively knocks over buildings and creates loud sound effects. The earthquake destroys the entire city, including all the people, buildings, and city life. Ronald says, "Everything is dead." Ronald places people in corpse-like positions and devastates the entire town. All the broken houses consist of heaps of wood. Ronald says, "All the horses are dead and nothing is alive." Ronald places all the animals in corpse-like positions as well, and quiet fills the scene (long pause). Ronald draws a picture of the ruin with a burned airplane (Figure 1). He says, "The airplane got burned and fell down." Ronald looks over this devastation for a long time and begins rocking back and forth. He then starts humming quietly as he takes all the pieces from the devastation and begins rebuilding a new city (an alternative story). New buildings and people fill the streets, and animals appear back in the farms. Ronald continues to hum and sing as the rebuilding continues. People line the streets, and animals appear plentifully on the farms. As Ronald observes the transformed picture, he appears peaceful, content, and calm.

I ask Ronald if he thinks a change has happened. He agrees. I inquire whether he would like to sit in the *Transformational Circle* with me to acknowledge the change. He sits in the circle and draws a picture of beautiful colors (Figure 2).

Ronald's transformation of everyday reality into dramatic reality creates a change and an observable shift in experience. I think of this as a shift in his body and spirit at a nonconscious level. A dominant story of being "Out of Control" and being powerless to control himself or his life experiences is momentarily transcended by a story of rebirth and hope. As I reflect on his picture of beautiful colors, I wonder about creating a "Rebirth" ritual or some kind of transformational ritual to help this story endure. Ronald's drawing begins this process.

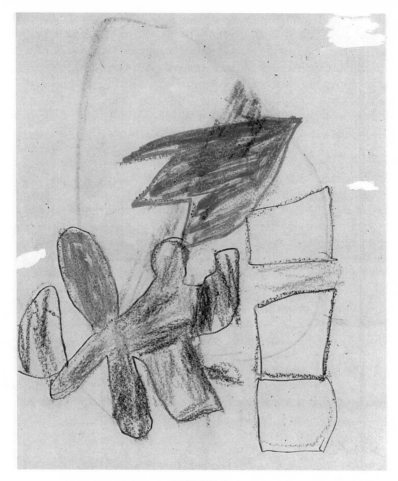

FIGURE 1

3. *Alligator and Dinosaur Attacks, and Invitation of the Fabrics*

Ronald enters the therapy space with strong emotions and energy. He takes some of the cute and playful puppets, such as the bunny and dog, and places them in a special configuration on the floor. Ronald's progressive play then begins as he takes the aggressive-looking puppets (i.e., the alligator, dinosaur, and tarantula). The alligator becomes the leader of the pack, and "Out of Control" appears to be present. Immediately upon placing his hand in the mouth of the alligator puppet, Ronald rages. As the alligator, he destroys all the other puppets and dwellings.

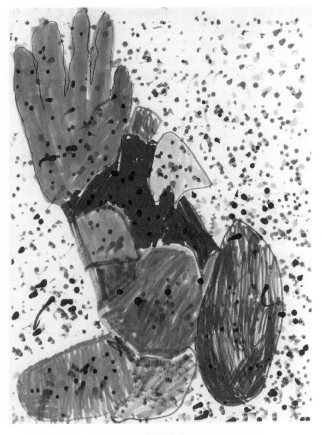

FIGURE 2

This theme of destruction revisits the therapy space. In another part of the story, Ronald sets up a dinner scene of a family of animal puppets. This dinner, interrupted by an attack from the alligator and the appearance of the witch, becomes chaotic. The alligator attacks the dinner table scene while the witch leans in the window. Then the dinosaur puppet threatens to destroy the homes of the children. The children run inside to escape the dinosaur. The dinosaur finally tires of scaring everyone and falls asleep. Ronald says, "Everyone needs to be quiet and ignore the dinosaur."

As I reflect on this story, I think about many things, I wonder if this might be how Ronald expresses his anger at being taken away from his mother. I also wonder about the wisdom in "be quiet and ignore the dinosaur." My silent wonderings continue as Ronald asks to play with the fabrics. Spontaneously, Ronald quietly spreads out and organizes the fabrics to create a special place. He selects each fabric individually and places it in the configuration that he wishes. It appears that the sensory quality of the fabrics invites Ronald to participate in a quiet and more peaceful state. This is a type of embodiment play because of its strongly sensory component. As Ronald continues to interact holistically, his body communicates a calm peacefulness. Ronald continues to grow quieter and more peaceful. I wonder, as I interact with Ronald, if he has not himself spontaneously discovered a ritual of transformation. As he invites me to move in the fabric environment, his actions communicate a sense of stillness and peace. Over the next 15 minutes, Ronald continues to interweave the fabrics in this special place. This exploration leads to new interactions, resulting in new perspectives. This "fabric environment" becomes a continuing action ritual which Ronald often repeats.

Ronald enters the *Transformational Circle* with a piece of fabric from the fabric environment around his shoulders. As I observe how Ronald responds with all his senses (particularly the sense of touch), I wonder about other ways in which he may discover that his senses are a friend to him. I also wonder to myself how Ronald in the future may invite the help of his senses when "Out of Control" tries to influence him. A shift takes place, and Ronald leaves the session in control.

4. *Three* Action Rituals

Ronald bounds into the play space, upsetting some of the objects and pulling objects, puppets, Legos and play food out of the bags. He empties all the fabrics in a big heap. Some small containers catch his attention and he begins an *Action Ritual* of "Dismantle and Fix," which involves taking all the tops of the containers and putting them back again. He completes this *Action Ritual* a number of times and appears happy with his accomplishment. Ronald seems to regulate his own play, rather than his play's regulating him. This is in contrast to some previous enactment and play experiences, in which Ronald appeared to be unable to resist the influence of "Out of Control." In these experiences his play looked more chaotic and destructive, and it seemed as if the play objects rather than he himself were controlling the scene. In this session, through the use of an *Action Ritual,* he becomes the author of his own play and uses the objects and play materials in ways that he prefers and that provide a sense of calm.

Ronald then develops a story about a family preparing to have dinner. While telling this story with the objects, Ronald talks quietly to himself about what he's doing. This *Action Ritual* of "Self-Talk" creates an inhibiting effect on "Out of Control." The more Ronald talks quietly to himself, the calmer he becomes, and "Out of Control" receives no opportunity to be present. Next, Ronald develops the *Action Ritual* of "Ringing the Bell." "Ringing the Bell" signals that something significant is about to happen in the scene. Because Ronald initiates the ringing, he becomes an active participant and observer in the telling of his own story. Ronald delights in the ringing and begins announcing the changes in the scene verbally as well. When he rings the bell, he particularly wants me to observe what will happen next. Ronald enters the *Transformational Circle,* draws a shape and fills it in with bright colors, and appears content.

5. "Moving" Stories, Putting the Boat Together, and Masks

Ronald takes the colored fabric pieces and creates a costume. He says, "I want to be a man." Then he begins arranging small plastic figures (cowboys, Indians, horses, tents, covered wagons, trees, and canoes). These small figures fall over easily and require fine motor coordination and patience. Ronald uses the ritual of "Self-Talk" and creates different stories with the figures. As the figures fall over, he places them upright again, and "Out of Control" receives no opportunity to be present. His stories center on "Moving" themes. In the first story, the animals and people travel in the covered wagon and set up a new home by the river. In the second story, the animals and people travel in a canoe down the river to set up a new home.

Next, Ronald creates another method of moving, a Legos boat. The largeness and intricacy of the boat require Ronald to take exceptional care in moving it so it will not fall apart. Ronald continues the *Action Ritual* of "Self-Talk," and adds another one, "Singing." As the boat collapses, Ronald holds back impatience and puts the boat back together again. Ronald then takes the boat on a very difficult course, which to accomplish requires exceptionally slow movement around curves so as not to break the boat. Ronald repeats this movement a number of times, demonstrating his ability to exercise patience.

I move to the *Wonder Space* and wonder aloud: "I am curious, Ronald, that both of your stories are about moving. I wondered if you were thinking about your move to the other group home." Ronald tells me he doesn't want to move and likes it where he is. As Ronald and I talk more about moving, we find that we have both experienced anxiety about moving. Then Ronald goes to the art area and makes a mask. He calls this mask a "Happy Mask" (Figure 3), and then he creates a "Sad Mask" (Figure 4).

I move into the *Wonder Space* and wonder out loud what experiences belong with the "Happy Mask" and what experiences belong with

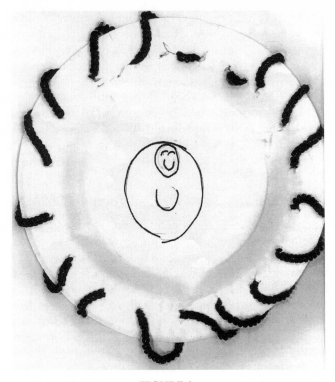

FIGURE 3

the "Sad Mask." Ronald says he is happy when he goes to McDonald's, but he is sad because he does not see his mother. Ronald continues to embellish the masks by making the downward mouth on the "Sad Mask" more pronounced. Ronald appears proud upon completion of this activity. I reflect out loud while Ronald is making the masks that I am curious about how he is able to hold "Out of Control" away while engaging in mask-making activities. Ronald says that he likes to make things and he thinks a lot about what he is making. I respond by saying, "It looks like you are using your 'Making Skills' and 'Strong Thinking' to keep 'Out of Control' away." Ronald continues to exercise his "Making Skills" and "Strong Thinking" by continuing difficult fine motor activities(i.e., attaching and interweaving of pipe cleaners) around the circumference of each mask. To engage in these activities requires making holes in the mask, running pipe cleaners through the holes, and tying the pipe cleaners together.

At the end of this session, Ronald returns to the fabrics and re-

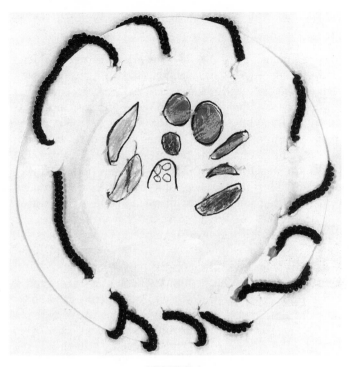

FIGURE 4

peats the "Fabric Environment" ritual. This ritual (spontaneously developed by Ronald in previous sessions) really appears to help Ronald in expressing his emotions and in keeping "Out of Control" away. I wonder (silently this time) how Ronald would describe his response to the tactile qualities of the fabrics. From observing his actions, it appears that he experiences these tactile qualities(embodiment play) as soothing, resourceful, and transformational. This ritual brings forth a tenderness and gentleness in the interaction between Ronald and the fabrics in the way he arranges them. I feel honored by the invitation to enter this environment, as I feel I am entering a very special place. A calm tranquility fills the scene. Ronald moves to the *Transformational Circle* and continues adding on to his "Happy Mask," with a special emphasis on the turned-up corners of the mouth.

I reflect silently about Ronald's ability to keep "Out of Control"away by using his "Making Skills," and "Strong Thinking," as well as the "Fabric Environment" ritual. Again, I feel honored to be a part of this experience.

6. *"Ringing the Bell," Food Rituals, "Making Skills," and "Strong Thinking"*

Ronald comes immediately into the therapy space, begins taking out the play food, and announces that he will be cooking a meal. He puts different foods in the pots and checks them as they are cooking. He announces that one pot contains the food being prepared for me. The other pots contain food he prepares for himself. Ronald continues to include me more and more in his play and role playing. He continues to use the "Self-Talk" ritual as he prepares the food. I reflect that "Self-Talk" seems to warm him up to increased interaction. Then using the "Ringing the Bell" ritual, Ronald announces dinner. He creates an attractive table setting and serves me the prepared food on a plate. We eat together. As I reflect to myself, I wonder if Ronald may have spontaneously developed a "Nurturance" ritual. The loving preparation of the food and interchange at dinner seem nourishing to both Ronald and myself. Then Ronald uses "Ringing the Bell" to announce the cleaning and drying of the dishes. During both the food preparation and cleaning rituals, Ronald keeps "Out of Control" from entering the scene. I reflect that in food preparation Ronald is also using his "Making Skills"to assist him. In calling on his "Making Skills," as well as other strengths he has developed (i.e., "Strong Thinking"), Ronald sometimes uses verbal commands such as "Stop" or "Go away" to show his preference; however, this usually, if it occurs at all, takes place in combination with the other strengths previously noted.

7. *Various* Action Rituals, *6 Weeks Later*

I next see Ronald 6 weeks later. As he enters the therapy space, he appears to be struggling with "Out of Control." He bounds around the room, trying to focus, speaking loudly. "Out of Control" appears to be influencing his behavior. I wonder if Ronald will remember some of the rituals he used previously to assist him in remaining in control. Ronald begins talking quietly to himself and takes out the play food ("Self-Talk" and "Making Skills"). As he starts meal preparation, he repeats a *ritual* ("Singing to Self" and "Nurturance" ritual). As he continues to sing and prepare food, his body and spirit quiet down. So, although we have not seen each other in quite some time, Ronald spontaneously remembers how to keep "Out of Control" out of the therapy environment. He prepares and serves me a special meal and plays with the puppets. He ends the session by repeating the "Fabric Environment" ritual and asks me to join in creating the environment. He shows me different cloths and demonstrates how he wants me to arrange them ("Making Skills"). The environment contains bright, beautiful, colorful fabrics

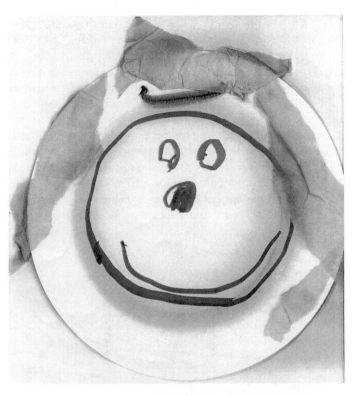

FIGURE 5

arranged in a small space. As the environment nears completion, Ronald and I wrap some of the fabrics around ourselves and sit quietly enjoying the tranquility of the scene. I reflect on the healing atmosphere I experience and on how Ronald's new abilities have contributed to this.

When invited to enter the *Consultant Corner,* Ronald creates a happy mask (Figure 5). He says he likes the masks, and the masks help him and may be helpful to other children. He says that this is a mask of me. Once more, I feel honored to be a part of this therapy process, and especially to be depicted in a mask.

Celia

1. "X'ing Out" Ritual

Celia, a lively and outgoing 6-year-old, enters the therapy space with strong emotions and boundless physical energy. Staff members describe Celia as a child who has been sexually abused. They report out-of-control temper tantrums and behavior. When asked what they appreciate about Celia, the staff members indicate that they appreciate Celia's outgoing personality and inclusion of other children in play activities. Caretakers show concern for Celia's sexualized behavior and are requesting therapy to look at those issues, as well as Celia's self-destructive tendencies.

Celia grabs the puppets and quickly discards them. She dumps all the objects, dolls, and playthings on the floor. She looks at an object or puppet and then eliminates it. This process keeps repeating itself. She seems unsure, unfocused, and agitated. I wonder to myself whether the freedom of the spontaneous play seems too much for her in the moment. I reflect on how structure might become a friend to her and invite her to play. I discuss the possibility of drawing, and she appears interested. She thoughtfully draws a picture and appears proud of her creation. However, as soon as she completes it, she destroys it by putting black marks

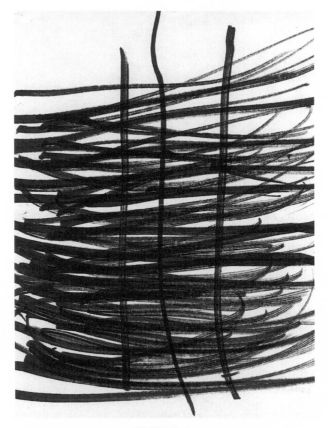

FIGURE 6

all over it. This happens again with another picture (see Figures 6 and 7). She X's it out, and the ritual of "X'ing Out" keeps repeating itself in later meetings. I wonder whether this ritual of "X'ing Out" serves as a witness to Celia's feelings and current perspective.

2. Doll Play and Improvisational Family Scene

Celia begins by taking out the small dolls. In playing with the dolls, she says, "Why did you pull her pants down?" Then she takes the two girl dolls, puts them on their heads, opens up their legs, and looks between their legs. She does this several times. She begins undressing all the dolls by removing every item of clothing. The dolls take a group bath together, and all hug and kiss and go through lovemaking rituals. This or a similar ritual appears over and over in therapy sessions. Then Celia says, "Pretty Mama."

Celia wants me to act out a family scene with her. She wants the family to be composed of a mother and a baby. She wants me to be the mother, and she wants to be the baby. In acting out this scene, Celia tries to be too physical and inappropriate (i.e., she tries to touch my chest and lifts up her skirt with sexualized gestures). I wonder to myself how she understands appropriate and inappropriate social behavior. I explain to her that I will be unable to continue the story if she fails to respect my personal space and act appropriately. We talk about personal space, but when she continues the scene, she again becomes too physically invasive. I stop the scene and remind her of the limits. She then continues playing the scene in a more socially appropriate way.

I think about Celia and other children I have seen like Celia. It feels to me that Celia wants to experience a nurturing relationship between a

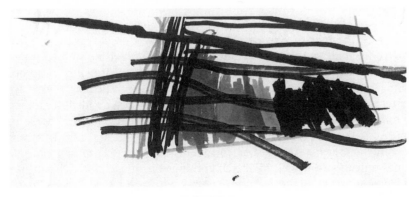

FIGURE 7

mother and a baby. She wants to experience being a baby peacefully sleeping, and when she cries as the baby, she wants a mother/therapist there to respond. This yearning for the consistency of a nurturing mother remains very strong. However, I wonder, based on Celia's background of sexual abuse, whether all this gets mixed up in her mind. She wants to experience the nurturance, but she doesn't know how to experience it in a socially appropriate way.

I think to myself that Celia has been more interactive by including me in the improvisational scene. I enter the *Wonder Space* and wonder out loud if Celia might like to draw her feelings. I am wondering what feelings she might draw. I continue to wonder out loud if she might later want to talk about what she is feeling or present a puppet show or doll play. The staff members have raised concerns about her temper tantrums and screaming, but I have noticed that art seems to assist her in expressing these strong emotions in ways that are not destructive to herself or others. I wonder to myself in what other ways art might be a friend and help to her.

Celia moves to the art area and begins drawing some pictures. She carefully removes the marker tops and puts them back on. She completes her drawings and then, as previously observed, she destroys all her pictures. On some pictures, she grabs the black marker and with strong emotional strokes goes through the "X'ing Out" ritual. On other pictures, she tears them up.

Celia ends up drawing a picture expressing anger. She holds the colored black pen so hard that the paper tears. She takes the tarantula puppet and speaks some angry words. She then creates a paper bag puppet (Figure 8) but again marks over part of her creation.

3. Baby and Mother Scene

Celia wants to play with the fabrics and wants to continue re-enacting a variation of the baby scene. She asks me to play her mother and cover her with the fabrics. She says, "You need to watch me go to sleep." I cover her and stay with her. She continues to wake up and tells me, "You need to be here when I go to sleep." I continue to sit close to her and watch her and say comforting words. I keep repeating, "You are safe, warm, and content." Celia wants me to get closer and closer to her. I move as close as I feel comfortable doing, and then explain to her as in previous sessions that I need some space for myself and that I am uncomfortable being too close in this scene. I keep trying to create a safe and appropriate place, while she continues to move closer. I stop the scene and say it cannot continue unless we respect each other's space.

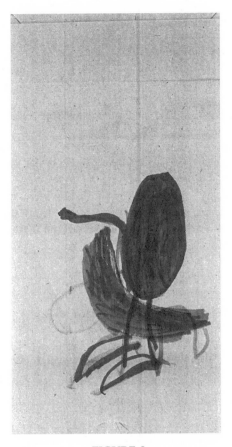

FIGURE 8

Celia begins making baby sounds; however, some of the sounds become sexual. These sounds only last for a moment, and she goes on to make normal baby sounds. I continue to interact with her in the scene in such a way as to introduce the idea of appropriate behavior and interaction, while still respecting her ideas. Then she wants me to reverse roles and play the baby. I agree to do this with specific conditions. She tries to get too close, and again I stop the scene. She finally agrees to the limitations, and we complete the scene.

Developing a scene like this creates an interesting challenge from a narrative perspective. It becomes important for me to assert more authority and direction than I normally would in a collaborative posture. However, I try to do this in a caring way, reminding myself that Celia's past has not provided her with an understanding of appropriate social behavior and that the therapy space will be a safe place to explore this. As I reflect to myself on the scene, I am struck by Celia's mixing of sexual and social behavior and by the way she goes in and out of these moments. I wonder privately what Celia may experience as helpful in beginning to separate these behaviors and to understand appropriate social behavior. I also reflect that once she accepts limits, she appears more at ease and content.

I move into the *Wonder Space* and wonder aloud about the change I am seeing in Celia's behavior. Celia agrees that she feels different, and so we move into the *Transformational Circle,* where Celia creates a beautiful piece of art by tracing her hands. She seems proud of her creation (Figure 9). She gives this artwork to me without going through the "X'ing Out" ritual. I reflect that as she leaves the therapy space, she appears more content.

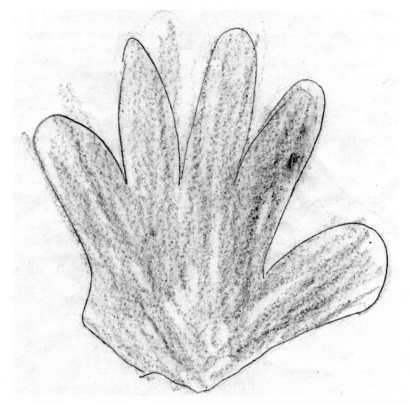

FIGURE 9

4. "Catch the Little Fish"

Celia takes the stretch rope and begins pulling and pushing motions, which she wants to do with me. These motions spontaneously develop to the point that Celia suggests that we play "Catch the Little Fish." She suggests that I cast a fishing line into the water, and she becomes the fish. I proceed to reel her in via the stretch rope around her waist. The first 10 times of doing this, she allows me to reel her in just a little bit. I respect this and let her go, and the game starts over again. Then Celia introduces a new element, weight. The fish becomes very heavy and is difficult to reel in. Then Celia becomes inappropriate in her behavior. She lies on the floor with her legs open, acting in a sexual way, and wants me to play the game. I explain to her that I cannot play the game that way, and I move away from the playing area. After we discuss the rules of therapy, a long pause occurs. Celia then drops the inappropriate behavior and continues with the game according to the rules.

After this activity, Celia wants to make a mask. She makes a face and asks me to help her in attaching tissue paper—a strip of green on the top and a strip of blue on the bottom. Celia then reverts to the "X'ing Out" ritual and destroys the face of the mask with a black marker.

I reflect to myself that Celia continues to deal with sexual behavior and images. It seems that through play she expresses this, but is also confronted with social appropriateness. It seems that the therapy space is providing a way to interact together to discover ways of acting appropriately on a social level.

5. "Catch the Little Fish" Again

Celia wants to begin with the stretch rope, and the activity starts with creating different shapes with the rope. Then Celia wants to play "Catch the Little Fish." I cast the line and begin reeling her in. Each time I reel her in, she lets me take her a little bit closer. I will only take her as far as she wants to go. Finally she allows me to reel her in a comfortable distance from me. She appears cheerful and peaceful and seems to enjoy that position. We each maintain our own individual space, but also respond on an interpersonal level. Then she repeats the ritual over and over, coming to the new enjoyed position. I sense that Celia seems to be exploring areas of trust, space, and distance. I feel honored that she chooses me to explore this with her. Celia delights in this game and wants to play it over and over. I think about Celia's ability to act appropriately in this game and in discovery of her own personal space.

Celia continues to play and concentrate very well in this session, and seems more content and less angry than she has in the past. It is encouraging that she is able to put "Anger" aside.

We move into the *Transformational Circle*, and Celia draws a picture to give to me. This session is the strongest statement of her ability to begin to control some of her impulsivity and over sexualized behavior. I think about "Catch the Little Fish," and wonder to myself whether this game may be assisting her to try out different degrees of closeness to another person, as well as different experiences in trust. Her calm and more focused actions seem to be holding "Anger" and "Impulsivity" in check, and assisting a softer, more sensitive side of Celia to make itself known.

6. Food Rituals

For most of this session, Celia plays with the play food and develops eating, cooking, and serving rituals while engaging my participation. She continues to relate to me in a friendly, social, and more appropriate manner. She also develops more characters to try out social relationships with. She places two dinosaur puppets in the play space and feeds "Thomas" (the dinosaur), improvising dialogue as she goes along. I notice she still wants to do art. Today she draws two pictures of her own hands in their natural simplicity. I reflect that this session shows me how she uses her art and her own artistic abilities as something to appreciate about herself. While she is appreciating herself and exercising her natural creativity, "Anger" seems less able to influence her.

There are no sexual themes or inappropriate behaviors this session.

Celia goes to the *Consultant Corner*. There she creates a collage of colors; she says these are happy colors (Figure 10).

Annie

1. Stretch Rope, Stories, and Rituals

Annie, a warm and friendly 7-year-old, enters the therapy space with curiosity, enthusiasm, and interest. Staff members inform me that she exhibits difficulty with gross motor skills, and they want her to have opportunities to develop in this area. The staff members also indicate that Annie acts very uncomfortably around others—they believe, because of negative feelings about her inability to move and take part in games as other children do. When asked what they appreciate about Annie, they respond unanimously with praises of her social skills, sensitivity, and kindness. Annie enters the therapy space showing awkwardness with gross motor skills, but giving 100% effort. I reflect to myself about Annie's effort and wonder how "Strong Effort" may become a help to her in other parts of her life.

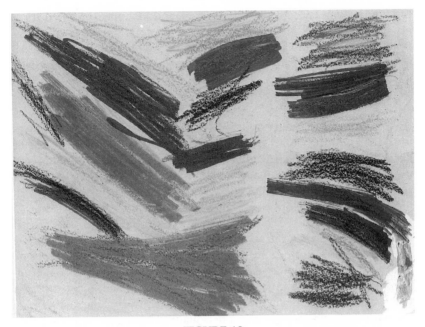

FIGURE 10

I take out the stretch rope, wondering aloud whether Annie may want to try using it. Her curiosity about the rope becomes apparent, and we begin some simple movements with the rope. The creativity of the rope seems to assist her with exploring gross motor movements without self-consciousness.

Then Annie sits on my play mat (a contained space) and develops an angry story. She takes out the angry-looking puppets, grabs the dinosaur puppet, and begins killing people. This killing goes on for a long time. Annie then appears to want to stop the killing and asks if all the angry puppets can be put in a trash bag with a cinch closure. She then places each angry puppet in the bag and says, "Now cinch it up so they can't get out." I ask, "Do you want to do it, or do you want me to do it?" Annie cinches up the bag, and a long pause follows.

Annie takes some of the containers and wants to employ all of them. She gathers up a bunch of small objects, puts them in the containers, and closes the containers. She repeats this *Action Ritual* ("Empty and Fill Containers") over and over. I wonder what holds her gross motor skills back, while her fine motor skills appear so developed. Annie remembers not only the number, but the shapes and sizes of all the small objects she puts in the containers. If one object is missing, she knows it. Annie's entire time becomes occupied with this ritual, and she appears pleased at her accomplishment. Her warmth and friendliness communicate an invitation to play, increased social interaction, and a sense of give and take. All of this activity takes place within a very small and defined area, however.

2. "Picnic"

Annie begins the "Empty and Fill Containers" ritual, and then moves into "Nurturance"rituals, in which she utilizes the play food, utensils, and dish sets. Her quiet friendliness invites me to participate. Annie continues to remember how many small pieces and shapes from the earlier session are now in the containers.

Annie next develops a story of a "Picnic." We are going to a special place and to a picnic. She dresses both of us in fabrics (a simple scarf and fabric belt). Then she takes all the food (play food) and utensils we will need. Annie creates a car by using a couple of chairs. She wants me to drive the car. She continually asks for my participation and collaboration in all parts of the story. She wants me to play many roles—driver of the car, friend, at a movie theatre, and friend enjoying lunch with her in the park. She continues to allow her qualities of creativity, resourcefulness, and playfulness to come forth. Since the previous session, she now uses half of the large room rather than a confined mat space. I reflect privately on how her natural playfulness invites her to explore more body movement.

3. "Going to a Special Place" and Masks

Annie wants to play a variation on the "Picnic" story—a "Going to a Special Place" story. This story takes on even more significance, I reflect, because all the children in the group home will be moving soon to another facility. Annie has lived in the present location for about 4 years. In this "Going to a Special Place" story, a character called "Boogie Man" enters. Annie packs all the objects and things and says she wants to go to church and then to a picnic. It is interesting to note that this time when she packs, she includes everything (not just items for a picnic). I reflect that this may relate to her forthcoming move. This "Going to a Special Place" ritual appears to be very important to her. We get in the car, and this time she insists on driving the car. We can't drive up to the park because of the "Boogie Man." When the "Boogie Man" finally leaves, Annie feels comfortable enough to go to the picnic. She also speaks about locking the doors to be sure she is safe.

Annie moves to the art area and begins playing with some of the mask materials. She makes two masks; one is called "Wooper" (Figure

11), and the other one is a mask of "Celia" (the child in the case example) (Figure 12). The "Wooper" mask is a primitive drawing of a person and shows imagination in the use of color—orange for the hair, which is strips of tissue paper, and two red legs. The "Celia" mask is particularly creative and detailed. Annie looks up to Celia and copies Celia's actions when they are together. Annie weaves black pipe cleaners to make the hair, and also uses black pipe cleaners to make legs for the "Celia" mask. She insists on putting ribbons in "Celia's" hair, which are made with red tissue paper. I reflect on her free display of imagination and see how imagination continues to be a really good friend to her.

4. Enlarging Space

Annie chooses objects, fabric pieces, and play food, and begins using the entire space of the room. Again, she wants to play "Going to a Special

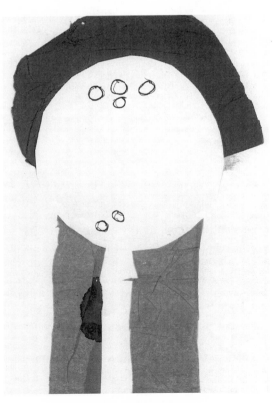

FIGURE 11

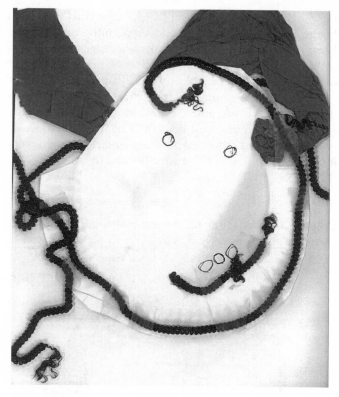

FIGURE 12

Place"—the circus and picnic, this time. She packs the bags with special objects, and we take off; she again insists on driving the car. The whole room becomes the playground for this story. Annie initiates all the dialogue and actions and remains totally committed to the scene. She creates costumes for both of us, which she assembles. This broad dramatic play offers an opportunity for Annie to continue to develop both gross motor and fine motor skills. I reflect to myself that "Creative Play" invites more comfortable and expanded movement. I wonder, as I watch her gross motor movement continue to improve, how she must feel about this accomplishment—progressing from staying confined to the play mat to moving across the entire room.

Annie wants to make a mask of how she feels sometimes with other people. The mask she makes consists of a veil (tissue paper), which covers her face or uncovers it as she desires (Figure 13). In the illustrated version, her face appears uncovered, with the tissue pulled back over the

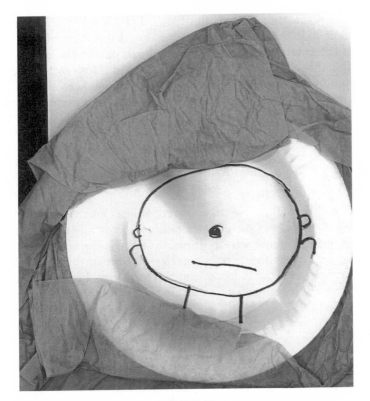

FIGURE 13

mask head. I wonder to myself about Annie's omission of eyes, and think that maybe eyes aren't as necessary when the tissue paper covers the face; however, now that Annie appears more visible, maybe eyes will become more important. As Annie continues to be friendly, interactive, and social, and more outward in expressing emotions, it seems to me she is acting as if she possesses greater "sight." Perhaps this may reflect itself at a later time in her artwork.

Susan

1. *Shut Down*

Susan (age 10) comes to the group home from being homeless and living in the streets with her brother, Mark (age 6). Fragments of information on her history indicate that her mother was killed. A review of the history shows some contact with the father, but no other information is forthcoming. When I first observe Susan and Mark soon after their arrival at the group home, their behavior shows qualities of anxiety, confusion, and sadness. They huddle together and refuse to be separated from each other for even a moment or to communicate with anyone else. They talk to each other through a stuffed toy, which they call "Herman." They appear blank and emotionless, and will not speak when I address them.

1 through 5. Rainbow Pictures and "Drawing" as an Action Ritual

My colored pens and new paper attract Susan's attention, and she begins slowly to draw a picture of a rainbow (Figure 14). Although she chooses not to communicate in words, her rainbow picture speaks to me of Susan's interests and gifts in art. Her pleasure at the completion of the picture gives witness to the energy created by the artistic process, and I wonder how Susan might take on the role of the artist in other aspects of her life. I also reflect on how Susan appears to want everything to be drawn in a specific way, and that "Perfect" seems to be restrain-

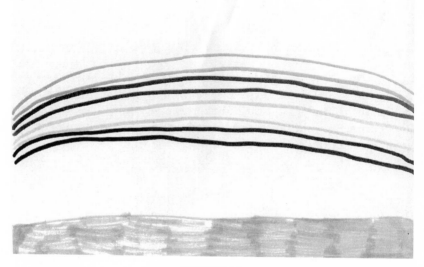

FIGURE 14

ing. Finally, I reflect to myself on the courage it has taken to make this picture, given how blank and emotionless she appeared the week before.

Susan communicates through art for the next four sessions, and "Drawing" becomes a pleasing ritual that captures Susan's attention and creativity. I appreciate the bright colors and energy of Susan's artwork, which usually consists of rainbows or nature images. "Perfect," continues to restrain some of the artistic process, but I notice that Susan is beginning to venture out more. In one session Susan draws her family. She includes in this picture of her family her mother, whose death she witnessed (Figure 15).

At a later session, I am really surprised when Susan greets me with a wave and a smile. I offer opportunities each meeting for Susan to play with the objects, puppets, or masks but she continually prefers "art." Upon completion of her artwork, Susan appears pleased and happy with her accomplishment. I continue to wonder to myself how the role of artist may influence other aspects of Susan's life.

On the fifth meeting, Susan continues to interact in a friendly manner by drawing a rainbow with balloons and a sun. Susan's verbal communication improves and consists of short phrases or yes–no answers. When asked a question, she pauses and thinks a long time before an-

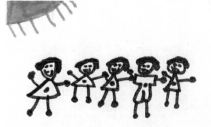

FIGURE 15

swering. I wonder how Susan's ability to contemplate and think may assist her as a strength; however, I also wonder if she perceives this as a strength. Susan's "Drawing" continues as an *Action Ritual* and offers Susan opportunities to view herself as competent and creative. She completes the fifth session by creating a short picture book with rainbow and nature pictures and a storm. In these five meetings, "Drawing" seems to be functioning as a friend to Susan and assisting her to express her voice, which later becomes expressed in a more verbal way.

6. *Puppet Stories*

On the sixth session, Susan's voice comes forth with spontaneity, and her ability to verbalize becomes much stronger. She becomes interested in the puppets and tells a story about the puppets she selects. Her language, use of words, rate of speaking, and ability to think and form ideas show great enthusiasm and sensitivity. In sharing the story with me, her spontaneity moves me. She loves the puppets, and it appears that through working with them the artist within Susan comes forth. Susan talks excitedly about school and tells me about her classes. Her pride and sense of self-esteem stand out to me. I hold my breath and marvel at Susan's spontaneity and life. Again, I wonder whether this is an extension of the artist voice present during the picture drawing from the previous give sessions. It appears that "Art" influences all areas (voice, language, emotions, and thinking process). I wonder how creativity can continue to blossom in Susan's life and what ripple effects it may have. Susan enters the *Transformational Circle* and draws a new book of rainbow pictures.

7. *More Puppet Stories and a Meal*

The seventh session brings the same spontaneity as the sixth meeting. Susan delights in choosing more puppets and eagerly approaches developing more stories. She chooses two puppets, a witch and snake, which she takes care to describe as good characters. She gives me the person puppet and the dog as my characters. The story involves a nice witch who gives candy to a little child. In the second story, Susan chooses the alligator and the spider as characters for me. She chooses to role-play the bunny and the pterodactyl (a dinosaur). There is a shortage of water in the forest, but the pterodactyl finds new water, and the animals move to the new location. In both of these plays, Susan improvises dialogue and seems to appear comfortable and spontaneous.

Next, Susan wants to play having a meal, and she chooses the foods she wants to eat. She invites me to the meal with her and asks me to choose the foods I want to eat. She also says she wants to play herself and wants me to play myself. Then we proceed to share a meal together. I speak to her about school, and it seems to be easier for her to talk about her life while play-acting this situation. She also really appears to enjoy this activity and expresses her feelings clearly. Susan continues to be appropriate in social interaction, to develop appropriate improvised dialogue based on the situation, to show an understanding of concepts, and to interact in creative and appropriate ways. Susan contributes to the Consultants Corner a journal of drawings. Susan Says "I feel happy when I draw; it takes my bad feelings away."

CONCLUSION

Ronald, Celia, Annie, and Susan have all responded positively to the invitations of drama and narrative. They have shown growth in self-esteem; in expression of emotions; and in the abilities to soothe and calm themselves, to communicate more fully with others, and to become authors of their own actions. By respecting and inviting collaborative processes, these children have discovered and made good use of the *Wonder Space, Transformational Circle, Consultant Corner,* and *Action Rituals.* On a bodily level, these children have experienced changes and shifts in themselves. Although they have not been able to articulate all of these changes verbally, they have experienced changes, and these new experiences have been articulated in their actions and behavior. In expressing the familiar, they have become increasingly willing to experience and embrace newness and change in their lives.

EDITORIAL QUESTIONS

Q: *(CS) One of the things that really impresses me about your chapter and your work in general is how you are able to utilize such a varied and large repertoire of drama and play therapy ideas and exercises without imposing these or allowing your own excitement with different techniques to silence your clients' small voices! You also weave a very unique tapestry of narrative and drama therapy, where each is enhanced by the other.*

I am intrigued with how you go about letting a child's actions guide you. You speak of not having a "predetermined . . . response," of being "moved by what the child is moved by." I think there are very subtle and yet powerful differences between doing this and doing conventional play therapy. Therapists who use a more traditional approach may appear very similar to what you have described. A traditional approach may incorporate and utilize the child's language, metaphors, and play activity as you do, but this is often done in order to steer the child to talk about or to enact certain predetermined topics the therapist thinks will help this child.

Thus I wonder if you could help us get a clearer sense of what your moment-to-moment, relational approach looks like and sounds like. Do you sometimes find it tempting to privilege your understanding of what is being expressed or to restrict the play conversation? If so, how do you return to a more open, relational focus? Are there times when it might be useful to steer the conversation in certain ways?

A: In my theatre training, I learned the concept of "moment to moment." When you act out an improvised scene with another, rather than having a predetermined idea of what will happen, you try to live each moment spontaneously in a "moment-to-moment" way. This has helped me stay "in the moment" with children. To invite spontaneity and multiple choices in a session. I find it helpful to have creative materials visibly available, such as art supplies (for masks, pictures, etc.), puppets, a sand box, life-size dolls, fabrics, and simple musical instruments—all of which may open space for communication. Children speak in many ways, through conversation, pictures, movement, music, poetry, and other creative forms. I believe it is important with children not to enter the therapy session with the conception that verbalizing is the preferred method of communication. I try to privilege a child's way of relating.

Sometimes there may be an occasion where I may wonder if a particular topic or topics may be helpful to explore. I may introduce this verbally or through dramatic action (e.g., by starting a dramatic scene or introducing a character with the small objects or puppets) to see if it is of interest to the child. If it is important, the child will take the idea and develop it. If it is not of interest to the child, the child will usually drop it and go on to something different.

When I find myself falling in love with my own ideas, I get myself back into the child's world by taking a long pause, listening, and interacting with the child in the moment, and/or by taking the child's physical posture.

Q: *(CS) What sorts of things go into your decision simply to remain silent and serve as a witness to the child's dramatic play? What sorts of cues might you use to decide to say or do something rather than remain silent? Perhaps we can take Ronald as an example. In your first segment on Ronald, you describe the therapy space as allowing him "to tell the story of losing his mother" (i.e., to stay for the moment in his more familiar world). There are long pauses. You experience some sadness and notice how his play evolves. At some point you begin reflecting on creat-*

ing a ritual called "Mother's Love," and you enter the Wonder Space *to ask Ronald about the qualities and characteristics of his mother's love. If it's possible for you to recall these interactions, or perhaps other similar ones, what sorts of internal or external things happen for you to decide to stay silent? To break this silence?*

A: I find pauses to be very helpful in therapy. Pauses allow time to think, to witness. As to whether to speak or remain silent, I look for the child's preference. I might ask, "Do you want me to watch or join in? If I join in, do you want me to play a role or to assist in some other way? If you want me to play a role, what role do you want me to play?" Pauses help me to enter the child's space. Some readers may be familiar with the concept of "doubling," a psychodramatic term. The double is a mind/feeling reader. The double tunes in to the other person's thoughts and feelings and expresses them. In order to be a double, respect for the person is primary. It is also important to take a posture of openness and to set aside preconceptions so that you may receive the other's inner and outer thoughts and ideas. I learned with children that in pauses and moments of stillness, I find it easier to enter their world by taking on some aspects of their physical posture. Although I do not double this (out loud) like a traditional double, it helps me to stay "moment to moment" in the child's world. I do this when I am on a reflecting team watching through the mirror. I pretend I am sitting right by the person. I often mirror her/his posture. I pause and try to enter the person's world. This assists me to reflect and wonder. This helps me with the wondering questions and with deciding whether to wonder out loud or to myself. If I have doubts as to wonder aloud or to myself, I ask the child. I am not hoping for a particular response. Sometimes with children—as in the case of Ronald—I find it helpful to use sensory language, as children often speak through their senses (i.e., color, weight, taste). Therefore, a question like "What texture is mother's love?" opens space to communicate more about mother's love through a drawing of it, or a conversation, or some other way.

Q: *(CS) To continue with this same example, in your second segment on Ronald, you note his performing a new story (rebuilding a new city). You describe his nonverbal calm behaviors. You point to this nonconscious shift in his body coinciding with a new story of rebirth. Here you seem to be mostly in the role of witness. Do you think that sometimes it is enough for therapists simply to be witnesses to a shift in narrative? How might a therapist gauge when it might be useful to go further and invite a child to acknowledge the change? What advantages might either of these directions have? When you think about working with young children's narratives and expanding their possibilities, how do you decide when to ask narratively oriented questions, as compared with inviting play and drama therapy activities or simply witnessing their own spontaneous play journeys?*

A: When change happens, it is not always necessary to privilege a verbal recognition of that change. The body has already witnessed the change and experienced it. There is no set way to recognize change. With a more verbal child (or older child), the child may prefer to acknowledge change by talking about it.

I see narrative and drama therapy in a more integrated way. Taking a role opens space the way a question does, as the person playing the role experiences a different perspective and often sees alternative possibilities. I think it is important not to privilege questions, but to invite a process of exploration and take a posture of curiosity and openness. I find it helpful to invite space to be expanded through a scene, a role, a mask, a picture, a conversation, and so on. Sometimes I may do a "shopping list": "Would you prefer to talk, do a scene, make a puppet, or create a mask? Or would you prefer something else?"

Q: *(CS) I was impressed with how carefully you are able to note your varied internal conversations and reflections as different children are playing. What role do these internal conversations play in your collaborative therapy? When do you decide to speak these out loud, and when do you decide to keep them to yourself?*

A: I may be likely to speak it out loud if I feel it is not intrusive and if it appears that speaking it out loud might open space. I may be more likely to wonder out loud if the child appears to be at a crossroads.

Q: *(CS) I know that the present chapter's examples come from a group home setting. When parents or caregivers are available for therapy conversations, do you like to involve them? If so, how? Do you sometimes include them in the session? Do you find this useful? If so, how? Are there times you prefer not to involve adult caregivers in sessions? If you don't include them in a session, do you find it helpful to involve them in other ways? Do you sometimes include other family members or nonfamily members when these are available?*

A: I very much prefer to involve parents or caregivers in many ways—as witnesses, participants, or audience members. It is important to understand a child's preference for the role that a family member or caregiver takes. Does the child want the parent to witness (or serve as audience), to participate as a helper, or to take an actual role in an improvised scene?

I have found that children in a group home prefer to share their masks, pictures, and puppets with caregivers and sometimes with the other children. Because the caregivers at the group home are so occupied with caring for many children, they are usually not available to participate in the sessions; often at the conclusion of a session, however, I like to allow about 5 minutes for the child to share with a caregiver what the child prefers. Children usually share something they have created, such as a mask, a puppet, a picture, a fabric environment, or a costume piece or prop. Sometimes they will talk to a caregiver about what they did, and sometimes just sharing the creation is sufficient.

REFERENCES

Andersen, T. (1996). Workshop presented at the California Family Studies Center/Phillips Graduate Institute, Los Angeles.

Anderson, H. (1993). On a roller coaster: A collaborative language systems approach to therapy. In S. Friedman (Ed.), *The new language of change.* New York: Guilford Press.

Barragar-Dunne, P. (1988). *The media in drama therapy.* Los Angeles: Drama Therapy Institute of Los Angeles.

Barragar-Dunne, P. (1992a). *The narrative therapist and the arts.* Los Angeles: Possibility Press. (Drama Therapy Institute of Los Angeles).

Barragar-Dunne, P. (1992b). *Drama therapy activities for parents and children: An exercise handbook* (2nd ed.). Los Angeles: Drama Therapy Institute of Los Angeles.

Barragar-Dunne, P. (1993a). *The creative therapeutic thinker* (2nd ed.). Los Angeles: Drama Therapy Institute of Los Angeles.

Barragar-Dunne, P.(1993b). *The fundamentals of drama therapy and narrative [Audiotape series].* Los Angeles: Drama Therapy Institute of Los Angeles.

Barragar-Dunne, P. (1995). *The creative journal.* Los Angeles: Drama Therapy Institute of Los Angeles.

Barragar-Dunne, P., & Barragar, K. (1997). *Double stick tape: Poetry, drama and narrative as therapy for adolescents.* Los Angeles: Possibilities Press (Drama Therapy Institute of Los Angeles).

Cattanach, A. (1992). *Play therapy with abused children.* London: Jessica Kingsley.

Cattanach, A. (1994). *Where the sky meets the underworld.* London: Jessica Kingsley.

Fogel, A. (1993). *Developing through relationships.* Chicago: University of Chicago Press.

Landy, R. (1986). *Drama therapy: Concepts and practice.* Springfield, IL: Charles C Thomas.

Landy, R. (1993). *Persona and performance*. New York: Guilford Press.

Landy, R. (1996). *Essays in drama therapy: The double life*. London: Jessica Kingsley.

White, M. (1989). *Selected papers*. Adelaide, South Australia: Dulwich Centre Publications.

White, M., & Epston, D. (1990). *Narrative means to therapeutic ends*. New York: Norton.

4

Narrative Therapy and Family Support

STRENGTHENING THE MOTHER'S VOICE IN WORKING WITH FAMILIES WITH INFANTS AND TODDLERS

PEGGY SAX

Writing this chapter has given me the opportunity to pause and reflect, to take stock of what I do, and to assess what I have to offer others doing similar work. I write from the perspective of ordinary life as a family therapist in private practice in a small rural New England college town. I am influenced by the family support movement (Carnegie Task Force, 1994; Garbarino, 1992; Family Resource Coalition, 1996) and the field of prevention (Lofquist, 1989; Pransky, 1991), which have been evolving in the United States since the mid-1970s. Feminism (Goodrich, 1991; Hare-Mustin & Marecek, 1994; McGoldrick, Anderson, & Walsh, 1991) and the shift toward collaborative approaches within the field of family therapy (Andersen, 1987, 1991; Hoffman, 1993) have also had a great impact on my work. More recently, narrative ideas and practices have become invigorating sources of education, training, and provocation for me (White & Epston, 1990; White, 1989, 1991; Epston, 1989; Epston & White, 1992). My aim in drawing links between these movements is to highlight shared philosophical premises and preferred practices, with the ultimate goal of further developing a unifying commitment to supporting families through highly stressful times.

NARRATIVE THERAPY

Several recent publications provide excellent descriptions of White and Epston's narrative therapy and its philosophical foundations, clinical applications, and relationship to other therapeutic approaches (Friedman, 1993; Freedman & Combs, 1993, 1996; S. Gilligan & Price, 1993; Nicholson, 1995; O'Hanlon, 1994; Parry & Doan, 1994). The focus is on helping people discover new stories about themselves—stories that are based on strengths, hopes, dreams, preferences, and new possibilities. This puts the accent on a different psychotherapeutic syllable, orienting therapists toward understanding the meaning people give to experiences, and how these stories structure lives. A narrative perspective also looks at cultural contexts, and at the effects on people's lives of such discourses as gender, class, race, and ethnicity. The therapist listens carefully to a client's or family's problem story, and follows the influence of the problem on the lives and relationships of family members. Times in everyday life when a person moves beyond the constricted lens of the problem are highlighted. In realigning with their hopes and preferences, clients develop strategies and countertactics to resist problems' getting in their way. Therapy, as a rite of passage, becomes a place where people can experience themselves as authorities on their own lives and where they can become established as consultants to themselves, to others, and to the therapist. Clients are encouraged to develop other supportive relationships in which their newly emerging alternative stories can blossom.

My work is influenced by two co-emerging narrative traditions (Smith, 1995): by the externalizing/deconstructing work of Michael White (White, 1991; White & Epston, 1990), and by hermeneutics/collaborative language systems (Andersen, 1991, 1993; Anderson & Goolishian, 1988, 1992; Anderson, Goolishian, & Winderman, 1986; Friedman, 1995; Hoffman, 1993). I value each heritage deeply, and I am troubled to sense a pressure to choose camps. In everyday practice, I draw from each, depending on the situation. Sometimes, holding both involves a creative tension that challenges me to grapple with conflicting choices about how to proceed. Ironically, my family therapy training has taught me to struggle with ways of moving beyond either–or think-ing toward creating openings for new dialogue. Both sets of theories are evolving, and, regardless, life goes on.

THE FAMILY SUPPORT MOVEMENT

Discovering the world of narrative ideas and therapeutic practices in the past several years has been like "coming home" again. Since the 1970s, I have been involved with a community of professionals and consumers guided by similar principles, a commitment to best practices, and a shared passion for developing supportive services for families of young children.[1] The family support movement is a multidisciplinary, multicul-tural perspective that for over 20 years has supported the evolution of such programs as home-based services for parents and infants with de-velopmental special needs, parent–child centers, and Head Start. What makes this field unusual is the interplay between theory and practice, supporting a research-based field of inquiry into the ecology of human development and a grassroots advocacy movement. This movement continues to gain recognition and momentum, and currently represents literally thousands of community-based programs throughout the Unit-ed States (Family Resource Coalition, 1996).

The family support philosophical framework orients families and their helpers toward fostering positive parent–child interactions over time (Sameroff & Chandler, 1974), within their interconnected social, cultural, and historical context (Bronfenbrenner, 1979, 1986). In recog-nizing that contexts can have positive and/or negative influences on de-velopment, the family support movement shares a fundamental commit-ment to creating supportive and healthy communities for families with small children (Garbarino, 1992). This perspective is connected to a sol-

---

[1]In British Columbia, I spent a decade home-visiting families with infants with develop-mental special needs, developing a family-focused infant development program, and con-sulting with the emerging network of British Columbia Infant Development Programmes. I focused my graduate studies on inquiries into parent–infant interactions and the phe-nomenon of turn taking between infant and primary caregiver. I gleaned from what was known about normal development to help guide professionals and parents in living with infants with developmental disabilities and delays. Upon moving to Vermont in 1983, I became involved with the Addison County Parent–Child Center and the family support movement. I decided to become a family therapist and to expand my repertoire beyond the birth-to-age-3 population and beyond a developmental focus on special needs. Since then, I have worked in community mental health; as an outpatient clinician; and as the co-ordinator of an intensive family-based services program, the Family Advocate Project. In 1992, I went into private practice as a family therapist and consultant.

id research base on enhancing parent–infant interactions through adverse conditions (Field, 1983, 1984, 1992), as well as the growing literature on coping and resilience for "vulnerable but invincible" kids who overcome enormous obstacles and environmental risks (Werner & Smith, 1982; Werner, 1988a, 1988b; Garmezy & Rutter, 1983; Losel & Bliesner, 1990). All of these studies acknowledge contributions by both caregiver and young child, addressing individual differences such as temperament, special developmental needs, and emotional distress (e.g., trauma, maternal depression). Family support focuses on family members' strengths and fosters mutual feelings of efficacy (Goldberg, 1977). For a caregiver, this means gaining self-confidence in reading, predicting, and responding to a young child's cues. For an infant or young child, this means developing an increasing sense of mastery and social competence, with ongoing supportive feedback from the caretaking environment.

The theoretical base for family support is strongly linked with the field of prevention. Lofquist (1989, p. 1) defines prevention as "an active process of creating conditions and fostering personal attributes which promote the well-being of people." Familial conditions, sociocultural conditions, and personal attributes are thus viewed as inseparably intertwined, contributing both to personal growth and development and to community development. Thus, facilitating change involves not only the remediation of specific problems, but the active creation of healthy, nurturing environments. The family support movement is a primary prevention approach relevant to all parents, not only those who are identified as "at risk" or who have problems. It normalizes parents seeking help and assumes that all families have both needs and strengths. Services are focused on engaging parents in developing their own resources and linking them to communities, not only as recipients of services but as active contributors to their communities. The guiding light is a shared vision of creating a national commitment to supporting families.

Within the family support movement, an active parent advocacy movement encourages parents to take on leadership, to build useful services responsive to family needs, and to hold professionals accountable to the folks they serve. Much has been written on the need to demystify psychological services and to enhance support systems and natural helping networks (Dunst, 1983; Featherstone, 1980; Turnbull & Turnbull, 1985; Whittaker, Garbarino, & Associates, 1983). Parent–professional partnerships are expected to address families' needs and priorities. Community building takes place through support groups, parent advocacy, and community playgroups. The advocacy movement also addresses the development of social policy that supports families and children at every level of local, state, and federal government.

In addressing the question of how best to provide services to families with infants, the field of infant mental health has emerged (Bromwich, 1985; Fraiberg, 1975; Levine, Garcia-Coll, & Oh, 1985; Partridge, 1987, 1991; Pawl, 1987; Trout, 1981; Weston, Ivins, Zuckerman, Jones, & Lopez, 1989). This multidisciplinary field assists families of infants struggling with special needs, such as developmental disabilities, developmental delays, drug exposure, severe postpartum depression, adolescent parenthood, and/or acute environmental stresses. Infant mental health practitioners are informed by family support principles and offer specific tools and information. Practitioners listen carefully to parents' specific concerns and requests in attending to the often grueling daily details of parenting. They provide gentle coaching about ways for a parent and child to get "in sync" with each other. The goal is not "perfect" parenting, but a relaxation into a mutually efficacious style of interaction.

I am struck by the enormous similarities and "fit" between the family support movement and narrative therapies. Although sharing a passionate, common-sense commitment to healthy families and communities (Duvall & Beier, 1995), they haven't yet really discovered each other. My hope is that these two communities, guided by a generosity of spirit, a contagious curiosity, and mutual respect, can work together in the future. This linkage has enormous power and possibility; the communities have a lot to learn from each other and their rich heritages.

STRENGTHENING THE MOTHER'S VOICE

In *Of Woman Born*, Adrienne Rich (1976) speaks of mothering as "the most exquisite suffering." She eloquently describes anger and tenderness as common experiences, thereby removing the veil from the ambivalent, nitty-gritty realities of living with children. Our culture has created a "good mother–bad mother" split that silences the untold story, the mother's voice (Weingarten, 1994). Mothers often blame themselves for not living up to the idealized, all-powerful image of the good mother. As a cultural assumption, "mother blame" can haunt mothers with a constant, insidious barrage of guilt and self-blame. Unfortunately, the culture of psychotherapy has done much to contribute to the omnipresence of mother blame and to pathologize mothers. As therapists, we must take responsibility for helping loosen "blame's" grip on mothers' feelings of efficacy (Caplan, 1989; Walters, Carter, Papp, & Silverstein, 1988). This is a guiding belief in my work with families.

Feminist theory raises serious concerns about the myth of motherhood and the cultural bias toward holding mothers exclusively responsible for the rearing and development of children (Lerner, 1988; Braverman, 1991). In work with mothers and young children, feminist therapists' observations and inquiry go beyond mother–child dynamics to address the larger social context. This includes addressing the structure of family and work life so that responsibility is more evenly distributed, and building healthy support networks of family, friends, and community. It also involves looking at how our dominant culture tends to define the institution of motherhood as a polarization between blame and idealization.

A cornerstone of feminism is the belief that every woman is the authority on her own experience, and that her experience is to be believed as personal truth (Hare-Mustin, 1991; Hare-Mustin & Marecek, 1994). Many women share struggles in developing a sense of personal authority—an intricate intertwining in the development of a sense of voice, mind, and self (Belenky, Clinchy, Goldberger, & Tarule, 1986; Rampage, 1991). Since the early 1980s, much has been written regarding women's growth in connection and the women-in-relation theory of development (C. Gilligan, 1982; Jordan, 1991; Surrey, 1991). This theory contributes to a broadened understanding of how women find meaning and identity in relational contexts. It informs feminist therapists' definitions of power and their ways of conducting therapy, highlighting mutuality, connectedness, and empowerment (Avis, 1991; Miller, 1991). Many women resonate with these ideas, and find affirmation, support, and self-confidence in their discovery. At the same time, feminist theory continues to raise consciousness regarding the portrayal of gender differences as objective, biological givens beyond social reform. Because I am a woman of my culture, my work reflects this dilemma. Naming it doesn't solve it. I continue to grapple in my work and in my life with affirming the mother's voice while fostering changes in how we perceive the responsibilities and structure of family life.

MY PROFESSIONAL AND PERSONAL CONTEXT

Narrative ideas and practices have become a dominant thread in the tapestry of my work, and have contributed to a personal resurgence of commitment and passion. Becoming part of a larger narrative community of like-minded people has transformed the isolation of private practice into a supportive web of connections and resources. However, I am reluctant to call myself a narrative therapist, since I am cautious about contributing to an unintentional exclusivity. Narratively oriented therapists need to be careful about developing exclusive tendencies, and tolerant in approaching colleagues with different ideas. The enthusiasm for new discoveries can create the illusion of having arrived at the therapeutic "promised land." All of us need to remember that we are not in competition for the therapeutic Holy Grail, but in great need of collaborative leadership to help guide us through difficult times.

Fortunately, my clients don't seem to care what I call myself, as long as I can help and don't have to waste time explaining my approach. In Vermont, high value is placed on resourcefulness, down-to-earth common sense, and durability, coupled with an interesting blend of community-mindedness and self-sufficiency. People tend to be suspicious of newfangled gadgets and of what can be construed as "holier than thou" presumptions. It takes the test of time for newcomers to be trusted; to do so, they must demonstrate a respect for existing land and traditions. Therapists aspire to the reputation of an honest mechanic: trustworthy, knowledgeable, giving good value for the dollar, and straightforward in approach. Professionals are held accountable to the community, and it is a privilege to be perceived as useful.

Vermont is a small state with much pride in her cultural heritage. It is possible here to imagine how the pieces of the puzzle fit together and to feel part of something larger than oneself. People wear different hats; expertise is defined contextually and with minimal hubris. Roles are more fluid and transitory than in the big city, so today's client can show up as tomorrow's emergency plumber when the pipes freeze, or in relationship with one's children at the local high school. Beyond the obvious ethical guidelines, role boundaries can seem arbitrary. This contributes not only to some interesting dilemmas, but to creative possibilities for creating bridges and building dialogues among clients, colleagues, and larger systems. This context can transform clinical practices into a learning lab for emergent new ideas, including a diverse blend of clinical practice, systems consultations, supervision, and teaching.

In Vermont, economic diversity is very apparent. I am acutely aware of my privilege in being an educated, white, middle-class professional. Many families have lived in poverty for generations. It is common for families to live in trailers with next-door neighbors in large colonial houses. Class issues are often unspoken influences on the opportunities available for families and on the choices made. It is an ongoing challenge to acknowledge the influence of class issues in our lives and relationships.

My context is also influenced by stresses inherent in the culture and in the work. Like so many other professional helpers, I am immersed in the daily details of clinical practice while attempting to navigate through turbulent times. The public perception of therapy is laced with a growing suspicion, with consumers rightfully wary of many of the assumptions and power dynamics beneath the traditional therapeutic relationship. Therapists risk isolation and losing the satisfaction that comes from feeling part of a larger community. They face the dilemma of discovering ways of staying financially solvent while continuing a commitment to the values that brought them to their work in the first place.

As a therapist, I counsel families in my office. In working as a consultant with family support organizations, I facilitate groups' coming together to articulate and strengthen their shared vision and commitment, to build resources, and to take specific action steps toward implementing desired outcomes. Consultation keeps me grounded in a larger perspective, and I feel part of a movement that can influence social policy and affect change. In each of these situations, there is an active "re-storying" taking place, as individuals realign with underlying beliefs and values, bolster inner and outer resources, strengthen links with other like-minded people, and renew their commitment to taking charge.

CLINICAL APPLICATIONS

I have chosen to highlight clinical work with two young mothers of toddlers. This is not to minimize the important role that fathers play in children's lives or the fathers' responsibility in finding solutions to problems. However, my focus in each of these examples is on strengthening the mother's voice. Honoring the mother's voice means valuing the ambivalent presence of tenderness and anger. An affirming inquiry into the particulars of a mother's experience encourages connectedness, self-confidence, and new developments that are in alignment with a mother's best intentions. This can have multiple ripple effects on family, friends, and community, including shifts in power imbalances.

Narrative therapy accents the importance of asking questions in order to open space for new stories. In reviewing transcripts, I am aware that I also do a lot of talking. My first inclination is to make excuses or to quietly do some extra editing. However, the truth is that this is my personal style, and I believe it works for me and my clients. Indeed, there are times when I consciously resist the urge to make statements, focusing on questions. I also believe it is helpful to share affirming reflections when dealing with such parenting issues as confidence and isolation.

For the first session, I like to meet with the parent(s) alone. This way, I can hear each parent's story without being distracted or interrupted by the immediate needs of small children. If both parents are present, I listen carefully for the mother's voice. I strive to be sensitive to gender issues, particularly the ways in which a mother can become dominated and take a back seat to her partner's experiences. I want to make sure that both partners have the opportunity to speak up. I also listen for the impact of class, ethnicity, and privilege on a client's aspirations and on the dynamics between us. In subsequent sessions, I invite parent(s) and children to attend. In observing a young child, I highlight feelings of efficacy and connectedness, especially the sharing of joyful moments in experiencing autonomy and mastery ("Look at what I did! I did it myself"). My primary focus is on the parents and infant or young child together, noting their mutual strengths, and helping them discover each other in new ways. As a new story becomes strengthened, I like to invite others to join us who can witness the new developments. This includes extended family members, friends, and others in a growing community support network.

Amy,[2] age 27, is a single parent of Matt, age 3 years. Amy separated from Matt's father a year ago, after moving back to Vermont to be closer to Amy's mother. Amy is in a new relationship with John, age 40. They are both very worried about Matt. This is an abridged version of our conversations. In choosing to leave out parts of the interview(s), I do not want to contribute to a therapist mystique; I believe that these transcriptions realistically portray the quality of our interactions. The following is a transcription of parts of conversations among Amy, John, and me (Peggy).

PEGGY: Tell me about your concerns. What prompted you to call me?

AMY: We are very worried about Matt. He has had a very rough first few years. I left his father a year ago when I realized it just wasn't going to work. He is a troubled, moody man who drinks a lot. He now lives 1,000 miles away, and we haven't heard from him in several months. He didn't treat Matt well, and used to strike him when he was angry. He used very harsh discipline. I was scared and didn't know what to do. Now Matt is acting in ways that make me think something is really wrong. He has been diagnosed with mild cerebral palsy. I worry that the physical punishments caused brain damage. He has these fits of rage that are very scary. I feel helpless, scared that the abuse has had permanent effects, and worried that he will be like his father.

PEGGY: Your story touches my heart, hearing how much you love this little guy, and how hard his first few years have been for you. I remember when we spoke on the phone how worried you sounded—to the point of desperation. It sounds like you've been living with a

---

[2]Names have been changed to protect confidentiality. I greatly appreciate the permission families gave me to include this material in this chapter.

lot of fear, discouragement, and worry for a long time. It can be so hard to find the courage to ask for help. What was it that helped you make the decision to reach out for help?

AMY: I am in a new relationship, which is wonderful (*looks at boyfriend, John, with a smile*. We knew each other 15 years ago, and now rediscovered each other. We want to be a family together. This has been confusing for Matt. And John has brought some things to my attention.

JOHN: Let me describe a couple of recent incidents. Amy isn't exaggerating when she describes Matt as going into rages. I would never hit him, although I am a lot firmer than his mother. The other day he was lashing out in a fit of rage while I was trying to hold him down to change his diaper. When I moved my arm to pin him down, I saw a look of terror in his eyes. I realized he thought I was going to hit him. . . . The other day in the laundromat, he saw a little boy a few years older, went up to him, and suddenly slapped him across the face, and then giggled. It was so inappropriate, and strange how he seemed to think this would be a good way to make a new friend. . . . He hits his mother a lot, and she doesn't know what to do. I think she needs to learn more about how to discipline.

AMY: I have also been getting reports at day care that Matt has been drawing attention to himself by hitting and hurting others. He plays a lot by himself, since the other kids avoid him. . . . But my biggest worry is how out of control I feel. I'm his mother, yet I just don't know what to do, how to handle him. I think I try to make up for the hurt he's gone through by being extra loving, but it isn't working.

PEGGY: Yes, it's hard to find self-confidence in your personal style as a mother when your son's behavior keeps reminding you of what's not working. Are there also times when you feel more in sync with each other?

AMY: Yes. He can be really sweet, and then we get along great. He loves to read books together. We build towers together. He's very smart and loves to build things and take things apart. He also has good times with my mother, who lives nearby. She loves to take him in the woods and to show him nature. I enjoy his company until he hits or flies into a rage. Then I get scared, worried, and angry.

PEGGY: This is the part of mothering that I also found the most challenging: learning to set limits, to detach, to not take things personally, and to avoid power struggles. I picture there is an imaginary mothering scale with an elusive balance between love and setting limits. Most mothers I know tip the scale one way or the other, and then learn to put a bit more weight on the other end to balance things out. It sounds like you're seeking information about how to discipline without resorting to the abusive tactics you witnessed his father use.

AMY: Do you have any books you can recommend? Or specific ideas? I want to feel good about myself as a mother again.

Two weeks later, Amy arrives with Matt for the second session. Matt is a wide-eyed, engaging 3-year-old who makes eye contact with me and then immediately heads for the shelves. As he moves about handling each enticing object in the room, the floor fills with scattered games, toys, and animal figures. Next time I will remove more from my room, but first I want to see his tolerance for stimulation and his mother's response. He stays with an object long enough to inspect it with his hands, then on to the next, all the while chattering away in short exclamations: "Look! See! What's this?" My first impressions are of a bright, curious, and social youngster, interested not only in the objects but in object play with adults, and showing the beginnings of imaginative play. The effects of cerebral palsy do not significantly hamper his fine motor control or ability to express himself in play. Amy is gentle and interactive, skilled at following his lead, distracting him when necessary. She clearly knows him well.

Amy takes my lead in sitting on the floor, together with several animal figures, a small doll, and some blocks. We talk quietly, sharing observations, prompting Matt to join us with his chosen objects. He seems gradually to relax, settle down, and focus his attention. Matt invents a game of dropping blocks and wild animals into a compact disc tower, giggling while instructing us how to play: "Build tower!" With his mother's gentle coaxing, he then engages in a game of putting the baby doll to sleep in the Kleenex box, ever so carefully covering her with a tissue. I note out loud his tenderness and ability to empathize, and acknowledge how Amy continues to nurture this in their joint play. Next, Matt begins a game of peekaboo, hiding under the chair; Amy and I pretend we don't know where he has gone. We are all enjoying ourselves, and there is laughter in the air.

While Matt continues to play, I share with Amy some of my observations of her strengths as a mother: her gentle playfulness, her intuitive ability to read Matt's cues and to follow his lead, her attunement with his needs. I remark on his obvious intelligence, inquisitive nature, intensity, and ability to engage adults. We talk about the cerebral palsy, challenges of parenting a child with a handicap, difficulties in knowing what is age-appropriate, the need to become grounded in normal development. We also speak about challenges in single parenting, and in transitioning into becoming a blended family. Matt seems content to play next to us with his tower, occasionally requesting our participation, exclamations, and reassurances. I share my awe in the sanctity of play, observing that children express themselves through their play, and that the caregivers' role is to encourage expression within established safe limits.

Our conversation also revolves around the theme of discipline, with Amy identifying new limit-setting skills as her primary need. She describes how she has felt guilty saying no, and yet knows she needs to learn how.

We talk about new strategies for dealing with temper tantrums, using clear rules and time out as a consequence. She says that Matt's physical therapist recommended a couple of books by T. B. Brazelton, which she has begun reading and finds helpful. I write out for her another couple of suggestions,[3] cautioning her to read them only as long as she finds them helpful, and not to let the experts intimidate her. She seems relieved to have specific information and resources.

Three weeks later, I meet again with Amy and Matt. A difference is immediately evident as they settle onto the floor to play. Amy reports that she has been reading and thinking a lot about her parenting. She seems relieved to realize that her worries are shared by others. She is learning some new ideas in how to be firmer with Matt, and how not to let guilt and self-blame trick her into feeling sorry for him or always giving in to his tantrums. She also reports a big change in his behavior at home and in their relationship. They have been having much more fun together. Meanwhile, Matt is intensely engaged in play, and quickly draws us into his favorite hiding game.

Amy, John, and Matt are present for the fourth and final session.

PEGGY: Amy, you have a very clear-thinking and assertive partner. John, your presence is really helping balance the scales. Unless you guys are extremely unusual, and even if you are, I imagine there are times when you see things differently.

JOHN: (*Interrupts*) I'm strong, but I'm not domineering. I don't dominate anyone else. I do have a strong personality.

AMY: There are times when we do see things differently. When I think he is being too firm, I do stand up for myself. Sometimes we play "bad cop, good cop."

---

[3]I recommended Brazelton (1992) and Lieberman (1993). Another favorite of mine is Kurcinka (1991).

Amy has a new partner who treats her with respect and demonstrates a strong commitment to parenting. At the same time, she faces the challenge of learning to trust her own "mother's voice" while in the presence of a man who is so clear about his. As she gains self-confidence, she seems better equipped to assert her perspective, to engage in a parenting partnership.

I ask Amy to describe what has changed:

AMY: Matt was finding that he could scream his way around anything, and that's not an exaggeration. This simple tactic shut us down immediately. Until it stopped working, he kept using it. In the early part of his life, he was being handled physically by his father. Because of his father's extreme physical ways, I would try to overcompensate by being soft. His father was the disciplinarian. I ended up so softened up that there was nothing clear and consistent.

PEGGY: What do you do differently now?

AMY: Well, if I really get angry at him, he can go to his room. It works well. Now when he has a tantrum—say, he's not ready to go somewhere—we talk. He says to me, "Matt, no room any more," and he calms down. We found something that works. Another trick is [to] give him the choice of whether the door stays open or closed.

PEGGY: What goes on inside of you while this is happening?

AMY: It's horrible. I have to remind myself, "It's okay, it takes time."

Amy is overflowing with personal wisdom. Her knowledge is ripe for documentation (Epston & White, 1990) to pass along to other parents facing similar challenges. She gives me permission to record her words, and speaks into the microphone:

AMY: The biggest thing for us, and for me as a mother, that I've learned is that there needs to be a balance. My balance of the scale was all love. I thought that love would do everything, cure it all. It was like sickeningly sweet chocolate, all the time, constantly, and he was always pushing me away. He wouldn't want me to touch him. He wouldn't let me kiss him. He would hit me. It was almost like he was saying in his own way, "This is too much. Back off." My response to that was to give him more love, thinking then he would love me. I would have big tears in my eyes. But now, just . . . balancing the love part with the discipline part has helped me find my confidence. Now I get the hugs and kisses and I get the impromptu snuggles. And I still get to have times just to love him. He's still my baby; it's natural to be protective.

PEGGY: You're describing to me, how when you respond to him in a more confident, positive way, he responds back to you in a more positive way.

AMY: I thought I was being firm before, but everything I was saying was falling on deaf ears. Now there must be something different in my tone of voice. For the most part, when he'll push it, it won't affect me. My button won't get pushed. Before, if we'd be in the store, and he would get out of control, I would just give in.

PEGGY: I'm very interested in how your confidence as a mother has been affected.

AMY: I don't know if I know exactly how I got the confidence. I just know when I look back how things have changed. Now I know "that feeling"—what it feels like to feel too far pushed out, and what to do about it.

PEGGY: If you are pushed too far out, what do you do?

AMY: First I see it.

PEGGY: And then what do you do?

AMY: Well, I used to get caught up in the whys. "Why, Mommy, why?" Now I see to stop *before* I get my buttons pushed. I just say, "Because Mommy wants you to." After a while, I just say, "That's enough"—no more point for discussion. Usually he rages for a minute afterward, and then he stops. I just set the limit. I'm not going to get pulled in. It just happened, but I don't know exactly when. I think if you have a game plan, something to follow, even if it doesn't feel like it's working at the time, if you just keep sticking with it, it gets easier. It helps also to have a strong relationship. My mother is even softer and doting than I am, plus she has extra license to be loving, since she has the grandmother role. She's had to learn along with us, which has actually made their relationship a lot stronger.

PEGGY: I am taking delight in watching the gradual blossoming of your confidence as a mother. How do you keep your confidence and your voice as a mother alive? For example, what's your support system like with other moms?

AMY: I've been hanging out more at day care. Instead of not saying anything, being afraid of the answer, I will ask, "How have things been going here?" I'll also describe what we are doing at home in using time outs, and ask that they do the same there.

PEGGY: It sounds like you are initiating more connections with others, being part of a larger network.

AMY: I realize I'm not the only one, and I can put things in perspective. Before, I felt like I was the only one in the whole world who had a kid out of control. Now I know it's normal. I can say, "You have that problem too. What did you do?"

PEGGY: Let's say a family came in here to see me who was in a very hard place, feeling like their toddler was out of control, and sick with worry. What would you say?

AMY: When you're right in the center of a crisis, you have no clue that others could possibly know what it's like. You need a little bit of hope, just to know that even though other parents also have rough times, that things can change. It's very tough, especially if you're alone, trying to be a single parent.

PEGGY: What helped you find the courage to ask for help?

AMY: It took me a long time to acknowledge that there was a problem. It took some reminders from other people—being told, "We're having some problems at day care," hearing back from people that there was a lot of inappropriate behavior going on. It took that feedback to get me to finally do something.

PEGGY: So you feel good about some of the ways you're handling things differently?

AMY: Yeah, We're not 100% there, but we're on our way. He's happier. Before, he was inappropriate. I'm still learning, but I'm more open to learning new things with him. Going to bed at night used to be one of the worst things, and getting him up in the morning, getting him dressed. Now we just have token struggles. I'm sure we're not at the end. There will be new hurdles ahead. He will be going to a different setting for preschool. We'll need to figure out how to help him handle having two fathers. And we'll need to figure out how to handle the unknowns ahead.

PEGGY: I hope you know I am here in the future if I can be of any help. Just give me a call.

I may indeed hear again from Any, John, and Matt as they face new challenges in the years ahead. I hope that asking for help has become more "normal" for them and will be easier in the future. I am pleased to be part of their support system—a network that will grow in providing family support and in witnessing a new narrative based on this family's many strengths.

Tanya is a single mother in her early 20s. Her daughter, Mandy, is 2½ years old. Mandy's father has not been in touch since before her birth. For generations, this family has lived in Vermont and has struggled with poverty and economic survival. The following conversations involve Tanya and myself.

PEGGY: What prompted your decision to call me, and how can I best be of help?

TANYA: I want to know what to do with my daughter, Mandy, who is 2½. I was in counseling before, but all I remember the therapist doing is listening. I want some advice about how to handle things better. I need to make sense of why I behave the way I do, and to know what to do. What part do I play, and what can I do differently? I'm afraid I'm going to ruin it for her. I've always been a very sad and angry person. I don't want her to be growing up having the same experiences I did. I need to know what to do, and what to do with what's not feeling right.

PEGGY: And what is not feeling right?

TANYA: I find myself being like my mother was with me, and I hate this. I want to be my own individual. My mom never took the time to get to know me, and still doesn't listen to me. Now I don't sit and play with Mandy. I know I should, but I just don't do it.

PEGGY: What seems to get in your way?

TANYA: I have a bad phobia. I try to be perfect, and I want my place to be perfect with everything clean. I am always thinking about what needs to be cleaned. I am always cleaning up after my daughter. I get so ugly, I want to scream and punch the wall. I feel like my mother made me think I'm not okay, so I try to make everything else perfect. I try to make my daughter perfect (*tearfully*). She is a wonderful child. But I can't let her make a mess. I keep telling her, "Go play, go play." But she just wants to be with me. I love her, but I want her to do what I want to do when I want her to do it. All I do is holler and scream. Then my daughter screams back. This scares me. I don't want to do that. I feel like I am ruining her life.

PEGGY: You are somehow finding words to express the difficulties and worries that challenge many mothers, and especially single mothers. Your description reminds me of my own memories of how stressful life can be when living with a 2-year-old. What strikes me most is watching you tear up when speaking about your daughter, your obvious love for her, and your commitment to making things better for her than life has been for you. Who in your life knows about this commitment of yours?

TANYA: The girls at work. They listen to me, and see me as a single mom who deals with a lot and who has strength. I feel good when I'm at work, and I miss my daughter a lot. But then when I see her, I stop feeling good. I always let her have her way; she makes me feel like I need to keep giving and giving. All she probably needs is for me to love her. My mom never told me I'm doing a great job. She just buys me things. She never gave me positive feedback. Now I try to buy Mandy presents. But I know this isn't helping. I give her absolutely everything. Whatever she wants to wear or play with, I let her have it. She knows I'm going to give it to her. When I stick to my guns, she gets out of control—hits, digs, slaps me. I've been having a really bad time at bedtime. Ever since she was a year old, she won't go to her bed. She yells, "I hate my room." She wants to sleep with me. I don't mind, but then I know it's not right. So we have screaming matches.

PEGGY: You are describing a tough situation. I have a strong belief that we're not meant to do the important work of raising children alone—that we need each other, and "it takes a village to raise a child." This is especially true for single parents. Otherwise, it's too much to bear, and it's hard to feel good about yourself as a mother, to remember your strengths, and to forgive your imperfections. Who can you count on in your support system?

TANYA: No one, really. I don't have anyone else except my family. My mother thinks everything is okay and that I'm just making too big a deal out of everything.

PEGGY: Do any of the women at work have small children?

TANYA: Yes but mostly their children are older. I did recently meet an old friend from school in the grocery store. We had lost contact, but we talked, and I could see she really understood since she went through something similar. Now I want to stay in better contact with her. I also would be interested in a support group or other ideas you have.

PEGGY: I can tell you about the local weekly playgroup in your community run through the Parent–Child Center. . . . You are also reminding me of several young mothers I know who are facing similar struggles. Would you be interested in forming a group together?

TANYA: Yes! I know I need to do something. I also need some help learning more about children. This is my first child. I don't know what they do, what I'm supposed to do, what are the phases of development, how to discipline, what is right or wrong. I don't know what I'm doing. For example, my mom said I should potty-train my daughter at 1 year. She said, "You're wasting money on diapers, just make her go on the pot." But I didn't make her. I also let her eat what she wants. I try to treat her like an individual who has likes and dislikes. I don't make her eat her whole meal, I let her make her own decisions. But my mom gives me heck, says I should have her eat the whole thing before I let her down. And I let her choose what she can wear, at least some of the time.

PEGGY: How are you finding the strength to follow your intuitive sense of what you believe is right, especially when you seem to get so little support?

TANYA: Well, sometimes I feel guilty. But then when I go to the doctor, he says I'm right. I also remember gagging on food, detesting being forced to eat, being made to wear my hair in hideous ways, feeling like I shouldn't be forced to do something that makes me so unhappy. I have always been unhappy. I don't want my daughter to grow up unhappy. I want her to love life and herself.

PEGGY: Can you hear your commitment to wanting your daughter to live and to love? It's ringing through loud and clear, despite all the obstacles in the way.

TANYA: Yes. I try to listen to it, but stuff gets in the way. I still want my daughter to do it my way. My mom wasn't an alcoholic, she gave me what I needed. Now she doesn't think I have any problems or need help. I'm a very lovable person. I like to kiss and hug. She tells me I'm too old, to stop. I don't think you're ever too old. I think there's nothing wrong with it. I tell my daughter 50 times a day that I love her. When I discipline her, afterwards I try to say, "Mommy loves you. I'm sorry I was mad at you." I'm so afraid she'll think I don't love her. I worry that she won't want to live with me. She hates the word "No." She keeps pushing till she knows she's got me. I can be relaxed at work, but then so uptight at home.

I hate to say this, but I don't know if I had "the bond" with her. I held her at birth for a minute, but then my mother did. I thought she was beautiful when someone else was holding her. And I miss her when we're apart. After I had her, I got depressed. I wondered if I should give her up, since I can't be the perfect family. But I decided to keep her. As long as she has love, we can do it. But it's the hardest job I ever had. I don't like the responsibility. It's very different than I imagined. I was 20 when I had her. I still feel like a kid. I hate the fact I never got to be something. I should have gone to school. I wish I could have waited more years. Still, I am determined to be there for her so that she can go through school.

In a subsequent session, Tanya talks about her desire to have others appreciate her, and her struggles with isolation:

TANYA: I need other people to tell me I'm okay and doing an okay job. I'm always looking for this in anything I do.

PEGGY: Yes, you're describing something that many women express, and that is now being written more about as women tell their stories. We like to feel in connection with others, and it matters to us what other people think. The challenging part is not to blame yourself for caring. It's also hard work developing confidence in yourself, especially when your way is different. It takes determination and practice.

TANYA: I don't know why I don't interact with other people. I love people, but when I'm with my daughter, I don't like to go out. I worry that others will see how I take care of my daughter and they will think it's not right. I have a big thing about discipline. I know we're not supposed to spank or [we] can get in trouble with the state. I worry that someone will see me with her and try to take her away if I correct her. I'm very afraid I'll lose her or that an accident might happen, and she'll get hurt. I'm afraid she will die. I think about death a lot.

PEGGY: It's so hard being a single parent, feeling alone with your worries. How else does isolation take over?

TANYA: I've never been able to keep a relationship. Instead, I end relationships before I get hurt. This is true with friends also. I get close, but the first time I get hurt, I don't do things with them any more. I have a hard time getting close, afraid of getting hurt. I'm always sad. I don't know what it's like to not be in pain.

PEGGY: What do you imagine the women at work would say to you if you confided in them?

TANYA: I do confide in them. Girls at work tell me I'm dealing with a lot of pressures and I need to find some new ways to make myself happy.

PEGGY: And who else out there do you think might understand your worries?

TANYA: My grandmother. She listens to me, tells me it's okay. I've told her about my mom, and how angry I am. She knows my mom and knows where I'm coming from. She's the mom I didn't have. But she wasn't there for my mom.

PEGGY: It's striking how grandparents are able to sometimes be there for grandchildren in ways they weren't able to parent their own children. Who knows? Maybe your mom might be able to be there for your daughter in ways she wasn't able to be there for you?

TANYA: Yes, when I was growing up, we were poor. My mom didn't work and we had to make do. Now she plays with Mandy and buys her things. This makes me mad. She still doesn't treat me well (*tearfully*). I guess I'm still hoping she'll tell me she loves me, but I know she won't, and I've been crushed. I'd love to tell her how she has hurt me, but I know we'd get into a huge fight. I'd like to be able to forget about my mother, and to just go on, but I can't.

PEGGY: It's like you've had the accent on the sad syllable, now wanting to shift it. It's hard to train ourselves to notice some of the good stuff when we're in the habit of noticing the hard stuff. So many of us are trying to learn how to do this, and it's hard to retrain ourselves. What are some of the little moments of joy you experience?

TANYA: I don't know. Maybe I don't recognize them, so it's hard to remember. I really enjoy it if my daughter tells me she loves me, wants to hug or kiss . . .

PEGGY: These changes take time.

TANYA: My happiest dream is to get married. I know it won't happen right now. I'm just too ugly. No one could do anything right. I need to just enjoy life. I'd like to be able to move beyond being so angry and hurt at my mother. My mother is unhappy with herself. She didn't graduate, never got her [driver's] license, has always had other people do things for her. She doesn't even do her own bills, and has never opened a checking account, [but] instead fills out money orders. I tell her, "I will help you get your GED," but she thinks she's not smart enough.

PEGGY: I'm amazed at how you have found ways of being there for your mom even when you have been so hurt. This must be very challenging! How have you been able to accomplish things beyond your mother's grasp and without her apparent help?

TANYA: I was so proud when I got my license, but my mom acted like it was no big deal. Same thing when I got my checkbook. She is always telling me I'm just like her, but I don't want to be like her. She's always picking on me, so that I just keep thinking about all that's wrong with me.

PEGGY: How have you managed to keep the discouragement from taking away your determination?

TANYA: I barely passed school, but I didn't really care. I didn't play sports. My parents didn't care, so why should I? I almost quit high school just to piss my mom off. But then I saw I'd just be hurting myself. I see with me and my brothers and sister what we lost, and I can see a lot of my mother in me. Now I am bound and determined to break the cycle.

PEGGY: So once again, your determination shines through. How does this affect your relationship with your daughter?

TANYA: I am determined to do things differently with my daughter. I want her to do sports, to always know how beautiful and smart she is. She seems so happy, loves to sing to herself, "My mommy loves me." Sometimes just to make my mother mad, I'll try doing things differently—like I don't give my daughter a bath every night, even though my mother insists I must.

PEGGY: And what's it like for you when you choose to do things your way, even when your mom disagrees?

TANYA: It makes me feel good like I'm a separate person who can do things differently than my mom. I'm laughing inside when I get back at her. If I'm excited and proud about something, my mother doesn't care. But when she buys Mandy something, we're all supposed to make a big deal about it. But I just ignore it, I don't say anything. . . . I'm so determined.

PEGGY: How do you keep that vision alive of what you want for your daughter?

TANYA: My anger toward my mom helps. She never went to my musicals, field trips, open house. I would be so proud, feel so hopeful, and then she wouldn't come. It felt like she would just slam the door. Maybe she's upset because she didn't get to do these things. Still, it hurts a lot.

PEGGY: How does your grandmother help?

TANYA: I see her every day. Normally, I work from 8:30 [A.M.] to 5:00 P.M. Then I go over to my mother's and have supper with her and my father. After dinner, Mandy and I go over to my grandmother's to sit and visit. We also go shopping together. I saw her every day growing up. She helped us out a lot when we were poor. She gave us Christmas and meals. Now my mother thinks we don't need her any more.

PEGGY: I haven't heard you talk about your father before.

TANYA: My dad is very important to all of us. I love him to death. He lets Mom do all the talking. But he wants the best for me. He is pushing me to go to cosmetology school, and says they'll help me. The girls at work are also pushing me. I'm just afraid of taking the whole 9 months. . . . He's not my real dad. My real dad is a real loser who had eight kids who he never supported. He never tried to be my father and has never kept a job. Both of my parents were losers, but I don't have to be. Just because they are, doesn't mean I have to be. I am so determined, I want to be something, to prove to my daughter that life is more for us.

Tanya's determination is inspiring. It is gratifying to witness her awakening to personal strengths and resources, and getting out of the grip of isolation, self-blame, and discouragement. Her commitment to parenting is a good foundation upon which to build confidence in herself and her parenting skills. I hope that she will be able to take pride in her quest for creating a life for herself and her daughter, and to appreciate her unusual ability to articulate her truth. I am touched by my encounters with her, and decide to write her a letter—a practice used by many narrative therapists (Epston, 1994; Epston & White, 1990; Nylund & Thomas, 1994).

> Dear Tanya,
>
> I'm writing to share with you some of my lingering thoughts as I am getting to know you. Fortunately, I have been able to refer to the notes I have been taking to keep your words alive. Writing a letter like this helps me gather my impressions and gives you an opportunity to reflect upon our words, by reading this letter as often as you like.
>
> I am both moved and impressed by your ability to speak your truth in describing your struggles as a mother. You put into words the anguished self-doubts that haunt many mothers. I imagine your words would provide comfort to other mothers who feel alone in their struggles, as though no one else could possibly understand. You say, "It's the hardest job I've ever had. I don't like the responsibility. It's very different than I imagined. . . . I also need some help learning more about children. This is my first child. I don't know what they do, what I'm supposed to do, what are the phases of development, how to discipline, what is right or wrong."
>
> Isn't it strange how our culture expects parents to confidently know what to do in raising healthy children when it's the hardest and most important job, with only hit-and-miss

prior training? Most mothers I know don't feel prepared for the stresses, relentless responsibilities, ongoing decisions, and constant demands—especially if you feel like you can't rely on your own mother as a resource. If we ask for help in learning other skills, this is seen as a sign of intelligence and earnest interest in attaining new knowledge and skills—like for you in learning about products, perms, the latest styles, going to that New Hampshire show, all toward becoming a hairdresser. Yet with mothering, there are so few supports and little guidance in place, and it can feel so embarrassing to ask questions, as though we should already know it all.

It takes real determination and courage to rise above these expectations and to keep self-blame from tricking you into believing you should go into hiding when needing support. Circles of support are very homemade, and it looks like you've already begun to create yours. You say, "The girls at work listen to me, and see me as a single mom who deals with a lot and who has strength. . . . My grandmother listens to me, tells me it's okay. She's the mom I didn't have. . . . I love my dad to death. He is pushing me to go to cosmetology school, and says they'll help me. . . . Sometimes I feel guilty. But then when I go to the doctor, he says I'm right. . . . I did recently meet an old friend from school in the grocery store. We had lost contact, but we talked, and I could see she really understood since she went through something similar. Now I want to stay in better contact with her. . . . I also would be interested in a support group or other ideas you have." These are the words of a determined woman just beginning to discover her own resources and to take charge of her life.

This determination also shines through in your commitment to wanting to be your own individual, and to raise your daughter differently than how you were raised. Somehow, while under enormous stress and pressure, you still struggle to follow your intuitive sense of what you believe is right, even while getting so little support. You say, "My mom said I should potty-train my daughter at 1 year. She said, 'You're wasting money on diapers, just make her go on the pot.' But I didn't make her. I also let her eat what she wants. I try to treat her like an individual who has likes and dislikes. I don't make her eat her whole meal, I let her make her own decisions. But my mom gives me heck, says I should have her eat the whole thing before I let her down. And I let her choose what she can wear, at least some of the time."

You also say, "I have always been unhappy. I don't want my daughter to grow up unhappy. I want her to love life and herself. . . . I remember gagging on food, detesting being forced to eat, being made to wear my hair in hideous ways, feeling like I shouldn't be forced to do something that makes me so unhappy. . . . I am determined to be there for my daughter so that she can go through school. . . . I'm a very lovable person. I like to kiss and hug. My mother tells me I'm too old, to stop. I don't think you're ever too old. I think there's nothing wrong with it. I tell my daughter 50 times a day that I love her. When I discipline her, afterwards I try to say, 'Mommy loves you. I'm sorry I was mad at you.'"

You also raised several areas of concern in dealing with specific situations toward gaining self-confidence as a mother. I hear your request in wanting to be able to feel good about yourself and to relax at home with your daughter like you are able to at work. Here are your words:

"I find myself being like my mother was with me, and I hate this. I want to be my own individual. My mom never took the time to get to know me, and still doesn't listen to me. Now I don't sit and play with Mandy. I know I should, but I just don't do it. . . . I've been having a really bad time at bedtime. She wants to sleep with me. . . . I don't mind but then I know it's not right. So we have screaming matches. . . . I try to listen but stuff gets in the way. I still want my daughter to do it my way. . . . I worry that she won't want to live with me. She hates the word 'No.' She keeps pushing till she knows she's got me. I can be relaxed at work, but then so uptight at home."

Again, your words reflect the mother's voice and struggles. As you get from under the grip of self-blame and isolation, I imagine you like a sponge soaking up guidance from your growing support system—always checking in with yourself, to get clear about what makes sense to you and what doesn't. I am happy to be on your team.

I'm delighted to hear about your recent decisions: to focus on the positive with Mandy, to take some more space with your mom, and to go to cosmetology school. It sounds like you're embarking on a new chapter in your life. I know it won't be easy, but I also know you've got the determination to make it happen! And to quote you once again, "As long as she has love, we can do it."

See you next month!

Peggy

I imagine I will continue to meet intermittently with Tanya and Mandy. I like to think of myself as a member of their support team. When the next mothers' group begins, I will invite Tanya to join us. She has a tremendous amount to offer other mothers, and to reap from the mutual support that comes from mothers' hearing each other's stories.

CONCLUSION

I have highlighted the influences of narrative therapy, the family support movement, and feminist theory on my work with families with small children. As helping professionals, we must find ways to open space for new parenting stories that strengthen the mother's voice. In this endeavor, I am interested in creating bridges and building dialogues between fields of inquiry so that we can all learn from each other.

Mothers frequently come to see me with anguished senses of failure and self-blame, frightening bursts of anger, frustration, fear for the future, images of their children as monsters that they have created, heartache over treating their children in ways they wish were different. Therapy can become a safe place in which to re-author new stories and for mothers to find their own voices—ones that embrace their personal style, honesty, commitment, and best intentions. Within this quest for self-confidence and personal authority, the courage and self-respect to ask for help are affirmed. Parenting challenges and stresses are normalized. Cultural discourses like "mother blame" and "supermom" are deconstructed in order to develop ways of detaching from their influence. Instead of the person's being the problem, obstacles such as "self-blame" or "discouragement" are externalized as the problem. We can work on building healthy support systems that will witness each mother's newly emerging alternative story. This means plugging into existing community-based services such as playgroups, and sometimes creating something new. This is a process through which a mother and child can rediscover each other in a new, more favorable light. It is gratifying to witness.

As therapists, we are also being invited to rewrite our stories: to debunk expectations of ourselves as neutral experts, to uncover our underlying beliefs and values, and to hold ourselves and each other accountable. Change is in the air. Our years of therapist training are now being challenged in how we highlight and interpret pathology, minimize sociopolitical influences, and take on an expert persona. We, too, need our friends, colleagues, and clients to help keep us honest and accountable. This is a time of tremendous promise.

EDITORIAL QUESTIONS

Q: *(CS) I'd like to ask you more about your highlighting of "the mother's voice." You include this term in your title and also speak eloquently about this in your introduction. Can you say a few things about your journey toward highlighting this voice? Has this been smooth or complicated? From your title, I imagine you see a link between "family support" and "strengthening the mother's voice." How do you see this? In families where you've emphasized this, how have husbands/partners responded?*

A: Strengthening the mother's voice holds a lot of meaning for me. I could easily write many pages about this, but I will try to be brief. Our culture has a long-standing tradition of valuing men's voices over women's. The particulars of women's experiences are often minimized, pathologized, or ignored. Mothers also carry great cultural expectations of themselves, so that no one can ever quite measure up to the idealized mythical mother. Mother blame is lurking behind every corner. This has a silencing effect, so that mothers often devalue their own experiences, blame themselves for problems, and ignore their own needs. This erodes self-confidence and fosters an undercurrent of self-blame and resentment. No one benefits from this. When mothers realign with their best intentions, their love for their children, and their commitment to take care of themselves, everyone benefits—including partners. Sometimes taking such steps creates additional transitional stresses, as relationships need to regroup in making room for the mothers' strengthened voice. Occasionally, there isn't enough room in a relationship for the mother's voice, which thrusts the relationship into crisis. But usually, I believe relationships emerge with increased health and vitality.

I have shared a draft of this chapter with my mother, and this has broadened my understanding of the history of my interest in strengthening the mother's voice. In reflecting on her own struggles as a young mother in the early 1950s, my mother described how hard it was to get supportive help. An otherwise accomplished woman, she was over-whelmed by the challenges of mothering—"totally unprepared, petri-fied, and afraid to expose my weaknesses." Her mother, my grandmoth-er, had been greatly influenced by the child-rearing practices of the North American behaviorist John Watson, who preached the impor-tance of strict discipline, feeding, sleeping, and toileting schedules, and not responding to the infant's cry (Watson & Rayner, 1920). My mother was taught to see dependence as weakness, to fight her own battles, and not to ask for help. As a young mother, she didn't have confidence in her voice, and her experiences were devalued. In her community, friends didn't share their troubles with each other, which contributed to a sense of isolation and self-blame. Dr. Spock's manual was her main resource; it was somewhat supportive in reassuring mothers, "Don't worry, every-thing will be all right." Counseling meant subjecting herself to a thera-pist's interpretations and contributed to her feeling judged and inade-quate.

My mother was wistful in imagining how her family life might have been different if she had consulted a therapist who had focused on strengthening her voice: "My therapist was more supportive of me than anyone else, but she never communicated that she understood how difficult my situation was, that she admired how hard I was try-ing. It wasn't done. In the '50s and '60s, the therapist was supposed to be a neutral background who helped the patient see the reality. But the patient couldn't help feeling that they were figuring you out, looking for your weaknesses. It's as though the patient had no insight, only the therapist did. If you were the patient, it made you afraid to expose your real self."

I have carried my mother's lament into my own history as a mother. I wonder how my life might have been different if my mother and grandmother had found support in strengthening their voices. As a mother, I've had my own struggles in gaining confidence in myself, trusting my personal style, forgiving my errors, and speaking up for my-self. Fortunately, I have discovered much mutual support in the compa-ny of other mothers. There are many parenting resources that I have ex-perienced as supportive, informative, and nonthreatening. These resources weren't as available to generations past. For me, this realiza-tion is bittersweet.

Q: *(CS) I value how clearly you have honored your different therapeu-tic heritages. You also have helped legitimize a mutually inclusive ap-proach with narrative therapies and other approaches, rather than feel-ing obliged to be a full-fledged, card-carrying narrative therapist! From these transcripts, it seems that both families really benefited from this creative integration. Your transcript vignettes offer us a view of your heritages in action, and I imagine that these vignettes don't encompass all the things you do with different clients in different situations. Among other things, I see you at varying moments offering empathy and support, being honest and self-disclosing, externalizing problems, curiously searching for "unique outcomes" and using these to help re-author, doing exploratory play therapy, offering parents specific advice and resources, offering invitations for mothers to connect and be supported by other mothers, and documenting/letter writing.*

In my own experience, it sometimes is challenging for me and for my clients to know which hat I'm wearing if I shift from one way to another. For example, am I opening space for new voices and stories, or am I providing information with something particular in mind? Is this ever a struggle for you? Are you sometimes steering people toward some specific answer or response? How do you combine this with a more "not-knowing," curious posture? What are your current thoughts about this potential confusion?

A: Usually, I don't see a conflict between providing ideas and creating space for parents to reflect on their own preferences. Parents of infants and toddlers live in the real world of sleepless nights, power struggles, temper tantrums, blowups, mealtimes, and countless worries. They want the knowledges and skills to make informed decisions in building healthy relationships with their children. Over and over again, parents have communicated to me their desire for concrete suggestions, as long as these are given respectfully and with the freedom to choose. I believe I can be useful by sharing some of what I have learned from other families, written resources, and my own experiences. However, I do try to be especially sensitive to the context and spirit in which these suggestions are given. I offer resources as possibilities that may or may not be helpful. I don't want to set up assignments that are burdensome and contribute to feelings of inadequacy and guilt. I am most interested in hearing the parents' reflections on what is and is not helpful. I believe this augments the process of generating their own ideas.

Recently, I have been thinking a lot about the balance in therapy of expressions of curiosity, affirmative statements, and specific ideas and suggestions. We therapists each have our own personal style—a unique blend of asking questions, making statements, and giving ideas. Writing this chapter has provided an opportunity for me to witness my work, my strengths, and my growing edge. Through my questions, I want to deepen my understanding of the lives of the people who consult me, and to value their experiences. Michael White (1996) describes this process as moving beyond thin conclusions to contribute to lives' becoming more richly described. I want to remember to continually consult families about their experiences of therapy, and how I can best be of help. It is my hope that my work will reflect this ongoing commitment. I see this as a work in progress.

I am increasingly aware of how our parenting resources are culturally bound. For example, in North America in the 1900s, expertise has evolved from John Watson (Watson & Rayner, 1920) to Benjamin Spock (Spock & Rothenberg, 1985), and now to Penelope Leach (1976) and T. B. Brazelton (1983). In the 1990s, there is a growing appreciation of diversity, the roles and responsibilities of fathers, and the importance of building supportive communities. Although I find these trends promising, I am also distressed to witness the simultaneous deterioration of the North American commitment in public policy to supporting families and children. I wonder what comes next as we approach the new millennium. The suggestions I give families are inevitably given within this historic context. Ideally, therapy is a safe place in which to explore these influences on how we approach the tasks of parenting. Families can then pick and choose what fits best with them in moving forward with specific steps and increased self-confidence.

Q: *(CS) You mentioned that you are interested in creating bridges and dialogues between different approaches. Can you say some specific things you hope narrative therapists could learn from other approaches? What do you think therapists working within these other approaches could learn from narrative therapists?*
A: We have a lot to learn from the people who consult us, who find ways of connecting with others in advocating for their families' needs despite numerous obstacles. We are more experienced at drawing distinctions between approaches and working in isolation than at thinking collectively and creating connections. Collaboration between approaches can be a mutually supportive and creative process of continual learning, and one of the best antidotes to professional burnout. I get excited when I envision creating bridges and building dialogues between folks who share core beliefs and values, yet who come from different cultural and intellectual heritages.

In writing this chapter, I sought feedback from colleagues with narrative and family support backgrounds.[4] I was encouraged by their ability to put their own ideas aside, and to listen with an earnest openness. This is contrary to our cultural orientation toward dichotomies and debates.[5] Folks knew little about each other's perspectives, so that provocative questions were often posed from a position of not knowing. In turn, these expressions of curiosity sparked new ideas. Being in dialogue with people from different perspectives also helped keep me honest and accountable. Constantly, I was challenged to explain concepts in plain English and to minimize professional jargon. This informal structure of accountability stretched me to act in alignment with my espoused belief in the co-authoring process. Through these conversations, my awareness grew of the constrictions of my own assumptions, and of the lure of professional arrogance. Already there are some subtle changes I wish I could make in these transcripts. More importantly, this process has helped enliven my ongoing work with people who consult me.

For therapists, isolation is an occupational hazard. Often our work separates us from the community, and it is difficult to find ways to share our work with others. Although the ethics of confidentiality and dual relationships restrict our choices, the need remains for finding ways to feel part of something larger than ourselves that unites us in our shared commitments to families and children. The family support movement can orient us toward becoming more actively involved in community development and knowledgeable about the politics of fostering changes in larger systems. Narrative therapists can benefit enormously from the family support movement's years of experience in working toward becoming consumer-driven, community-based, depathologized, and family-centered. By studying family support's theoretical foundations, we can broaden our perspective to see our work as part of a larger social history that reflects shifts in philosophies and attitudes over decades. This abundant literature highlights the need for fostering mutually efficacious interactions between parents and young children, and for programs that take on an empowerment approach.[6] It challenges many of the implicit assumptions underlying the power dynamics in the helping professions, and it supports a growing paraprofessional movement. I hope readers will find the time to explore some of this literature, including references provided in this chapter.

---

[4]My heartfelt appreciation to the following people for their support and input into this chapter: Lyndall Bass, Mary Brevda, Carl Bucholt, Hope Cannon, Mon Cochran, Randye Cohen, Sydney Crystal, Eileen Fair, Edith Fierst, Eva Fierst, Herb Fierst, Beverley Kort, Bill Lax, Peter Lebenbaum, Dario Lussardi, Chip Mayer, Chris McLean, Maggie McGuire, Lee Monro, Cheryl Mitchell, John Pierce, Jack Pransky, Valerie Ross, Sallyann Roth, Darden Rozycki, Shel Sax, Pat Schumm, Shoshana Simons, Craig Smith, Penny Tims, Anne Wallace, Nancy Webber, Marc Werner-Gavrin, and Michael White.

[5]This reminds me of the message I received this week in a fortune cookie: "Ideas are like children: There are none so wonderful as your own."

Most people I know who identify with the family support movement are suspicious of therapists. They have had too many experiences of making referrals that have resulted in families' being pathologized, interpreted, and disempowered. Parent–child centers, Head Start, and other community support services are frequently searching for family therapists with whom to collaborate with families; yet they lack ways of knowing whether a suggested therapist shares their philosophical assumptions. I hear a collective sigh of relief as these folks discover narrative therapy. Narrative therapy decenters the therapist's role as a member of the family's support team, and fuels a renewal of hope and possibility for therapist involvement in community based programs. A shared vision emerges of therapists working in connection with paraprofessionals and families' informal support systems. Upon hearing about narrative therapy, one member of the Best Practices Project of the Family Resource Coalition[7] spoke enthusiastically of developing an international roster of narratively oriented therapists as a readily available resource to communities.

Narrative therapy also provides specific practices, such as documentation and letter writing. One colleague who consults with schools regarding communication challenges for children with multiple handicaps called me with excitement in discovering the possibility of letter writing as an alternative to traditional paperwork. In documenting with families their experiences and specific steps toward implementing desired changes, she described some of the ripple effects. Not only do she and the families benefit, but some of her school colleagues have become inspired to explore similar practices. This is also enhancing the valuing of families' experiences by coworkers, and the ways in which families are spoken about in the staff room. Everyone benefits, and the learning is continual.

---

[6]"Empowerment" is defined by the Cornell Empowerment Project as an intentional, ongoing process centered in the local community, involving mutual respect, critical reflection, caring, and group participation, through which people lacking an equal share of valued resources gain greater access to and control over those resources.

[7]The Family Resource Coalition "builds networks, produces resources, advocates for public policy, provides consulting services, and gathers knowledge to help the family support movement grow" (1996, p. ii). I highly recommend their recently published *Guidelines for Family Support Practice*. This document is the culmination of a 4-year Best Practices Project, which compiled input from hundreds of programs, practitioners, and leaders in the field, as well as focus group discussions. It clearly articulates shared philosophical premises, underlying values, and principles for implementation. The commonalities with narrative therapy are uncanny. For information, contact the Coalition at 200 S. Michigan Ave., 16th Floor, Chicago, IL 60604. Phone, (312) 341-0900; fax, (312) 341-9361.

REFERENCES

Andersen, T. (1987). The reflecting team: Dialogue and meta-dialogue in clinical work. *Family Process, 26*, 415–428.

Andersen, T. (Ed.). (1991). *The reflecting team: Dialogues and dialogues about the dialogues.* New York: Norton.

Andersen, T. (1993). See and hear, and be seen and heard. In S. Friedman (Ed.), *The new language of change: Constructive collaboration in psychotherapy.* New York: Guilford Press.

Anderson, H., & Goolishian, H. (1988). Human systems as linguistic systems: Preliminary and evolving ideas about the implications for clinical theory. *Family Process, 27*, 371–393.

Anderson, H., & Goolishian, H. (1992). The client is the expert: A not-knowing approach to therapy. In S. McNamee & K. J. Gergen (Eds.), *Therapy as social construction.* Newbury Park, CA: Sage.

Anderson, H., Goolishian, H., & Winderman, L. (1986). Problem-determined systems: Towards transformation in family therapy. *Journal of Strategic and Systemic Therapies, 5*(4), 1–13.

Avis, J. M. (1991). Power politics in therapy with women. In T. J. Goodrich (Ed.), *Women and power: Perspectives for family therapy.* New York: Norton.

Belenky, M. F., Clinchy, B. M., Goldberger, N. R., & Tarule, J. M. (1986). *Women's ways of knowing: The development of self, voice, and mind.* New York: Basic Books.

Braverman, L. (1991). Beyond the myth of motherhood. In M. McGoldrick, C. M. Anderson, & F. Walsh (Eds.), *Women in families: A framework for family therapy.* New York: Norton.

Brazelton, T. B. (1983). *Infants and mothers.* New York: Delacorte Press/Seymour Lawrence.

Brazelton, T. B. (1992). *Touchpoints: The essential reference. Your child's emotional and behavioral development.* Reading, MA: Addison-Wesley.

Bromwich, R. M. (1985). "Vulnerable infants" and "risky environments." *Zero to Three, 6*(2), 7–12.

Bronfenbrenner, U. (1979). *The ecology of human development: Experiments by nature and design.* Cambridge, MA: Harvard University Press.

Bronfenbrenner, U. (1986). Ecology of the family as a context for human development: Research perspectives. *Developmental Psychology, 22*(6), 723–742.

Caplan, P. J. (1989). *Don't blame mother: Mending the mother–daughter relationship.* New York: Harper & Row.

Carnegie Task Force on Meeting the Needs of Young Children. (1994, August). *Starting points: Meeting the needs of our youngest children.* New York: Carnegie Corporation of New York.

Dunst, C. J. (1983, April). *A bibliographic guide to measures of social support, parental stress, well-being and coping, and other family-level measures.* (Available from the Family, Infant and Preschool Program, Western Carolina Center, Morganton, NC 28655)

Duvall, J. D., & Beier, J. M. (1995). Passion, commitment, and common sense: A unique discussion with Insoo Kim Berg and Michael White. *Journal of Systemic Therapies, 14*(3), 57–80.

Epston, D. (1989). *Collected papers.* Adelaide, South Australia: Dulwich Centre Publications.

Epston, D. (1994). Extending the conversation. *Family Therapy Networkers, 18*(6), 30–37, 62–63.

Epston, D., & White, M. (1990). Consulting your consultants: The documentation of alternative knowledges. In D. Epston & M. White (Eds.), *Experience, contradiction, narrative, and imagination.* Adelaide, South Australia: Dulwich Centre Publications.

Epston, D., & White, M. (1992). *Experience, contradiction, narrative and imagination: Selected papers of David Epston and Michael White, 1989–1991.* Adelaide, South Australia: Dulwich Centre Publications.

Family Resource Coalition. (1996). *Guidelines for family support practice.* (Available from the author at 200 S. Michigan Avenue, 16th Floor, Chicago, IL 60604)

Featherstone, H. (1980). *A difference in the family: Life with a disabled child.* New York: Basic Books.

Field, T. (1983). High-risk infants "have less fun" during early interactions. *Topics in Early Childhood Special Education, 3*(1), 77–87.

Field, T. (1984). Early interactions between infants and their postpartum depressed mothers. *Infant Behavior and Development, 7,* 517–522.

Field, T. (1992). Infants of depressed mothers. *Development and Psychopathology, 4,* 49–66.

Fraiberg, S. (1975). Ghosts in the nursery: A psychoanalytic approach to the problems of impaired infant–mother relationships. *Journal of the American Academy of Child Psychiatry, 14,* 387–421.

Freedman, J., & Combs, G. (1993). Invitations to new stories: Using questions to explore alternative possibilities. In S. Gilligan & R. Price (Eds.), *Therapeutic conversations.* New York: Norton.

Freedman, J., & Combs, G. (1996). *Narrative therapy: The social construction of preferred realities.* New York: Norton.

Friedman, S. (Ed.). (1993). *The new language of change: Constructive collaboration in psychotherapy.* New York: Guilford Press.

Friedman, S. (Ed.). (1995). *The reflecting team in action: Collaborative practice in family therapy.* New York: Guilford Press.

Garbarino, J. (1992). *Children and families in the social environment.* New York: Aldine de Gruyter.

Garmezy, N., & Rutter, M. (Eds.). (1983). *Stress, coping and development in children.* New York: McGraw-Hill.

Gilligan, C. (1982). *In a different voice: Psychological theory and women's development.* Cambridge, MA: Harvard University Press.

Gilligan, S., & Price, R. (Eds.). (1993). *Therapeutic conversations.* New York: Norton.

Goldberg, S. (1977). Social competence in infancy: A model of parent–infant interaction. *Merrill-Palmer Quarterly, 23*(3), 163–175.

Goodrich, T. J. (Ed.). (1991). *Women and power: Perspectives for family thera-py.* New York: Norton.

Hare-Mustin, R. T., & Marecek, J. (1994, August). Feminism and postmodern-ism: Dilemmas and points of resistance. In *Problems with postmodernism: Historical, critical and feminist perspectives.* Symposium presented at the meeting of the American Psychological Association, Los Angeles.

Hoffman, L. (1993). *Exchanging voices: A collaborative approach to family therapy.* London: Karnac.

Jordan, J. V. (1991). Empathy, mutuality, and therapeutic change: Clinical im-plications of a relational model. In J. V. Jordan, A. G. Kaplan, J. B. Miller, I. P. Stiver, & J. L. Surrey, *Women's growth in connection: Writings from the Stone Center.* New York: Guilford Press.

Kurcinka, M. S. (1991). *Raising your spirited child: A guide for parents whose child is more intense, sensitive, perceptive, persistent, energetic.* New York: HarperCollins.

Leach, P. (1976). *Babyhood.* New York: Knopf.

Levine, L., Garcia-Coll, C. T., & Oh, W. (1985). Determinants of mother–infant interaction in adolescent mothers. *Pediatrics, 75*(1), 23–29.

Lerner, H. (1988). A critique of the feminist psychoanalytic contribution. In H. Lerner (Ed.), *Women in therapy.* New York: Harper & Row.

Lieberman, A. F. (1993). *The emotional life of the toddler.* New York: Free Press.

Lofquist, W. (1989). *The technology of prevention workbook: A leadership de-velopment program.* (Available from the Associates for Youth Develop-ment, Inc., P.O. Box 36748, Tucson, AZ 85740)

Losel, F., & Bliesner, T. (1990). Resilience in adolescence: A study on the gener-alizability of protective factors. In K. Hurrelmann & F. Losel (Eds.), *Health hazards in adolescence.* Berlin: Walter de Gruyter.

McGoldrick, M., Anderson, C. M., & Walsh, F. (Eds.). (1991). *Women in fami-lies: A framework for family therapy.* New York: Norton.

Miller, J. B. (1991). Women and power: Reflections ten years later. In T. J. Goodrich (Ed.), *Women and power: Perspectives for family therapy.* New York: Norton.

Nicholson, S. (1995). The narrative dance: A practice map for White's thera-py. *Australian and New Zealand Journal of Family Therapy, 16*(1), 23–28.

Nylund, D., & Thomas, J. (1994). The economics of narrative. *Family Therapy Networker, 18*(6), 38–39.

O'Hanlon, W. H. (1994). The third wave. *Family Therapy Networker, 18*(6), 18–26, 28–29.

Parry, A., & Doan, R. E. (1994). *Story re-visions: Narrative therapy in the post-modern world.* New York: Guilford Press.

Partridge, S. (Ed.). (1987). *The awakening and growth of the human infant: A telecourse study guide for infant mental health practitioners.* (Available from the Child and Family Institute, Division of Human Resources, Univer-sity of Southern Maine, 246 Deering Avenue, Portland, ME 04102)

Partridge, S. (1991, May 17). *Infant mental health practices: Pitfalls and path-*

ways. Keynote address presented at the Fourth Annual Conference of the Maine Association for Infant Mental Health, Portland.

Pawl, J. H. (1987). Infant mental health and child abuse and neglect: Reflections from an infant mental health practitoner. *Zero to Three, 7*(4), 1–9.

Pransky, J. (1991). *Prevention: The critical need.* Springfield, MO: Burrell Foundation.

Rampage, C. (1991). Personal authority and women's self-stories. In T. J. Goodrich (Ed.), *Women and power: Perspectives for family therapy.* New York: Norton.

Rich, A. (1976). *Of woman born: Motherhood as experience and institution.* New York: Bantam Books.

Sameroff, A. J., & Chandler, M. J. (1974). Reproductive risk and the continuum of caretaking casualty. In F. Horowitz, M. Hetherington, S. Scarr-Salapatek, & G. Siegel (Eds.), *Review of child development research* (Vol. 4). Chicago: University of Chicago Press.

Smith, C. (1995). *One way of incorporating two different narrative therapy approaches: "Collaborative language systems" and "deconstructive-externalizing."* Paper presented at Narrative Ideas and Therapeutic Practices: The 3rd Annual International Conference, Vancouver, B.C., Canada.

Spock, B., & Rothenberg, M. B. (1985). *Dr. Spock's baby and child care.* New York: Pocket Books.

Surrey, J. L. (1991). The self-in-relation: A theory of women's development. In J. V. Jordan, A. G. Kaplan, J. B. Miller, I. P. Stiver, & J. L. Surrey, *Women's growth in connection: Writings from the Stone Center.* New York: Guilford Press.

Trout, M. (1981). Potential stresses during infancy: The growth of human bonds. In S. Tackett & M. Hunsberger (Eds.), *Family-centered care of children and adolescents.* Philadelphia: W.B. Saunders.

Turnbull, H. R., & Turnbull, A. P. (1985). *Parents speak out: Then and now.* Columbus, OH: Charles E. Merrill.

Walters, M., Carter, B., Papp, P., & Silverstein, O. (1988). *The invisible web: Gender patterns in family relationships.* New York: Guilford Press.

Watson, J. B., & Rayner, R. (1920). Conditioned emotional reactions. *Journal of Experimental Psychology, 3,* 1–14. Reprinted in R. Ulrich, T. Stachnik, & J. Mabry (Eds.). (1966). *Control of human behavior, vol. 1.* Glenview, IL: Scott, Foresman.

Weingarten, K. (1994). *The mother's voice: Strengthening intimacy in families.* New York: Harcourt, Brace.

Werner, E. E. (1988a). Individual differences, universal needs: A 30 year study of resilient high risk infants. *Zero to Three, 8*(4), 1–5.

Werner, E. E. (1988b). Resilient children. In E. M. Hetherington & R. D. Parke (Eds.), *Contemporary readings in child psychology* (3rd ed.). New York: McGraw-Hill.

Werner, E., & Smith, R. S. (1982). *Vulnerable but invincible: A longitudinal study of resilient children and youth.* New York: McGraw-Hill.

Weston, D. R., Ivins, B., Zuckerman, B., Jones, C., & Lopez, R. (1989). Drug exposed babies: Research and clinical issues. *Zero to Three, 9*(5), 1–7.

White, M. (1989). *Selected papers.* Adelaide, South Australia: Dulwich Centre Publications.

White, M. (1991). Deconstruction and therapy. *Dulwich Centre Newsletter,* No. 3, 21–40.

White, M. (1996, November). *Informal presentation of current ideas.* Intensive workshop presented at the Dulwich Centre, Adelaide.

White, M., & Epston, D. (1990). *Narrative means to therapeutic ends.* New York: Norton.

Whittaker, J., Garbarino, H. J., & Associates. (1983). *Social support networks: On informal helping in the human services.* Hawthorne, NY: Aldine de Gruyter.

5

Lists

JILL H. FREEDMAN
GENE COMBS

We were visiting with some friends and asked Sarah and Eli to tell us about their trip to the zoo that morning. "We saw monkeys and giraffes and snakes," Eli said. "Yeah, monkeys and alligators and a zebra," amended Sarah. "And we ate hot dogs and Cokes and popsicles and popcorn."

Lists seem to be a natural way of keeping track of experience, especially for young people. When we first began to use narrative ideas (Combs & Freedman, 1994; Dickerson & Zimmerman, 1993; Epston, 1989; Freedman & Combs, 1996; Laird, 1989; White, 1995; White & Epston, 1990; Zimmerman & Dickerson, 1996) in working with children (Freeman, Epston, & Lobovits, 1997; White, 1984), our tendency was to take a list such as Eli's or Sarah's and ask questions to develop it into a storybook-like narrative of their trip to the zoo. While some children are astonishing in their memory of detail and can spontaneously provide rich narrative accounts, many others seem to prefer to recount their experience in the more condensed and efficient manner that lists make possible. Lists are a great way of working with these children's experiential worlds.

The section "Erica: A Therapy Story" is reprinted (with very minor revisions) from Freedman and Combs (1996). Copyright 1996 by Norton. Reprinted by permission.

A list of accomplishments can bring forth vivid and meaningful experience of those accomplishments. In making a list with a child, the therapist helps to identify and name things that are worth listing. The process of writing these things down and reading them back makes them more "real" and more memorable. Once written down, a list becomes a document (White & Epston, 1990) that can be displayed, consulted, and circulated. A child can read a list and re-experience the knowledge it contains. She/he can see how big it is and count the number of items on it. If a list is worked on over the course of therapy, the child can see it grow. (See Freedman & Combs, 1996, pp. 232–236.)

We offer the following story to illustrate several ways in which lists may be brought forth and used. We have used this story previously (Freedman & Combs, 1996) to illustrate other ideas.

ERICA: A THERAPY STORY

Although the school had indicated that 9-year-old Erica[1] should be seen weekly by the school social worker, his caseload and Erica's class projects seemed to get in the way all too often. Grant and Diana, Erica's grandparents, worried that Erica might be "depressed." They decided to take matters into their own hands and brought Erica to see me (JF).

In a phone conversation before the first meeting, Ron, Erica's father, told me that he thought Erica needed something because she seemed to "always be cowering and not speak up," and her grades had plummeted. However, he and Erica's mother, Clarisse, and Erica's younger sister, Hannah, could not regularly attend our meetings because the couple worked different shifts, they were already in couple therapy, and Ron was in individual therapy and night school. The family had tried family therapy once and believed that it didn't work. Ron said that it was okay with them if Erica came to see me with his parents. We agreed to stay in touch by phone, and Ron indicated that the family would consider coming to occasional meetings.

The First Meeting

At the first meeting, I began by asking Erica what she liked to do. She mumbled, "I don't know," but did not disagree with her grandparents' list, which included art, drawing, singing, working on the computer, ice skating, swimming, and rollerblading. Erica did volunteer that she didn't

---

[1]Names have been changed to protect confidentiality. The family described here has granted us permission to use this material.

like her 7-year-old sister, Hannah. She didn't know if there was a problem, but listened quietly as Grant said, "She doesn't give herself credit for anything. She never brags. She's always saying she's sorry—for nothing." Diane added, "She's very quiet. Hannah tells all of Erica's good news. Erica has nothing of her own because Hannah is always in on it."

I asked Erica what she thought about what her grandparents said. She said she didn't know. When I asked several more questions, she finally said that she guessed she didn't give herself credit. I asked if she would be interested in making a picture to show what she didn't give herself credit for. She quietly drew on a large piece of newsprint a framed picture to represent her art, a report card, a bell to represent the bell chorus she was part of, a Taekwondo uniform because she was taking Taekwondo, a math book, and six friends.

I asked her about each of the elements of the drawing. She reluctantly told me that her grades in math were pretty good. Her grandparents agreed. She said that she didn't know whether the six kids she drew really were her friends or not, but in answer to questions she decided it was better to think they were because that would make her "act on the other side," acting friendly instead of shy.

Erica did not seem interested in conversation about what kept her from taking credit for these things, so I asked her, "If you could wave a magic wand that would help you start taking credit, what do you think you would notice that you are not noticing now?

Erica quickly answered, "I would be thinking on the happy side." She explained that she would be seeing brighter colors, like a rainbow. She added a rainbow to the picture.

With further questioning she said that she'd feel better about going to Taekwondo and would be saying to herself, "I'll do better than usual. I'll get my pattern right."

Erica seemed to know so much about this that I asked her if the words she would say to herself were familiar ones. It turned out that just a few days before, she did a whole song in bell chorus without messing up once! She had said to herself, "I'm going to do good," and she did. She thought that saying to herself, "I'm going to do good," helped set the mood that would make her chances for "doing good" great!

Erica's grandparents were delighted to hear that Erica already had taken a step toward giving herself credit. They knew she could do it, because she had in the past. To back this up, they recounted some experiences that they were delighted to hear about when Erica told about them in past years.

As they were getting ready to leave, I asked Erica if she wanted to take the picture home to remind her of what we had talked about. "No, I want you to keep it," she said, looking down. "But could I borrow the magic wand?" On my desk, she had spied my telephone companion, a clear tube full of glittering confetti suspended in a thick substance. I gave it to her.

The Second Meeting

At the second meeting, Erica was much more talkative. She told me that immediately after our first meeting she had forgotten about our conversation, but when she saw the magic wand she remembered. Then she reminded herself to take credit. The forgetting and remembering happened a few more times, and then she decided to carry the wand with her. She found out that " . . . it could make life better to give yourself credit. Then you won't always be mad at yourself."

In the course of our conversation, we began calling the problem "self-blame." Erica saw that she was getting the best of the self-blame already. We developed the following list of ways that giving herself credit was making a difference in her life:

- It made it possible for her to keep doing what she already could do.
- It made her feel good about what she could do, rather than not letting it make any difference.
- It made her happy.
- It let her see that she was really good at Taekwondo.
- It helped her do a biography of her grandfather.
- It made her teachers notice and comment on how she was working harder.
- Maybe (she wasn't as sure about this one) it let her parents notice that she was doing better, because she had been feeling happier at home.

Grant and Diane added the following item to Erica's list:

- It helped her smile and talk to other kids, rather than stand quietly by herself when they picked her up from school.

We all wondered about where this project would make itself known next. Erica thought it might be with her sister. She told me, "I might not always fight with her. I might stop getting mad at her for stuff she doesn't do."

"So do you think the self-blame turns into blame against others sometimes?"

She nodded.

"And it gets you in fights too, huh?"

She nodded again.

"Wow. I didn't know it was so stressful. And you've already turned it around this much?"

Again she nodded.

"Do you think as you turn this blame around even more, you'll be more in touch with loving your sister?"

Erica nodded.

"Then what will happen?" I asked.

"Well," she confided, "probably my parents will stop telling me I'll get coal in my stocking." (It was December.)

I wondered if maybe the blame was messing up Hannah's life too. Diane and Grant thought maybe it was. We all agreed that it would be good for the whole family to know about how Erica was turning self-blame around and feeling better about herself. We agreed I would phone Ron and Clarisse and invite them and Hannah to the next meeting. We agreed that we would show them Erica's picture and fill them in on her "feeling better about yourself" project.

The Third Meeting

Erica, Hannah, Clarisse, and Ron attended the third meeting. I had expected Diane and Grant to come as well, but the family worked it out for just the four to come.

After I got to know Hannah, Clarisse, and Ron a bit, we unveiled Erica's pictorial list. Together, Erica and I described what the different images meant, and went over the list of what she had accomplished in regard to feeling better about herself.

Ron had already noticed a big difference in Erica. "Erica has always tried hard," he said. "But now she seems to be taking big steps." He noticed that she had become more involved with kids her own age, whereas before she always seemed to be alone or with younger kids. He noticed her interacting more at the bell choir practice and Taekwondo. She began having guests over for the first time. Both he and Clarisse were happy about these developments.

I asked Ron what he thought this said about his daughter. He answered, "She's becoming more mature." He then added that she was also standing up for herself. He noticed her standing up for herself both with other kids and with Hannah.

Clarisse agreed in part, but said that she still hoped that the fighting, arguing, bickering, and whining between Erica and Hannah would stop.

I turned to Hannah and told her that Erica and I had had a conversation about how Erica thought that blame had come between them.

She agreed. I wondered what effect the blame had on their sisterhood and whether this was something they might work on together.

Erica blurted out, "I don't want her coming. This is for me."

"Would it be okay if you fill Hannah in on what we talk about that has to do with her, and the two of you see how you could work together?" I asked.

Erica nodded.

The Fourth Meeting

At the fourth meeting with Erica, Grant, and Diane, Erica updated me on areas she was feeling better about herself in. She added these items to her list:

- She got promoted to a green belt in Taekwondo.
- She got an 89 on a report she had done.
- She felt happy most of the time!

As there was now more that she was taking credit for, she updated her picture. She added a stage for being in a play, a snowflake for sledding, and "NUBS is the best and so am I!" (NUBS was the name of a group she belonged to at her church.)

I asked a number of questions to fill out the story of how all of these changes were happening, what steps Erica was taking, what the turning points were, and how she was advising herself.

Erica shrugged in response. "I still carry the magic wand. I remember the picture, and I look at my list."

"What do they mean to you?" I asked.

"That I can do it," she said. "That I can turn self-blame around."

Again my attempts at co-authoring detailed narratives with Erica fell flat. Yet it was clear that she was progressing rapidly and that the therapy was helpful to her. I stopped asking re-authoring questions and invited her to develop some more lists.

I asked her if she would like to show me how much ground self-blame had before and how much it had now. I said, "First, you could draw a box that would hold all the self-blame from before."

She drew an oblong box.

"And what would be in it?" I asked. Erica made this list inside the box:

Getting bad grades.
Pictures aren't good.
Fighting with sister.

My parents fighting.
Because I don't have any friends.

"So those are all the things that self-blame blamed you for?"

"Yes," said Erica, writing "Before" in the box.

"How big of a box would it take to hold the self-blame in your life now?"

Erica drew a much smaller box.

"What's in it?" I asked.

"Fighting with my sister," she answered, filling the words in and adding "Now." She then drew a line through "Getting bad grades," "Pictures aren't good," "My parents fighting," and "Because I don't have any friends" in the first box, leaving only "Fighting with sister."

I showed the representation to Grant and Diane. "Did you know Erica had shrunk self-blame this small?"

They had wondered but hadn't known for sure. We all speculated about the relative sizes of the two. The change had happened over the course of 9 weeks, so we wondered how long it would take to shrink the "now" box, or if it was okay to leave it the size it was.

The Fifth Meeting

The fifth meeting took place 3 weeks later. In a phone call with Clarisse before this meeting, I discovered that Erica and Hannah were getting along much better and that Grant and Diane were on vacation. Clarisse volunteered to bring Erica to the meeting. I assumed we would meet together, but Clarisse dropped off Erica, so I saw her alone.

Erica told me that the most important thing that happened since the fourth meeting was that she made a lot of new friends. At this point in the therapy, I was quite aware of Erica's preferred style of communication. Rather than attempting to draw her out about an experience with a friend or asking questions about how she was going about making friends, I joined her in making this list of new friends:

Alison	Heather	Demetria
Emily	Vera	Antonio
Ilana	Stephanie	Reed
Brooke	Hannah	Sam
Enid	Melissa	Matt
Natalie	Dawn	Aaron
Shannon	Yukiko	Hayden
Morgan	Christina	Frank
Mara	Ginger	Robert
		Sean

Once the list of friends was documented, I asked Erica a few questions to fill in some detail. I learned that Erica was able to make all of these friends just by being herself. What she learned was "Don't act like you're somebody else." The self-blame got her to try to act like somebody else. The work she began in therapy helped her be herself.

We made a list of the main differences between this year and the last for Erica:

- Now she felt better about herself.
- She appreciated herself more.
- She had better grades.
- She had more friends.

She said that her parents and teachers noticed and that her grandparents would notice when they came back from vacation.

When I turned the conversation toward the relationship with Hannah, Erica said, "But I told you. Now she's one of my friends." I hadn't realized when she listed "Hannah" that she was talking about her sister. Erica was very matter-of-face about the old news that blame no longer was coming between her and her sister.

She thought that our work together was finished. We decided to meet one more time with the whole family to celebrate. I felt confident in making this suggestion, because of my previous conversation with Clarisse, who had confirmed that Erica was doing great.

The Sixth Meeting

At the sixth meeting, I announced that we were there to celebrate Erica's turning around self-blame and achieving the project of feeling better about herself! Erica showed the picture list again, describing it and pointing out the additions. She then read the list of accomplishments and the list of her friends' names. Hannah beamed when her name was read. After the reading was completed, Hannah confirmed that blame was gone from their relationship. She thought that Erica was mostly responsible, because she had been "nicer and happier." Everyone agreed this would make a big difference in family life.

Ron added that at the time the therapy began, the school was very concerned about Erica's performance. There had been talk of her possibly repeating the year. This prospect had been extremely distressing to Ron. He and Clarisse had contacted a Catholic school about the possibility of Erica's going there. They hoped that this would forestall her repeating a grade and that in a more structured program she would catch up. The Catholic school was not willing to admit Erica at grade level unless reports improved. Ron was relieved that at a parent–teacher conference just 2 days before, Erica's progress was characterized as excellent. He wondered if the therapy was responsible.

I said that we hadn't talked about school problems. I had known that Erica's grades were lower than in previous years, but I hadn't known the extent of this. I had spoken to the school social worker twice, but he had not mentioned academic problems. I said that it sounded to me like Erica was responsible for turning this around all by herself! She beamed.

We all had cookies that Diane supplied, and we congratulated Erica.

As the family was getting ready to leave, Erica handed me back my "wand."

"You can keep that," I said.

"I don't need it any more," Erica told me. "The magic is here now," she said, patting her heart.

This therapy illustrates the use of a number of lists—the "picture list," the list of ways in which giving herself credit was making a difference in Erica's life, the lists in the "then" and "now" boxes, the list of friends, and the list of differences between this year and last year. In the therapy with Erica, the lists were read and reread. They were shared with other people, and she reviewed some of them between meetings. They served as concrete representations of portions of the work that seemed to make it more real and graspable.

AN EXERCISE

We offer the following exercise as a way of directly experiencing the usefulness of lists—even for adults. We hope that if you take the time to do this exercise and to become experientially involved in it, you will have some ideas about how you might use lists in working narratively with children.

This exercise will probably work best if you do it with another person, allowing her/him to guide you through it, talking with each other about your experience as you go. You can then switch roles and assume the guide/witness role for your partner. However, since you are probably reading this piece to yourself, we have written our suggestions as if you were doing the exercise by yourself.

Step 1. Begin by identifying a problematic situation in your current life—a set of circumstances in which you experience yourself as stuck, unduly restrained, or not quite measuring up. Then set this situation aside for a few minutes. We will return to it later in the exercise.

Step 2. Remember what your life was like 5 years ago. Can you recollect what was going on in your life back them? Where were you living? What projects were you involved in? What were the important personal relationships in your life? What problems were you struggling with? (It is not important that you answer all these questions, or any of these specific questions. What is important for this exercise is that you remember your circumstances 5 years ago clearly enough to contrast them with your present circumstances.)

Step 3. Reflect for a few minutes on some of your experiences in moving from your circumstances of 5 years ago to those of today. We would guess that certain experiences stand out as memorable or important. For example, what do you know how to do that you didn't know how to do 5 years ago? What places are you familiar with that you weren't 5 years ago? Who do you know that you didn't know then? What have you accomplished? List these as they come to mind. As you look at the first few experiences on your list, do others come to mind? Add these to your list. What knowledge or skills did you learn in each experience on your list?

Step 4. Hang on to your list while you remind yourself of the situation from your present life that you identified in Step 1.

Step 5. If you really acknowledge and take ownership of the living knowledge that your list represents, what difference does that make in your experience of the problematic situation? What new possibilities do you see for how you will deal with that situation in the future?

Step 6. Reflect on the exercise and the helpfulness of using lists.

In both our therapy story and our exercise, we have hoped to illustrate the usefulness of lists in documenting "story-worthy" experiences, Do you think you will keep lists on your list of ways to work in doing therapy with children?

EDITORIAL QUESTIONS

Q: *(CS) Among the things that jumped out at me in this chapter and that impress me about your work in general are your flexibility and creativity! For instance, throughout earlier sessions you co-constructed Erica's externalized "self- blame." In response to your question of what her next step might be with this "self-blame," she threw a new twist in by saying that her next step was wanting not to get as angry with her sister. But you were adept enough at this transition to ask her if her "self-blame" sometimes turned into "blame against others." In another similar instance, Erica had understandable worry that her sister might assume too large a presence in her therapy. She suddenly declared that she didn't want her sister coming to therapy any more. Rather than become adamant that she come or completely dismissing her sister's participation altogether, you respectfully asked whether it was okay if Erica told her sister only what pertained to her sister and their relationship together.*

Another example of your creativity is your emphasis on list making with children. From my reading, it appeared that you chose this emphasis with Erica as a way to honor her matter-of-fact communication style with you. Is this so? You contrast list-making questions with "co-authoring detailed narratives," which could involve such things as asking "meaning questions" (Freedman & Combs, 1996, pp. 136–139) about her personal characteristics or values enabling her to do the things on her list. As you think about your work with children currently, how might you go about deciding whether to focus more on different verbal and pictorial list-making questions, and when to attempt to thicken clients' stories by asking "meaning" and other questions? Do these two emphases (list making and story-developing questions) overlap at times?

A: Thank you for your appreciation of our work. I (JF) did choose list making because it matched Erica's style. We hope that our decisions to ask questions or invite children to make lists or other symbolic representations follow from their styles. We move into particular ways of working simply by trying one way and moving to another if the first doesn't work. We are both "talkers," so we usually start by inviting people to talk with us. If we notice that a child responds in lists, we will probably start thinking in terms of list. If he/she tells stories, we will think more in terms of story development and meaning questions. If a child gives very brief answers to our questions or seems uncomfortable talking very expansively, we will usually think more about lists or using symbols (see Freedman & Combs, 1996, pp. 224–236). We do find that sometimes when we have developed more of a relationship with particular children, they talk more and in more detail. Then we might move from making lists to asking more story development and meaning questions.

Q: (CS) One frequent thing that supervisees ask is how to respond when children give a host of "I don't knows," shrugs, or all-too-brief answers to all our efforts! I noticed you did a variety of things in Erica's therapy at these times. You turned to her grandparents in the session and asked them to provide examples of things she liked to do, which helped join with her as a human being rather than as a "patient." You sidestepped verbalization by inviting her to draw the territory of "self-

blame" in the past and currently, and then to make a written list of what was in these boxes. You also asked a hypothetical, future-oriented question at one point.

Can you share what sorts of things you think about when a child is reluctant to talk in therapy? Are there other things you have done at these times as well? Is there any pattern or similarity in the things you might attempt to do at these times? How important do you think it is to try to involve family and other "audience" members when children are more reserved or in general? If this is significant for you, can you share a couple of ways you might go about this?

A: Perhaps the most important things we think about when a child is reluctant to talk in therapy are the prevalence and power of discourses that work to rob children of their voices: the "Children should be seen and not heard" discourse, the "Father knows best" discourse, the "Children's knowledge is primitive knowledge" discourse, the "Good students sit still, don't talk, and obey all the rules" discourse, and others. These discourses are insidious, and can very easily overwhelm our belief that children have lots of knowledge that is worth listening to.

It is a rare child who hasn't been silenced to some degree by these discourses, so it is no surprise at all to us when children are reluctant to talk—we expect this to be the case, especially in the beginning of therapy. However, we don't believe that this means that children have nothing worthwhile to say, or that they will *remain* reluctant to talk. Usually a child just needs a little proof that we are really interested in what he/she has to say.

Our earlier work was using Ericksonian therapy, and Milton Erickson believed that whatever the person said or did was a "perfect" response. That early training was helpful in keeping us from feeling rejected or hopeless when someone doesn't show much verbal response. When a child is reluctant to talk in therapy, we wonder both how and what she/he is communicating and how we can adjust our communication style to be more compatible with hers/his. One of the things we might do in addition to introducing lists is to offer some possibilities ourselves and ask the child if we are right, or to choose from a number of possibilities. We do think audience is important for all of us, and particularly for children. One way I (JF) included the family with an 11-year-old who wanted to be seen alone was at the end of therapy to make a tape reflecting back on our work, which the child then shared with her family.

Q: *(CS) I know that a lot of your work with adults involves respectfully opening space for them to consider whether various sociocultural ways of being are currently useful in their lives. Erica was initially described as struggling with self-blame and not feeling entitled to much of a voice. If Erica had been 16 instead of 9 years old, do you think you might have tried asking her about whether she perceived her struggles as related to larger gender issues? If so, how might you have tried to do this?*

If she didn't find these questions helpful and gave matter-of-fact replies once more, might you have let the more overt sociocultural questions go for now and returned to your list- making questions or other sorts of questions, or might you have persisted with the former questions? What sorts of indicators might you use to determine whether you want to pursue sociocultural issues with children and adolescents (e.g., age, maturity, etc.)? In this or other situations, could you envision yourselves combining these sociocultural and list-making questions?

A: Before we answer any of these questions, we want to respond to your presupposition that the way we address sociocultural issues in therapy is directly, by asking questions that attempt to tie people's particular problems to general social issues such as gender inequality. Although we sometimes do this, we are more concerned that we be *thinking about* limiting or oppressive discourses as we sit with people.

We believe that it is our responsibility to be aware of as many of the potentially problematic discourses that affect people as we can, and to facilitate life narratives that are relatively unencumbered by such discourses. (See Hare-Mustin, 1994, for an excellent discussion of this.) For example, we are aware of at least two commonly encountered discourses that might have been depriving Erica of her voice—the "Adults know and children don't" discourse that we discussed in responding to your second set of questions, and those gender-based discourses that you refer to in this set of questions. The main way that we challenged these discourses with Erica was by not letting them make us deaf to her knowledge.

We didn't try to get her to link self-blame and voicelessness to either of these discourses; we used our knowledge of them to help us avoid their tricks. To the degree that we were able to avoid being tricked by them, we were able to believe that Erica had a voice and to find ways to help her use it. This would have been our basic stance, whether Erica was 9, 16, 32, or 64.

If she had been 16, we *might* have invited her to examine self-blame and voicelessness in the light of her experience of patriarchy, and she might have found this useful, but what was of most importance to us about sociocultural issues would still have been whether or not *we* were aware of them and striving to keep them from closing down possibilities for how Erica might live her life. If we did decide to ask her whether she perceived her struggles as related to larger gender issues, we might do so by asking a direct and simple question, such as "Do you think self-blame is a gender-based issue?" Alternatively, we might ask something more indirect and complex: "Do you know anyone else who has trouble speaking up at times? Who? Do you know anyone else? Do you know more women or more men who have trouble speaking up? Why do you think it is that, among the people you know, more women than men have trouble speaking up?" And so on and so forth. If she didn't find our questions helpful, we would let them go.

As to your question about indicators of when we would and wouldn't want to pursue sociocultural issues, we *always* want to pursue sociocultural issues. However, we don't always pursue those issues directly and out loud. What is more important to us is that we situate our experience of people's problems within a complex and rich understanding of the discourses (such as those surrounding race, gender, class, sexual orientation, and age) that might be working to sustain those problems. Only to the extent that we ourselves can escape the clutches of sociocultural issues can we help the people who consult with us escape them. In light of this, can you see how all list-making questions are *already* sociocultural questions, in that they help people who are being storied as voiceless to have a voice?

REFERENCES

Combs, G., & Freedman, J. (1994). Narrative intentions. In M. F. Hoyt (Eds.), *Constructive therapies.* New York: Guilford Press.

Dickerson, V. C., & Zimmerman, J. L. (1993). A narrative approach to families with adolescents. In S. Friedman (Ed.), *The new language of change: Constructive collaboration in psychotherapy* (pp. 226–250). New York: Guilford Press

Epston, D. (1989). *Collected papers.* Adelaide, South Australia: Dulwich Centre Publications.

Freedman, J., & Combs, G. (1996). *Narrative therapy: The social construction of preferred realities.* New York: Norton.

Freeman, J., Epston, D., & Lobovits, D. (1997). *Playful approaches to serious problems: Narrative therapy with children and their families.* New York: Norton.

Hare-Mustin, R. (1994). Discourses in the mirrored room: A postmodern analysis of therapy. *Family Process, 33*(1), 19–35.

Laird, J. (1989). Women and stories: Restorying women's self-constructions. In M. McGoldrick, C. Anderson, & F. Walsh (Eds.), *Women in families: A framework for family therapy.* New York: Norton.

White, M. (1984). Pseudo-encopresis: From avalanche to victory, from vicious to virtuous cycles. *Family Systems Medicine, 2*(2), 150–160.

White, M. (1995). *Re-authoring lives: Interviews and essays.* Adelaide, South Australia: Dulwich Centre Publications.

White, M., & Epston, D. (1990). *Narrative means to therapeutic ends.* New York: Norton.

Zimmerman, J. L., & Dickerson, V. C. (1996). *If problems talked: Narrative therapy in action.* New York: Guilford Press.

6

Miserere Nobis

A CHOIR OF SMALL AND
BIG VOICES IN DESPAIR

TOM ANDERSEN

Traditionally, clinical chapters begin with a theoretical overview and introduction to the clinical transcript. I have chosen to write this chapter in such a way as to show how certain immediate, urgent, and unexpected events created an uncertain and challenging therapeutic situation. Thus, I share orienting information in the way I learned it as events were unfolding.

A CRESCENDO AT THE BEGINNING

We—three women and four men—met for a day's work in a country far from my own. The other six belonged to a therapeutic team at an open consultation center. I was the only stranger. I had not been informed about any plan for the day, so we started to talk about how we could best use the time we had together. Maybe just have a discussion, or maybe do a consultation with only the team and no clients present?

As our discussion went on, Marco, one of the team members, went to check the telephone answering machine. His quick and heavy footsteps when he returned alerted us that something was going on. "Why in hell didn't she call?" he sighed in anger. The others understood immediately. But I did not.

The rest of the team members forgot me as they engaged very emotionally while talking about someone named Sara. Some were angry as they spoke; some cried. It took me 15 minutes to understand that Sara was *not* Marco's daughter, but a client at the center.

Sara,[1] in her early 30s, had a history of drug addiction, which had led to her losing custody of her two older children (from earlier relationships). Being connected to the team, particularly Marco, had helped her stay "clean" the last 4 years. The team members were not family members, but a friendly and safe group to be with. It was Sara's current husband, José, who had left the message on the phone. An old friend of Sara, still heavily hooked on drugs, had touched base with her, and the two women were somewhere out there—on the streets.

As I listened, I had my own ongoing inner dialogue:

"The Russian Mikhail Bakhtin (1993) has said that life is a chain of once-occurring moments, and that every moment is 'Once occurrent, Being-as-event.' The moment we are in *now* is the only one we can influence. The moment 1 second ago is gone, and the moment ahead is only there as many possibilities, not yet turned into life. In *this* moment, the voices that inhabit us make us the persons we become. And these are both inner voices (which talk in our internal dialogues with ourselves) and outer voices (which talk in our external dialogues with others). Bakhtin and another Russian, Lev Vygotsky (1983), both hold the opinion that 'We are the voices that inhabit us' (Morson, 1986, p. 8). We are like constantly shifting shelters, formed from moment to moment by the voices that have taken up residency in us.

Our utterances include words *and* bodily movements. As we allow these to be seen and heard, they are not only informative but also formative. As we speak, we become who we are at that moment.

How do drugs influence our utterances?"

NO MOMENTS TO LOSE

What would happen when Sara's language was contaminated with drugs? Would her protecting herself increase or not with drug use? We

---

[1]Names have been changed to protect confidentiality. The family described here has granted permission to use this material.

all knew that people who have been off drugs for a while often resume drug use with amphetamines before going to heroin. Because they are not used to being back on drugs, they can easily overdose and die.

We needed to act quickly, and we needed to create a "problem-dis-solving system" (Anderson, Goolishian, & Winderman, 1986). Who would be interested enough to come? We called her husband, José, who said he would be there as soon as he had cleaned and fed their 10-month-old baby, Teresa. We also called her brother, André, who said he would be there in 20 minutes.

André arrived first, shouting, "She has betrayed me. Damn her! We need to lock her up somewhere." Marco, knowing Sara's great sensitivi-ty to being imposed upon or dictated to, disagreed with the idea of lock-ing Sara up, and a quarrel between the two men broke out.

This was what I could hear in my inner dialogue:

"When fear or anger or sadness overloads a person, she/he easily feels that her/his perspective should be given priority. When two persons think this, conflict easily breaks out. Two monologues that never reach each other easily emerge. A monologue is charac-terized by being conducted from only one party's perspective. A dialogue is embedded in both parties' perspectives" (Seikkula et al., 1995).

One of the other team members had probably grasped this differ-ence as well, and was able to talk first with Marco and then with André. André's idea of locking Sara up was explored in more detail until André gave this idea up, as his own answers convinced him that it would create more difficulties than it would solve.

INNER VOICES WITHOUT THEIR OWN WORDS

André said that he was 13 and Sara was 3 when their mother died of a drug overdose. They had two different fathers, who also both died of overdoses. "When Mom died, I was determined to do my best to keep the rest of our family together," André said. The rest of us listened as our thoughts traveled in different directions. What happens to a 3-year-old child who suddenly loses both of her parents? We could imagine her crying, "Mom and Dad, where are you?" When Mom and Dad never showed up, what happened? Maybe only a shivering, small body wept until no more sound was heard. How long did this take? What was left? A scar? An emptiness? A black hole?

Here are some more of my thoughts:

"Lev Vygotsky (1988) has some interesting thoughts about how language emerges. He thinks differently from Jean Piaget, who believed that language grows and matures from inside the person. Vygotsky believes that a small child first learns to imitate adults' words. At first, the child's words are imitated sounds. But during the period from about 2–3 years of age until 6–7 years, the child plays in a distinct way. He/she plays alone, while talking loudly as the play unfolds. This play has a stronger tendency to occur if there is an adult present. The adult does not participate in the play, but is just there to witness. When the child is 6 or 7, this play stops as the child establishes inner dialogues and the words become personal. They are not private, as they come from and belong to the community, but they become personal through being said outloud while the child plays."

If Sara did not yet have her own words when she lost her mother and father, was she able to carry with her the memory of this loss? Or did the loss just disappear or dissolve? Another excerpt from my ongoing inner talk:

"Mark Johnson (1987) proposes that a person first experiences circumstances with the body. What the body senses is 'transformed' and made meaningful through the use of learned metaphors. Gunn Engelsrud (1995), a Norwegian physiotherapist, is in agreement when she refers to Charles Peirce and Maurice Merleau-Ponty. I think similarly about this: The body perceives circumstances by sensing the shifts in its own respiration. This feeling is 'worked on' by inner and outer talks until a meaning is reached (Andersen, 1995).

It is possible to think of this movement from sensing to meaning as a characteristic that develops gradually in a person's life. At first, a baby has its ability to sense the environment. Then it develops the ability to make movements and utter sounds; then it becomes able to imitate words; and then, as an older child, it becomes able to reach meaning through its own words. When bodily reactions to an event are painful and breathing is suppressed, does this diminish the feeling of pain—and, in turn, the ability to express pain? (The question mark indicates that these are unfinished thoughts on my part.)"

How did Sara manage to suppress her painful cry ("Mom and Dad, where are you?")? Did this loss of her mother and father make her less prepared to protect herself later in her life when her circumstances were threatening? Or did this lack of protection occur later? Could an embracing arm of one of her brothers have contributed to her safety?

We listened to André talk about Sara's childhood, and I could imagine that an inner protesting voice in each of us cried, "Oh, my God!" How old were we when these inner voices of ours were born? Probably very young. Each of us had at least a protesting inner voice. Did Sara have inner voices that protest? Or were such voices not available to her? Protesting inner voices tend to protect.

If Sara now had no words for her loss, maybe the loss of her mother and father resided in her body as a shivering wave of the far past—a bodily reminder of a disaster?

If there had been a therapist there at the time when Sara lost her parents, what would have been the best thing to do? If Sara had not yet found her own words, maybe bodily touches from an embracing adult who repeated the words "I am here to take care of you. Don't be afraid. Just cry!" would have sufficed? If the words had been repeated sufficiently over time, until they became part of Sara's own inner talk, would that have contributed to protecting inner voices for her future life? Maybe family therapists have become too eager to reach small kids through words and "adult" talk? Maybe physical availability and touches are better for the small ones?

André said that he and Sara and another brother were dispersed when their mother died. They were taken care of in different places. Sara lived in several places, as one foster family after another gave her up. It was particularly hard for her to leave a certain foster family where she finally found safety, André said. However, when Sara was 7 years old, she was told that she had to leave this foster family to go to a certain clinic because she was too thin and had to gain weight. She stayed in the clinic for a year. During that year, she very much wished to come back to her foster mother, whom she loved greatly. Nobody had told Sara that she was sent away because her foster mother was ill. When she came home, she realized that her foster mother was dead. After that, Sara was never the same, André said. She became more bitter and angry, but rarely spoke of her sadness. Nobody saw her cry anymore. One of us in the group had once heard that a small child in the same position as Sara had decided not to cry any more, because it would take her 3 weeks to stop if she started to cry. This other child felt that it was easier to be angry, because her anger helped her stand and continue on, whereas crying made her fall apart.

What could we have done if we had been there as therapists when Sara realized she had lost her favorite foster mother? Could we have contributed in such a way that eventually she could have gotten past her feelings of being betrayed? Could we have interacted with her so that she, in anger, could have let the adults understand they should have told her that she was sent away to the clinic because her foster mother was dying? If she had had the chance to finish expressing her angry and sad feelings, maybe she would have found it less necessary to be angry later in life? Maybe she could even have cried when sad feelings were strong?

We listened quietly to André and thought of his profound wish to keep his family together. One person asked him, "Who helped you to protect your family?" "Nobody," he said. The silence in the room touched and moved us. We felt his despair when as a young teenager he could not fulfill his wish to have his family be together.

A male therapist in the group was particularly touched, as he was reminded of what he himself had experienced as an 11-year-old boy. His father was very ill. He was afraid that the father would die, and he went to the woods to find the most difficult trail to walk along. He climbed high trees and steep mountainsides, jumped from big heights, and swam through cold water. As he did so, he thought that if he did succeed in finding a very difficult trail and make his way along it, his father would overcome his illness. He made it through the pathways he chose, but when he came home he learned that his father was dead. His immediate thought was this: "I should have chosen a more difficult trail!" That thought had remained with him ever since in the form of inner voices: "Make it more difficult! Be more brave! Be more courageous!"

If we had been there as therapists with André when his family was first separated, what could we have done? What would André have wanted us to do? Maybe listen to him for a while, quietly? Maybe it would have been good for him to share his plans and thoughts? Maybe it would have been good if we let him feel that there was also space for his despair and worries to be expressed? Perhaps this would have meant shedding tears and sobbing? Would it also have been helpful for him if we expressed the admiration we felt for him? What about also saying that if he needed an adult to discuss his task of responsibility, we would be available? We would hope to be available for as long as he thought such company would be useful. What would these possibilities have been like for André?

SMILES WITHOUT WORDS

Sara's husband, José, arrived with their baby, Teresa—a smiling infant who exemplified a feeling of security as she crawled on the floor or sat on the various laps in the group. What story would she bring with her from today? Since she did not yet have words, how would her body remind her of today? If smells and touches and what she saw were more meaningful than words, what would be good for her now? Maybe to see her father's smile? If so, how could we help this happen? Maybe it would be good for Teresa to feel the constraint of the father's breathing slowly vanish? How does a child feel such vanishing? Does it smell it, or does the young child experience it in a different way? If Teresa could feel it, how could we contribute to her father's breathing so that it would be more free? Maybe the solidity of the warm hands embracing her as she sat on people's laps was soothing for her? What should therapists think about when a 10-month-old baby is in a therapeutic meeting like this? Being available to Teresa would undoubtedly be helpful.

If today made no mark on her memory, would she ever be told the story? If it were to be told, how could it be told in such a way that it would contribute to *her* feeling protected from harm in *her* life? Some of us in the group thought of this, and we even discussed it with André and José later in the meeting.

Teresa was born prematurely. She was so small at birth that one hand could enfold her. One group member who had also had a premature child was able to empathize with Sara's position. In her inner talk, she could imagine that Sara had probably asked herself over and over again, "Will I lose my baby?" Teresa was in intensive care for a long time at the hospital. Every time the phone rang or there was a knock on the door, Sara was prepared to be told that Teresa was dead. How much stronger that feeling must have been since the social authorities had forced her to give up her two children from previous relationships!

"Sara was so exhausted," José said softly. "We had hoped to go to the country for a few days' vacation, but we had no money. The rest of my family lives close to the mountains and they invited us to come there, but they had no money to give us for travel. We also asked the social authorities, but they also had no money to give us." We asked, "If Sara comes back, will she still want that vacation?" José thought she would. All of us in the group looked at each other and had the same thought: Today's consultation fee should go toward that vacation. José and André were asked whether they could accept this money, and they nodded their acceptance quietly. This was clearly a small relief to them, at least.

We reached the understanding that Sara was exhausted and needed time off. It was just by chance that the drug-using girlfriend came and offered her a form of time off. She had not intended to be on the streets. It was just one possible way to be in the world and to find some temporary relief. And Sara did not see any other possibilities for herself at that time.

A DRUMMING TEXT

The two men, José and André, said that the "jungle drums" had to be used to send the message "Sara, come home." No more words.

When we left, the two men said they would search the town separately, "because we will go places from which we may never return. If they try to kill us, they'll only get one of us."

DONA NOBIS PACEM

Handshakes and glances for farewell were exchanged. That was all. No words were heard. But there were choirs of inner voices in all of us. Mostly chaotic choirs.

We imagined all the voices that were engaged in Sara whispering in despair. Voices begging for light. Voices demanding justice. Small voices and big voices—most of them saying, "Please help us!"

I took a long walk through the town and ended up at a church where a choir called "Fifteen Voices" and a small orchestra performed Franz Schubert's Mass in G Minor. At one point the soloist sang, "*Agnus Dei, qui tollis peccata mundi, miserere nobis*,"[2] and the choir quietly echoed him: "*Miserere nobis.*" The soloist continued, "*Agnus Dei, qui tollis peccata mundi, dona nobis pacem*,"[3] and again the choir sang faintly in the background: "*Dona nobis pacem.*"

EPILOGUE

I called the leader of the team the next afternoon, to let her know that I was thinking of them. She said that Marco had just called and said that Sara had come home. Four weeks later I received a letter from their faraway land, saying that the vacation Sara, José, and Teresa had just taken in the mountains with José's family had created new hopes. Maybe hopes created by new voices could balance the old inner voices that hardly could believe in a future. I thought to myself:

"Peggy Penn and Marilyn Frankfurt (1994) underline the importance of balancing the inner voices, without eliminating any, not

---

[2] "Lamb of God, who takest away the sins of the world, have mercy upon us."

[3] "Lamb of God, who takest away the sins of the world, grant us peace."

even the nasty or critical or blaming ones. They talk about just adding more hopeful and friendly voices."

EDITORIAL QUESTIONS

Q: *(CS) Reading your chapter was like reading a very moving novel! I was drawn into the mystery and despair, and anxiously awaited each new unfolding in this human drama. From this chapter and from what you have said in your workshops (Andersen, 1994, 1996), I get the sense that you feel that reflecting processes can provide words for clients to "try on"—words that may provide new, more satisfying perspectives for clients.*

For example, you have a subhead here called "Inner Voices without Their Own Words." I'd like to explore this a bit. For example, I imagine that if Sara had been able to overhear the team's reflections (i.e., about her having a protesting inner voice or whether she had had the chance to finish expressing her anger and sadness), this could have had a very liberating effect on Sara. Would you think of these possible reflections as providing new words, new descriptions for Sara to consider and "try on"? Might this mean that if she resonated with these perspectives, she might have used these words to help her reply with a fuller, more satisfying voice in dealing with current situations? Is this one implication of clients' having "voices without their own words"?

A: Yes, the team could have talked about its reflections while Sara was in a listening position. For instance, one team member could have said: "If Sara is in a difficult situation and feels unprotected, would it be of any help to hear the voice of a person who, at some time in Sara's life, said something that made her feel safe? Who was that person? How can Sara get more in touch with that voice (or that person)?"

Q: *(CS) Let us suppose that Sara had come in for therapy with one of her foster mothers when she was about 8 or 9. Let's further suppose that her foster mother was concerned about Sara's making angry comments to her and to others. If Sara was not willing to talk during this meeting, can you say hypothetically how you might have thought about this and what sorts of things you might have done? Might you have tried to imagine what she might be experiencing and to reflect on this out loud with the mother, to provide some additional possibilities for talking about what was happening? Might you have asked the foster mother what she or other people imagined Sara was experiencing? I am trying to explore what you might do and how you think about a child with whom the parent or caretaker is concerned, but who isn't willing to talk during a meeting.*

A: If Sara was not willing to talk, I think I would first ask the foster mother what she thought would be best for Sara—to listen to the foster mother and me as we talked about Sara's anger, or not to listen. If Sara stayed to listen, I would ask the foster mother if she thought Sara's anger was anger only or if there were other feelings in it. Fear? Sadness? If fear, of what? If sadness, in relation to what?

Q: *(CS) I wonder if you could say a few words about what you have called "four ways of knowing" (Andersen, 1996)? I have found this an extremely helpful way for myself and for the people we train and supervise to think about our work with both children and adults.*

In the chapter, you point to the importance of "bodily knowing" for appreciating children's experience. You also underline the relevance of "relational knowing" in many ways. For example, you ask questions like these: "What would André have wanted us to do? Maybe listen to him for a while, quietly? . . . Would it also have been helpful for him if we expressed the admiration we felt for him?" Such relational questions seem to suggest that it is frequently helpful to ask ourselves (and our clients), "How would they [or you] like for me to participate with them [or you] right now? What would be most helpful?" Many times, it seems we therapists take these matters for granted and assume we know what would be best for our clients (i.e., asking certain types of questions, etc.). How do you think about the "four levels of knowing," and how do these influence your work?

A: The four ways of knowing are as follows:

1. "Rational": to reason, to think, to grasp meaning, and so on.
2. "Practical (technical)": to have agency; to practice a repertoire of methods for implementing rational knowing.
3. "Relational": to find a position in relation to one or more others so that these relationships are tolerable or not too uncomfortable for all to take part in. In other words, for a person to put himself/herself in the others' position in order to try to understand how it is for the others to be *here now,* which also includes being with the therapist.
4. "Bodily": to be able to notice one's sensory reactions in order to feel that something significant is being expressed, without necessarily knowing what the significance entails. Having a conversation with oneself and/or with other(s) will help this understanding unfold.

I prefer to think that all four kinds of knowing are important. In therapy, I think that we should start with the third (relational knowing) and fourth (bodily knowing) kinds, and let these determine how we think about what has occurred (rational knowing) and what methods we use (practical knowing).

Q: *(CS) In this chapter, I found myself identifying with your musings as you and the group wondered about what Sara, José, André, and baby Teresa might have found or would find helpful in the future. It also seems you are focusing on different ways they might talk about their life stories. For example, you wonder about Teresa's future telling about what happened during this meeting. If it was spoken about, would it be told in a way indicating that she experienced being protected from harm or abandonment, unlike her mother's experience?*

Could you say something about focusing on the "content" of clients' stories, as compared with "how or from what perspectives" clients talk about these stories? How is this distinction useful for you? Does this distinction connect to a therapist's trying to facilitate genuine dialogues and providing additional voices with clients?

A: I mostly concentrate on how people form(ulate) their stories. The act of form(ulat)ing is how we become the persons we become. So I am increasingly interested in co-discovering ways clients can nuance and increase their repertoires for how they express (utter) themselves. The "story" a client shares provides the vehicle for exploring various ways it can be expressed.

REFERENCES

Andersen, T. (1994). Workshop presented at the California Family Studies Center/Phillips Graduate Institute, Los Angeles.

Andersen, T. (1995). Reflecting processes; acts of informing and forming: You can borrow my eyes, but you must not take them away from me! In S. Friedman (Ed.), *The reflecting team in action: Collaborative practice in family therapy.* New York: Guilford Press.

Andersen, T. (1996). Workshop presented at the California Family Studies Center/Phillips Graduate Institute, Los Angeles.

Anderson, H., Goolishian, H., & Winderman, L. (1986). Problem created system: Toward transformation in family therapy. *Journal of Strategic and Systemic Therapies, 5*(4), 1–11.

Bakhtin, M. (1993). *Towards a philosophy of the act.* Austin: University of Texas Press.

Engelsrud, G. (1995, May). *Kvinner i bevegelse—mellom lengsel og lyst.* Paper presented at the Senter for Kvinneforskning, Arbeidsnotat, University of Oslo, Norway.

Johnson, M. (1987). *The body in the mind.* Chicago: University of Chicago Press.

Morson, G. S. (1986). *Bakhtin: Essays and dialogues on his work.* Chicago: University of Chicago Press.

Penn, P., & Frankfurt, M. (1994). Creating a participant text: Writing, multiple voices, narrative multiplicity. *Family Process, 33*(3), 217–233.

Seikkula, J., et al. (1995). Treating psychosis by means of open dialogue. In S. Friedman (Ed.), *The reflecting team in action: Collaborative practice in family therapy.* New York: Guilford Press.

Vygotsky, L. (1988). *Thought and language.* Cambridge, MA: MIT Press.

7

Destination Grump
Station—Getting Off
the Grump Bus

DEAN H. LOBOVITS
JENNIFER C. FREEMAN

Like the twin masks of comedy and tragedy, play reflects both the mirth
and pathos of the human experience. When children and adults meet together, playful communication provides a common language to express
the breadth and depth of thoughts, emotions, and accounts of experience. In this way, we are all bilingual. A child's comprehension of logical
and analytic communication varies with the child's cognitive development and maturity. Playful communication, on the other hand, is not
wholly dependent upon the child's development; lends itself to the ellip-
tical, magical, or fantastic; and has the capacity of being infectiously
lighthearted and inclusive in conversations with families (Freeman, Epston, & Lobovits, 1997).

When families with children tell about difficult problems, the therapist may be tempted to attend mainly to accounts that are told by the
adults in a linear and factual manner. The children's versions may be
judged irrelevant or illogical—or ignored altogether because they are expressed nonverbally. Subject to adult translation, their stories often un-

dergo interpretation and revision without their consent. This can happen when a professional offers "interpretations," when children are talked "down to" or "over their heads," or when they are talked about in front of others as if they are not present. Children's solutions to problems may be deemed irrelevant, insufficient, or infeasible. Their unique contributions, ideas, and solutions may be excluded by adult-centered language, limiting their full participation as authors and as contributors of change for themselves and for their families.

When family members communicate in a therapeutic conversation, they rarely share one point of view, or tell one version of a story. Typically, there are many stories and versions of stories being told simultaneously; each perspective is unique by virtue of the diversity of age, experience, and gender in a family. In family therapy the therapist must exert her/his attention actively, attending to and joining in the development of several stories simultaneously. The therapist's attention is guided by her/his own unique point of view, age, gender, class, culture, spiritual experiences, and so on (Pinderhughes, 1989; Rosenwald & Ochberg, 1992; Tamasese & Waldegrave, 1993). Since the therapist's attention is influential, she/he must carry both the moral and social responsibility to examine the consequences of various choices of what to attend to and what to focus on with the family (Lobovits, Maisel, & Freeman, 1995; Waldegrave, 1992).

It is especially important for a therapist to listen and be accountable to children, responding to their interests and getting suggestions approved. Communicating with children may require that the therapist converse in a language that is not usually used for serious communication—playfully entering realms of fantasy and humor; being willing to follow repetitive, tangential, and mysterious plot twists. Given a chance, children and adults can resolve problems together in unique and surprising ways, co-authoring new stories together in a relationship of respectful collaboration.

We are among those who acknowledge, nurture, and encourage the passage of change within a narrative metaphor (Adams-Westcott & Isenbart, 1996; Barragar-Dunne, 1992; Epston, 1989, 1997; Epston & White, 1995; Dickerson & Zimmerman, 1993; Durrant, 1989; Freedman & Combs, 1996; Nylund & Corsiglia, 1996; Stacey & Loptson, 1995; White, 1985, 1989; White & Epston, 1990). We have been engaged in an exploration of the ideas and practices that evolve when therapy with children and families is inspired by playful and inclusive narratives of transformation.

One analogy for a journey of transformation is that of the "rites of passage" (van Gennep, 1960). Co-authored narratives evolve when a child, family, and helper meet together in the preparation, trials, confirmations, and celebrations of life's passages. The rites of passage may be described loosely as having three parts. First is the evocation of a state of readiness or preparation for change. The second stage is liminal, and consists of experimentation with the new, strange, and different, as well as passing through the trials or tests of change. The final stage consists of the reincorporation of the new into the old, as well as the confirmation and celebration of a new identity.

HARBINGERS OF CHANGE

Unease, discontent, and pain are often the harbingers of change. The rites of passage for a child and family may begin with the acknowledgment of pain, betrayal, and injustice, but repetitive analysis of vicious cycles of thought, feelings, and interaction can bind a therapist and family collectively to hopelessness or limit their vision of possibilities. Carefully attending to the virtuous cycles that are already occurring or are on the horizon invites a readiness for change. When problems arise in the life of a family, it takes skill and persistence to identify nascent virtuous cycles. Those cycles contain the thoughts, emotions, behaviors, and interactions that lead toward transformation. Attention to virtuous cycles encourages renewed or novel efforts to amplify these cycles.

If the problem of Fighting, for example, has taken over family life to such an extent that it is the primary mode of interaction between family members, initial and validating steps would be identifying the Fighting interactions and acknowledging the deep pain, distrust, and destruction that accompany them. However, this is not a place to dwell indefinitely—nor is merely understanding the roots or workings of the Fighting and waiting until the problem works itself out. Instead, family members can be invited into a conversation that clarifies the family's preferences for communication—spotting and highlighting Fighting-free interactions, while contrasting their effects with the Fighting-dominated ones.

The benefits of Fighting-free interactions, such as mutual support, trust, and safety, can be contrasted with the pain, alienation, and destruction wrought by Fighting. These contrasts help to identify the effects of Fighting on family relationships. They set up an antagonist–protagonist relationship between Fighting and Peace, and invite the child and family to enter into roles consistent with their preference. Even if members of the family are simply ready to acknowledge that a preference for Peace exists, the rites of passage have begun. In the initial phase of family narratives built on such choices, bits and pieces of past experiences, exceptions to the problem, and future aspirations are gathered together to build the nest where further plans for change can be hatched.

For a fledgling change to take flight, each small accomplishment needs nurturing. Have the family members ever had a Fighting-free outing? If not, can they allow themselves to wish for one? Is there any safe place in their house? If not, is the family interested in creating a "safe house" or, for a start, a "safe room?" How will small changes such as these, if nurtured, eventually grow strong enough to stand up to the stresses that previously evoked the Fighting behavior? If peaceful moments lengthen, will they eventually bring the benefits of mutual support, trust, and safety to family life? If those qualities grow, how will they see the family through the next obstacle or transition, such as adolescence, job loss, or pregnancy?

MEETING THE CHALLENGE

When change occurs in the midst of serious problems, it is fragile, like a baby sea turtle facing an unrelenting tide of negative characterizations, attributions, and history. In spite of this fragility, it must immediately stand the test of life's hardships. Like the newborn sea turtle struggling across the beach and through a ring of predators, fledgling changes must face the testing and trials of the rites of passage. Fledgling changes become more resilient by being challenged, but challenged appropriately to their strength. A balance must be achieved between the test's being strong enough to be meaningful and the change's not being overwhelmed by the challenge.

Let's say a family recounts a visit to the zoo together last Saturday that took place without Fighting "for a change." To test the mettle of this exceptional moment of Peace, the therapist can ask questions about how Fighting could have destroyed the outing, find out how the family resisted looping back into the vicious cycle, and draw out each member's contribution to the event.

Another avenue is to inquire about how the skills or choices that created the Peace could be put to a test—or, less directively, how the family foresees these will survive when applied to another "Fighting zone." For example, how will the Peace skills the family displayed at the zoo translate to getting off to school and work in the morning? How will they stand up to the pressures of rushing and grumpiness?

The therapist can also invite the child and family to predict the inevitable hiccups of the problem's reasserting itself even after the alternative story of Peace in the family has taken root. How could Fighting make a comeback? What loopholes might the problem exploit to undermine the Peace process? What are the family's counterplans? The therapist can explore these issues playfully, remembering that serious problems detest lighthearted and especially humorous approaches.

The scenario above might also be initiated when a family member expresses skepticism: "Well, it's easy to have a good time at the zoo, but what about on a school morning?" This challenge creates an opening to explore similar questions: What would be the impact on the family and its members if Peace stood up to the rigors of getting off to work and school? If this occurred, would it prove that Peace not only had broken out for a moment at the zoo, but had found a place in the day-to-day life of the family?

CELEBRATION AND CONFIRMATION

When a virtuous cycle takes hold that can pass through these tests, it is time for reincorporation and confirmation that a meaningful change has taken place. In the example above, the therapist might ask: At what point can the family members feel confident in describing themselves as Peaceful rather than a Fighting family? When this has been accomplished, the therapist can ask: What will the future relationship with Fighting be? Reincorporation questions can define such new relationships with the problem. Sometimes the family may choose to include the problem in the new scheme of things: What role should Fighting play, now that it is no longer the dominant mode of interacting? Should the family members keep enough Fighting in themselves to express their point of view? Could there be "fun" fights or "fair" fights to handle disagreements in the family?

Sometimes oppressive problems (e.g., Abuse) are better left completely behind. Others, however, can be rehabilitated (e.g., a Temper that used to grow into a tantrum can become a beneficial ally when assertiveness is needed) or reformed (e.g., an attack of the Grumpiness that used to isolate a person might serve as a reminder to employ self-caring tools).

Finally, confirmation and celebration take place. How should the new Peace be celebrated? Of what should this celebration consist—a reminiscence about the journey, a ceremony of art making, or a party with speeches? Who should be in attendance? Who would be pleased to know that Peace has broken out? A teacher who was concerned enough to refer the family for therapy? The spirit of a Peace-loving grandparent who is no longer alive? Should there be a Peace proclamation, or a Peace party with a "Peace o'cake" for all?

CONSULTING YOUR CONSULTANTS

When children or families have taken the journey of transformation, they gain the knowledge and expertise that can only come from grappling with a problem firsthand. Epston and White (1990, 1995) have developed the art of consulting a child in order to document the child's knowledge of the problem and the skillful means the child has developed to resist the problem's dictates. They invite the child to share, during a retrospective interview, his/her unique narratives for his/her own benefit, as well as that of the family, the therapist, and others who face similar problems.

As we have written elsewhere (Freeman et al., 1997),

When engaged as consultants, children assume an unconventional role:

- They are consulted as authorities on their own lives.
- Their pre-existing and newly acquired knowledges and abilities are deemed effective and worthy of respect.
- Their ideas are considered significant enough to be documented and circulated to others. (pp. 126–127)

The case story below offers an example of a final collaborative meeting between a therapist (JCF—Jenny) and a child, Michaela, in what was primarily a family therapy focused on the reclamation of a mother–daughter relationship from Fighting. This meeting consisted of a "consulting your consultant" interview with Michaela. We hope that this interview will illustrate the reincorporative, affirmative, and celebratory aspects of family and personal change—in Michaela's own words and through the narrative she co-authored with her therapist.

MICHAELA

Background and Description of Therapy

Nine-year-old Michaela and her mother, Angela,[1] met with Jenny both individually and conjointly over a period of 3 months. Angela is of Chinese descent, and Michaela's father is European-American.

---

[1]Names and identifying details of the therapy portrayed here have been altered in order to safeguard the confidences of the participants. The participants have granted permission to use this material.

Most of the material that is presented here is drawn from the final meeting between Michaela and Jenny. The conversation at this meeting was a review of Michaela's progress; it shows how the forging of meaning is a continual process that takes place right up until the last words are exchanged in a farewell. But some backdrop to the conversation is needed first. This first section briefly describes the family's initial circumstances, as well as the family therapy that took place up to that point.

Angela had had primary responsibility for parenting Michaela since her birth. Unfortunately, because of the onset of a severe mental illness shortly after her birth, Michaela's father had been unable to continue in the marriage or participate fully in parenting. For many years Angela and Michaela's relationship had been a close and happy one. Then, when Michaela was 9, Hal entered their lives as Angela's boyfriend. Along with his arrival, Fighting and Grumpiness, more or less hand in hand, made a dramatic appearance in the mother–daughter relationship. It was this that brought them back to see Jenny.

Several years before, Jenny had seen Michaela for a while in play therapy to support her in coming to terms with her father's disability. This time, when she walked in the door, Michaela smiled briefly at Jenny and then flung herself down on the couch, turning her sullen eyes away from Angela, and sighing loudly, when her mother sat down beside her. Feeling uninhibited in the familiar setting of Jenny's playroom, they got right to the point of the disharmony in their relationship.

Jenny recalled out loud the harmony that had previously existed between the pair, and asked them if they could find a name for what had come between then now. The three pondered for a little while over naming the "culprit." "The Fighting" didn't seem to satisfy Michaela as an adequate term. But while discussing how the Fighting had interfered with their communication, Michaela suddenly exclaimed, "I know—it's 'The Uncommunication.'"

It seemed in review, that Uncommunication arose when Angela got involved with Hal, in the first serious dating relationship she had enjoyed for many years. The negative spiral of Uncommunication had swept both Michaela and Angela up in it, and there were few areas of their life together that were unaffected. The pressure of Uncommunication had Michaela refusing to be around Hal, talking back all the time, having tantrums, and slamming her body into her mother's in a hurtful way. The pain and bitterness in their mother–daughter relationship had escalated to the point where both were feeling rather hopeless about being able to get along, let alone resolve their differences over the new relationship.

Angela was alarmed by Michaela's apparent possessiveness and jealousy over her new friend, and had begun to despair that she would ever be able to have a romantic life and a close relationship with her daughter at the same time. She was also shocked by the effects of Grumpiness when it overtook Michaela. Her energetic and cheerful daughter, who would usually jump up off the couch to join her mother on an outing to the movies or a store, was now sulking and scowling much of the time. She had become clingy and was even having a hard time enjoying visits with her grandparents and her father.

Michaela sighed audibly and rolled her eyes while listening to her mother. She exclaimed that she didn't want anyone else in their lives, that Hal was a nerd, and that it was all very unfair. But after some more questioning by Jenny about "the unfair effects of the Uncommunication" on her life, Michaela was willing to admit that it was making her angry and sad, and that she missed the closeness with her mother.

For her part, Angela acknowledged that she had been pushing Michaela hard to accept Hal. She reflected that perhaps she could afford her daughter some time to maintain her distance, but she would also continue to expect her to treat Hal with civility. Angela and Michaela agreed somewhat wistfully by the end of the meeting that both wished to reclaim the humor, fun, and sweetness in their old relationship. These qualities were still present, but in scant supply! They were also ready to imagine that some new discoveries might be possible in the relationship that could unfold when the Uncommunication was ousted and good communication was restored at its center.

From this point, Jenny met with either Angela, Michaela, or both about eight times. These meetings were planned cooperatively, depended on who wanted to work or play the next time. Much happened in these meetings that would be of interest to review, in terms of both family and individual work. But for our purposes here, we will have to "fast-forward" to the final session. When it was clear that Michaela had gotten the better of Grumpiness, and that the pair had reclaimed the harmony in their relationship, a last meeting was planned.

LAST MEETING

A narrative of positive change for a young person is often affirmed by a celebratory performance of meaning in the last session. Even when a celebration is not preplanned, the meeting may have a jubilant flavor. In Michaela's case, she requested that her last meeting consist of a small party and a talk with Jenny. Several previous family meetings had entertained the spirit of confirmation, so Michaela, her mother, and Jenny agreed that she would come in alone and make a "consulting" tape with

Jenny. Since she had decided to come in alone, Michaela asked her mother to give her reflections for the meeting to Jenny by phone.

When Michaela arrived and sat down, Jenny offered to bring Angela's input into the conversation. Her mother had indeed phoned to catch Jenny up on the latest developments. Jenny asked Michaela if considering her mother's comments would be a good way to start. Michaela said that it was.

Angela had declared that she appreciated Michaela's newfound maturity, and was delighted to share the return of fun and respectful communication to their lives together. Michaela's monthly weekend visits with her father were turning to the better. Things were still somewhat "distant and rocky" between Michaela and Hal, but last Saturday they had gone out for breakfast and even had a laugh together. Angela had reduced Michaela and Hal's contacts with each other by seeing Hal mainly when her daughter was with either set of her grandparents (with whom she maintained a close relationship). A "key development," Angela felt, was that there was "more acceptance of each other's needs" in the mother–daughter relationship. Michaela listened, nodding sometimes, at times smiling, and at other points looking pensive. She did not wish to comment further, saying, "We talked about this stuff before here and at home." Then she added, "But it was just nice to hear it again."

Jenny offered some soda and cupcakes to celebrate. While they were sipping and munching, Michaela chose to sum up some of the developments she felt good about. She started by telling Jenny about her upcoming weekend. "I'm planning to stay with my grandparents in 2 weeks. I feel really okay at their house now. We played cards and football and dug up roots while Dad got food this weekend, and we also took a hike behind the house. I'm feeling more comfortable, and ready and confident to go to the movies. I don't feel weird any more." She paused thoughtfully. "I haven't been cooperative in the past. I decided I enjoyed being more mature now, except I like to play baby at recess with my friends. I like having laughter in my life, and I like Hal better. He's funny."

Jenny was writing as fast as she could to keep up. "I like having laughter in my life and Hal is funny," she managed to scribble. She wanted once again to confirm the contrast between the fun Michaela was now having and the misery of the Uncommunication, so she asked Michaela, "Before, when that old Uncommunication or some of that misery or uncooperativeness was stronger, you couldn't enjoy his sense of humor so much, right? Wouldn't it kind of get you grouchy?" Michaela readily agreed: "Yeah. And I was more jealous of him, rather than letting him into my life and having fun with him. I was just stuck on the jealousy and how it made me feel—like I should pay him back for doing it to me. Now

I feel like 'Michaela, what were you doing? You were going crazy. You should try to help the problem more than try to make it worse.' "

"You didn't like joining the problem?" Jenny asked. "You got bored with that?" "Yeah," said Michaela.

"Did you feel you were making the problem bigger before?"

"Yeah."

"And how did you decide to free yourself and your mind from it?" Jenny wanted to know. Michaela explained, "I thought about how people feel when you don't treat them nice. Sometimes people treat my friends and me really badly, and it doesn't feel good *at all.*" Jenny was moved by Michaela's capacity for empathy; it had helped her to put herself in Hal's shoes. "And you decided you didn't want to be like that?" Jenny inquired, confirming Michaela's ethic of caring. "You wouldn't like to be a person who makes people feel bad?"

"Yeah, because you would know how they felt," Michaela reiterated. "And you wouldn't want them to feel that way, because you wouldn't like how it felt. If you have some anger you should tell somebody, and not just try to hold it in by doing bad things like body-slamming my mom and stuff."

Jenny couldn't help but be impressed, this time with Michaela's insight. "Ah, ha! That was quite a turnaround!" she said with real delight. "That's really something! What you said fits with this maturity that your mom told us about and that you tell me you're interested in. Looking back, what inspired you to make this turnaround? I'm curious."

"I don't know. I just felt that it was okay to make that turnaround. I'm going to be happy with that, and I'm not going to let the Uncommunication or anything else bad get in my way."

Michaela's resolve made Jenny think of just how far she had come. "Mmm . . . the Uncommunication was pretty bad for a while, wasn't it? I can remember when it was really getting between you and your mom and making you forget how much you meant to each other. Do you remember that?"

"Uh-huh."

"Don't you think that was pretty unfair?"

"Well, yeah, it was!" Michaela continued. "And I think it's nice to do a turnaround once in your life! You know, I know some people who have moved away, who would probably feel really happy I can turn around my bad attitude and make it a good attitude."

Jenny considered asking a question about how the people who had moved away might now comment about Michaela's turnaround. Many such questions whirred around in her mind, but she was more interested in the possibilities for confirming Michaela's burgeoning expertise by pursuing the idea that Michaela's turnaround could inspire other young people, "Wow, maybe you can also inspire some other kids about this! Would it be all right if I find out more about it, so I can tell some other kids about how you turned that around by yourself?" "Okay with me," said Michaela, grinning. She continued to look at Jenny inquiringly.

"Umm, let me guess. . . . Did you make the turnaround because it was more fun and interesting for you to do?"

"Yeah."

"It certainly sounds like you're a lot stronger now, although the Uncommunication was strong before? Is that right?"

"I guess, yeah."

"And what do you think your strength lies in?" Jenny paused. "Is it in being more relaxed? I mean how do people make these turnarounds, once they decide to, and are inspired to?"

Michaela gave this some thought. "Well I don't know, but I have a lot to do, and I don't like spending my time with my mom arguing with her and trying to figure out the answer to the problem. I just want to be easygoing so I can just go and have fun and have a nice life. There's got to be some bad things, but at least you know you're not trying to make the bad things worse."

"You're not getting caught up in these things any more?" Jenny repeated. "Oh, that's great, and, well, I have the feeling that you could make other turnarounds—I mean, that is if you ever needed to. Now you really know that you can do stuff like that." Michaela didn't respond much to this, so Jenny tried another tack, although somewhat awkwardly. "Now that you're even stronger, is it like you're coming back to yourself in a new way?"

"I guess so," Michaela replied tentatively. "You know there was a lot going on then," she went on. "My friends were kind of pushy, and one of my friends got jealous of us 'cause we were in the talent show. I don't want to say it's their fault, but I just felt from seeing them be jealous, I guess, that I had the right to do the same with my mom. Except, you know, they didn't body-slam me or anything."

"Do you think it might have been catching . . . almost like a cold?" Jenny wondered. "Yeah," agreed Michaela, "but it got worse than a cold." "Did it turn into a fever?" Jenny ventured.

Michaela pondered this, nodding in agreement. "But I didn't catch too much from them. I just got the idea that maybe I should do this to punish my mom."

"Maybe just a little germ of it?" Jenny persisted, a bit more entranced by the play of metaphor than by what Michaela had just said. Michaela was graceful enough to humor Jenny by building on this: "And then it spread bigger and bigger and bigger. But I couldn't blame my friends," she said, returning to her own more mature interest in taking responsibility. "I thought, 'Maybe I can punish my mom,' and I kept on doing it—thinking it would work, not even knowing I was thinking this. Then the problem just got worse, and it didn't punish her; it punished me!"

"Mm, yes, you found that out for yourself, didn't you?" Jenny reflected, then paused to compose a question that would clarify Michaela's knowledge. "And of all the important things you have come to know, which is the most important to you?"

Michaela told Jenny the following maxim, with a grin: "Fighting will never help you get your way—it will just help you get in trouble!"

Jenny laughed in recognition. "How clever of you to see through it! I bet it didn't want you to see through it like that. You know how miserable you were; is that what you meant by 'it punished me'?"

"Yeah! If I went over to a friend's house, I couldn't watch TV. I was grounded and had no TV and couldn't go to a friend's house and stuff," recalled Michaela.

"Yuck!" exclaimed Jenny. "That's no way for a kid your age to spend your life, is it?" This time Michaela laughed out loud: "*No, it isn't!*" Then she continued, more reflectively, "I've been thinking—my mom isn't a terrible person. She was punishing me because I was trying to punish her and it didn't work. She isn't like that in real life."

"No, she isn't, is she?" Jenny agreed. "You remembered who she is to you, huh?" Michaela nodded for a while. There was a pause of shared appreciation for Angela. "And how special your relationship is to both of you?" More nods and smiles.

Michaela was quiet. As Jenny turned over the conversation in her mind, she just couldn't help thinking some more about the metaphor of catching a fever of negative emotions, and it reminded her of a story. She asked Michaela whether she wanted to talk more about her and her mom at the moment, or whether she wanted to talk about anything else. Michaela said, "I'm open."

"Well," Jenny said, "do you mind if I come back to something? You know, this catching stuff we were playing with reminds me of a time I caught a bus, and the bus driver was mean and rude to me when I came in, and I sat down hard and bumped the passenger next to me. They glared at me. I was growling and thinking 'People are so mean.' Then I realized that the bad-temperedness was catching. I decided to stop it and make some smiles instead, so I smiled to the person and they smiled back. That was catching too. So I thought, 'What do I want to spread around?' I wonder, did you ever notice anything like that?"

Michaela nodded. "I think it's nice to spread the nice things around, not the bad things, 'cause you don't want a whole busload of grumpy people."

"So you don't want to be on the Grump Bus?"

"Going to Grump Station!" Michaela giggled.

"Did you decide that your destination wasn't Grump Station?"

Jenny and Michaela were laughing so hard at this point that all Michaela could do was choke out, "No, no, no!"

"Well, what's your new destination?"

Michaela took a moment to think and responded earnestly, "I guess . . . trying to get along with people. And trying to have more confidence in myself, and to go to my dad's house, 'cause it is one side of my family and I can't just cut them out of my life. Also, I think I'm gonna sign up for acting, 'cause I think that will get out all my drama."

Jenny was excited about this last idea. "I love it!" she exclaimed happily.

Michaela grinned widely. "Yeah, so you don't have to stay in the house being grumpy and saying the same old lines over and over again."

"That gets boring, doesn't it? Could we share that idea too with some other kids? You're having so many good ideas. What allows you to have such good ideas?"

"Sometimes you may just be doing something and an idea just comes to your head, without even knowing it. It just says, 'Oh I've got an idea. Maybe I can solve this problem.'"

"What makes your mind open and ready to receive these ideas?" Jenny was curious about how Michaela got her ideas.

"I just see things that I figure were the problem." Michaela explained. "Like with my solution over mom and her boyfriend and me. I just pretended in my mind that we were different people, all getting along, and it was really happy."

"Do you mean that you used your pretending mind to imagine how it could be? You imagined it, then it could happen?"

"Yeah."

There was a pause. Michaela looked around the playroom. Jenny was somewhat surprised that Michaela had not said she wanted to play in the sandtray. It was one of her favorites among the play activities she had enjoyed in the past. Aware of the time, Jenny found herself wanting to summarize Michaela's accomplishments in her mind; Michaela had separated her mother from the Uncommunication and regained respect for her. She had also separated herself from the problem, and had done this while taking full responsibility for her own actions. Michaela had accomplished this by putting herself "in the other person's shoes" and inventing other helpful ideas. Jenny thought some more about what had probably been helpful for Michaela. Both Angela and she had been ready and willing to reclaim their old relationship from the Fighting. Michaela had contrasted the undesired consequences of going along with the problem with the kind of person she wanted to be and the kind of relationship she preferred to have with her mother. It seemed that she had been able to see what kind of life was in store for her if the Uncommunication continued. Jenny decided to ask Michaela more about what she had not liked about the effects of the problem, and what she appreciated about her freedom from it now.

Michaela listed the Uncommunication's consequences in review: She disliked not caring about others, punishing others, being miserable, getting grounded, and not watching TV. She liked being able to go out, watching TV, having fun with friends, and acting. As to what kind of person she preferred to be, she was interested in maturity, being easygoing, and having fun.

Jenny checked with Michaela to see if it would be okay for her to summarize the changes she had observed. Gaining Michaela's consent, she began: "When I think back, this is how I saw it. You and your mother got together and found out how the problem was making you both miserable. It was coming between you and making you forget how you usually work things out. After all, you're both usually very clever about getting together and working things out. Did you both decide that you really didn't want to get tricked any more into punishing, as you got tired of that?" "Yes," Michaela said emphatically. "I don't know any kid who loves punishment!"

"What started you thinking again and got you to wake up to what you care about and what really matters to you?" asked Jenny, recalling her own knowledge of the kind of person Michaela had been before the Uncommunication took over.

"I just saw my friends and we'd be happy together," Michaela explained. "We'd get together and have a good time, and I realized I wanted it to be that way with Mom and Hal. I mean, if you just do your best and it doesn't happen, it wouldn't be your fault, 'cause you were trying your hardest."

"Wow, that's an interesting thought! What gave you the idea to give it a chance anyway, to do your best to enjoy yourself?"

"I don't know," Michaela began. "I was just thinking. When I play with my trolls, I get ideas, 'cause its a relaxing thing, you know—it's like you're moving things around, pretending they're talking. I do this with my Barbies too."

Just then Michaela had a brain wave. First she paused, then her face lit up. "Hey, I just got this idea now. If you had a problem, you could pretend that one of them [the toys] was you and you had the problem, and you could act it out. You could play each character, and you could think of ideas and use them. You would have to think how the other person would feel . . . you may think it's a happy ending but you don't know how they'll react to it unless you try it out."

Jenny was delighted by this imaginative idea for figuring out both external consequences of "what would happen" and the internal experience of "how the other person would feel." She wished she had another meeting just to ask Michaela about these ideas, but with so little time remaining, she had to content herself with a few remarks.

"So you'd play it out and see what would happen with different ways?" Jenny repeated. "That's really clever! I wonder what would happen if you tried that." Michaela was already ahead of Jenny, "Yeah. We had a problem at school, and I'm gonna try that idea on it!"

"Well, congratulations!" Jenny said enthusiastically. "You helped yourself solve the problem in a fun way, and I really liked hearing about it! And now you're having even more creative ideas. Let's have a toast to that!" They sipped the last of the raspberry apple soda.

Michaela heard her mother at the door and stood up. "Thanks," she beamed modestly. "Oh, and by the way, thanks for your help."

FINAL THOUGHTS

This interview exemplifies an externalizing therapeutic conversation that wends its way through several significant events and issues in the life of Michaela and her family (Epston, 1993; Freedman & Combs, 1996; White, 1991, 1995). It mingles the discussion of problems in adult terms with playful and child-inclusive language. Many learners have expressed to us and to others (Dickerson & Zimmerman, 1996) their concern that linguistically externalizing a problem in a playful manner might offer an "easy way out" for children, deprive them of insight, and assist them in avoiding responsibility for their part in a problem. We have found it hard to reassure newcomers that what occurs is typically quite the opposite. Perhaps the interview with Michaela presented above can provide an example of this ostensibly counterintuitive occurrence. It is hard to miss how Michaela comfortably assumed responsibility for her part in the Uncommunication. Her re-found self-assurance and knowing perspective about her relationships are evident and endow her astute comments and keenness for celebrating this passage.

EDITORIAL QUESTIONS

Q: *(CS) Jenny and Dean, I was really warmed by the spirit of camaraderie, playfulness, and imagination that Jenny and Michaela em-*

braced! This reminds me of how therapy can be fun and still lead to solid, lasting changes. Among other things, I agreed with your statement about how Michaela accepted more rather than less responsibility with the nonconfrontational externalizing conversations. My sense is that her articulateness provided specific evidence of how she accepted this responsibility. She was able to furnish a lot of nuances and details concerning how she used to participate in the problem lifestyle and how she succeeded in gaining influence over it.

In workshops, my colleague Tom Hicks and I have shown video excerpts of a bright, articulate young boy who successfully and enthusiastically overcame Worry and Withdrawal with externalizing. Frequently workshop attendees comment about his articulateness, and they wonder aloud whether narrative therapies are more suitable for more verbally sophisticated children. I wonder if any readers might have similar concerns. How do the two of you respond to this reaction? Can you describe any examples of what you might have done if Michaela was less verbally expressive, or what you have done with other children who are expressive in "nonverbal" ways?

A: Craig, the two issues you mention in your question are analogous—that is, taking responsibility and verbal sophistication. We have found that when we find a way to communicate fluently with a child, the child is likely to express himself/herself with unique eloquence, as well as to take responsibility for his/her part in the life of the problem. We prefer not to make initial assumptions about a child's "verbal expressiveness," which may reside more in the particular circumstances of social interchange and in the perceptions of the beholder than in objective measures of verbal "abilities." This is not to say that some children are not more or less verbal than others, but that all children can express themselves on their own terms when the conversation is of interest to them, when they have means of communication that suit them, and when their audience is genuinely engaged and appreciative. Michaela, for example, did not strike me (JCF) as a particularly "verbal" child when she first came to therapy. Instead, she appeared rather shy and quiet. She tended to take her time responding to questions, and then to reply with brevity. Remember, Michaela had spent some time meeting with me when she was about 6, and in this earlier phase had chosen play, sandtray, and art therapy media to express herself. She had also enjoyed making conjoint sandtrays with her mother.

Many children "clam up" at the outset of a conversation with an adult, especially if they or someone they care about is in trouble and the adult is focused on that trouble. To label such a child as "verbally unsophisticated" would be an unfortunate error. It is easy to fall into the trap of trying to "pry" a child open to get at what hurts—an approach that the child is likely to resist. It is better to immerse the "clam" of noncommunication between adult and child in the warm and nurturing waters of externalizing play and imagination, and let it open up of its own accord. The onus rests on us to provide an environment that makes communication possible for children, whether by providing alternative means of expression or by our skill in meeting children with language that is developmentally well matched. As we do when conversing with a person of any age, instead of trying to get a child to "open up," we strive for a conversation that truly engages the interest of both parties.

Mutual immersion in fruitful conversation may include both verbal and nonverbal approaches. Expressive arts and family or individual play therapy methods include warmup games, drawing, cartoons, sculpting, sandplay, dramatic role play, movement, puppet theater, and so forth (Barragar-Dunne, 1992; Freeman et al., 1997). Scaling questions, which rate relative influence concretely, are also very useful. A therapist's questions, metaphors, stories, or pictures help provide new avenues, like a trellis for the vines of a child's imagination to grow on. Whatever media are employed should be intended to evoke a child's imagination and resourcefulness. When children open up in this way, their eloquence about their relationships with problems may really surprise us.

An avenue we have explored that starts conversational flow (Freeman et al., 1997) is to spend time getting to know a child apart from a problem, with questions such as these: "Would it be okay with everyone if I spent a bit of time getting to know [name of child] apart from his problem? We can return to the problem, but I'd rather get to know [name] naturally than have the problem define her [or him] from the start." Then we inquire about the child's interests, qualities, abilities, what others appreciate about her/him, and so on. Not only do we make a friendly connection with the child, but when we return to the problem we have information about resources (such as a wonderful imagination) that the child might have to tackle the problem, or that we might weave together into an alternative story.

Q: (DN) Jenny and Dean, in the chapter you mention that Jenny met with Angela, Michaela, or both about eight times. How do you decide who is going to meet with whom and for how long? I am asked this question a great deal with therapists I supervise/train—particularly as it applies to working with children and when to include or not to include parents.

A: The decisions of "who to meet with" and "how long to meet," like others in a narrative therapy, are made collaboratively. Our approach to this collaboration might generally be described as "child-focused family therapy." Both of us typically hold conjoint sessions with various family members. Even if an individual approach is agreed upon, regular collateral sessions with parents and communication with other significant people in a child's life typically take place.

Decisions about who shall meet together are made in consultation with the family. Usually, on first contact, we arrange to talk with significant caretakers on the phone about who is concerned about the problem and should come in. Conference calls are useful when there are two parents. The parents or other caretakers may then seek the child's preferences if this seems appropriate. We usually say that we meet with the whole family first, but are interested in meeting the needs of the family and would like to consult with them about what would be most useful. Many families have expressed appreciation for an ongoing flexibility in addressing their interests and needs. Sometimes the adults have strong opinions about who should be present throughout therapy or at a particular session; sometimes they want our opinion. The children may also express strong preferences. We try to respect people's wishes, and to trust their sense of what is appropriate. Persons of any age can be asked about the reasons for their preferences, and these should be addressed respectfully.

We think that who is included depends partly on the nature of the problem and where it occurs, although this may take some time to assess. If, for example, the problem is defined as Sibling Squabbles, it makes sense to have the siblings come in. If the problem concerns one child, and the parents think that this child would be too distracted by younger children in a first session, we would give seeing just the parents and this child a try. Parents may want to come in alone to address concerns that they would prefer not to discuss in front of children. At times, it is useful to meet alone with a child or her/his parent(s).[2]

Ideally, a child can "perform new meanings" in the presence of the family, but at times the child's transition from "being a problem" to "having power over the problem" is facilitated by a chance to meet first with just the therapist as an audience. Also, the parents' response to the

---

[2]We generally meet alone with a child if she/he was traumatized, particularly if the child is now living with a new family—foster parents or relatives (M. Rossoff, personal communication, November 24, 1996). Individual therapy provides a place for the child to talk about the trauma and focus on herself/himself without having to worry about the negative impact of the painful story on others. If the child has been placed in another family, individual therapy can provide a time for the child to talk about the loss of the original family without having to worry about hurting the feelings of the new caregivers. Even in this instance, periodic meetings with the child's new family that focus on supporting new developments are very helpful.

child's new status may be more welcoming if they have had a chance to revise a problem-saturated view of their child while meeting separately with the therapist.

Alternative narratives co-authored in therapy are typically circulated to the significant people in a child's life (White & Epston, 1990). The duration of therapy can be shortened by such "public practices" (Lobovits et al., 1995). Let's consider that when a child is brought to therapy, he/she is typically seen by the therapist for only 1 hour in the week. The rest of the time, he/she is in contact with different influential people in other settings. Places such as school or home are fostered as part of a "brief therapy" environment—for example, through phone contact or letters. Through their participation in the ongoing narrative, parents, siblings, and others can identify strengths and abilities the child may not have realized that anyone noticed. New understandings develop about the problem's influences and strategies for resisting it. Many of these understandings may have already emerged in the family, among friends, or at school, but were previously overlooked or taken for granted.

When we develop narratives collaboratively with parents, siblings, and teachers, even fledgling developments that emerge in therapy sessions can be made more notable to all concerned through the week. Conversely, if subtle transformations that take place at home and school are recognized and fed back to the therapy sessions, they can be celebrated and thus attain durability. Most importantly, others in the family and community have the opportunity to participate in reflections and rituals that support a family's preferred narrative (White, 1995).

ACKNOWLEDGMENTS

We wish to express our gratitude to David Epston for his invaluable assistance and inspiration, and to Margaret Rossoff for her help in answering the "Editorial Questions." We hope that through their consent to share their story in this public forum, Michaela and Angela gain the altruistic satisfaction of making a contribution to other mothers and daughters caught up in Uncommunication. However, we feel that through the inspiration and ideas they have provided to us, we may have been the primary beneficiaries of their generosity.

REFERENCES

Adams-Westcott, J., & Isenbart, D. (1996). Creating preferred relationships: The politics of recovery from child abuse. *Journal of Systemic Therapies,* *15*(1), 13–30.

Barragar-Dunne, P. (1992). *The narrative therapist and the arts*. Los Angeles: Possibility Press (Drama Institute of Los Angeles).

Dickerson, V. C., & Zimmerman, J. L. (1993). A narrative approach to families with adolescents. In S. Friedman (Ed.), *The new language of change: Constructive collaboration in psychotherapy* (pp. 226–250). New York: Guilford Press.

Dickerson, V. C., & Zimmerman, J. L. (1996). Myth, misconceptions, and a word or two about politics. *Journal of Systemic Therapies, 15*(1), 79–88.

Durrant, M. (1989). Temper taming: An approach to children's temper problems—revisited. *Dulwich Centre Newsletter*, No. 3, 1–11.

Epston, D. (1989). Temper tantrum parties: Saving face, losing face, or going off your face. *Dulwich Centre Newsletter*, No. 3, 12–26. (Reprinted in *Retracing the past: Collected and selected papers revisited*, edited by M. White & D. Epston, 1997, Adelaide, South Australia: Dulwich Centre Publications.)

Epston, D. (1993). Internalizing discourses versus externalizing discourses. In S. Gilligan & R. Price (Eds.), *Therapeutic conversations* (pp. 161–177). New York: Norton.

Epston, D., & White, M. (1990). Consulting your consultants: The documentation of alternative knowledges. *Dulwich Centre Newsletter*, No. 4, 25–35.

Epston, D., & White, M. (1995). "Ben," consulting your consultants: A means to the co-construction of alternative knowledges. In S. Friedman (Ed.), *The reflecting team in action: Collaborative practice in family therapy* (pp. 277–313). New York: Guilford Press.

Freedman, J., & Combs, G. (1996). *Narrative therapy: The social construction of preferred realities*. New York: Norton.

Freeman, J. C., Epston, D., & Lobovits, D. H. (1997). *Playful approaches to serious problems: Narrative therapy with children and their families*. New York: Norton.

Freeman, J. C., & Lobovits, D. H. (1993). The turtle with wings. In S. Friedman (Ed.), *The new language of change: Constructive collaboration in psychotherapy* (pp. 188–225). New York: Guilford Press.

Lobovits, D. H., Maisel, R., & Freeman, J. C. (1995). Public practices: An ethic of circulation. In S. Friedman (Ed.), *The reflecting team in action: Collaborative practice in family therapy* (pp. 223–257). New York: Guilford Press.

Nylund, D., & Corsiglia, V. (1996). From deficits to special abilities: Working narratively with children labeled "ADHD." In M. Hoyt (Ed.), *Constructive therapies* (Vol. 2, pp. 163–183). New York: Guilford Press.

Pinderhughes, E. (1989). *Understanding race, ethnicity, and power: The key to efficacy in clinical practice*. New York: Free Press.

Rosenwald, G. C., & Ochberg, R. L. (Eds.). (1992). *Storied lives: The cultural politics of self-understanding*. New Haven, CT: Yale University Press.

Stacey, K., & Loptson, C. (1995). Children should be seen and not heard?: Questioning the unquestioned. *Journal of Systemic Therapies, 14*(4), 16–32.

Tamasese, K., & Waldegrave, C. (1993). Cultural and gender accountability in the "just therapy" approach. *Journal of Feminist Family Therapy, 5*(2), 29–45.

van Gennep, A. (1960). *The rites of passage* (M. B. Vizedom & G. Caffee, Trans.). Chicago: University of Chicago Press.

Waldegrave, C. (1992). Psychology, politics and the loss of the welfare state. *New Zealand Psychological Society Bulletin, 74,* 14–21.

White, M. (1985). Fear busting and monster taming: An approach to the fears of young children. *Dulwich Centre Review.* (Reprinted in *Retracing the past: Collected and selected papers revisited,* edited by M. White & D. Epston, 1997, Adelaide, South Australia: Dulwich Centre Publications.)

White, M. (1989). Pseudo-encopresis: From avalanche to victory, from vicious to virtuous cycles. (Reprinted in *Retracing the past: Collected and selected papers revisited,* edited by M. White & D. Epston, 1997, Adelaide, South Australia: Dulwich Centre Publications.

White, M. (1991). Deconstruction and therapy. *Dulwich Centre Newsletter,* No. 3, 21–40.

White, M. (1995). Reflecting teamwork as definitional ceremony. In M. White, *Re-authoring lives: Interviews and essays* (pp. 172–198). Adelaide, South Australia: Dulwich Centre Publications.

White, M., & Epston, D. (1990). *Narrative means to therapeutic ends.* New York: Norton.

8

Listening with Your "Heart Ears" and Other Ways Young People Can Escape the Effects of Sexual Abuse

JANET ADAMS-WESTCOTT
CHERYL DOBBINS

Our work with families who have experienced child sexual abuse has evolved over the past decade. Ten years ago, our therapy was informed by family systems ideas that located problems in dysfunctional relationships. We assumed an expert stance and intervened by shifting patterns of interaction and creating more appropriate boundaries between parents and children.

Though we practiced family systems therapy, we agreed with feminist critiques about the failure of the field to adequately address issues of power (see, e.g., Flaskas & Humphreys, 1993). We were attracted to narrative approaches because they allowed us to address the patriarchal culture that supports abuse of women by men. Instead of locating problems inside people or in relationships between people, we began to locate the problem in restraining beliefs, patterns of interaction, and cultural expectations and practices that create vulnerability to abuse (Adams-Westcott & Isenbart, 1990).

We were immediately struck by the positive effects of this approach. Because it involves consideration of cultural expectations and practices, this new way of thinking allowed us to address issues of power in a way that invited accountability (Jenkins, 1990). Parents began to recognize that they could choose either to continue to cooperate with these restraints or assume personal responsibility for challenging abuse and its effects. The young people we worked with began to understand that although they had been victimized, they did not have to adopt a "victim" story. We quickly discovered that we could develop more collaborative relationships with people who consulted with us by giving up our expert stance and encouraging family members to develop their own expertise. As the focus of our work shifted from confronting dysfunction to highlighting strengths and progress, we began to access our own resources as people and experience new generativity as therapists.

This chapter demonstrates our use of narrative therapy to help children and adolescents challenge abuse-dominated stories and develop more validating stories about themselves. We are privileged to share the story of Krystal, who learned to listen with her "heart ears" and escape the effects of abuse.[1]

PRIVILEGING LIVED EXPERIENCE

Narrative approaches assume that all of us are rich in "lived experience" (White & Epston, 1990). Even people who have lived what others might perceive as extremely impoverished lives have a multitude of everyday experiences. Beginning in childhood, we begin to make sense out of these experiences by organizing them into narratives or stories about ourselves and our relationships. We interpret subsequent life events within the "plots" that develop from these stories. We ascribe meaning to experiences that support the stories. Experiences that contradict the stories are either not noticed or are interpreted in a manner consistent with the plots. Within the frameworks created by our stories, we interpret and respond to our experiences in ways that either open up possibilities or limit the choices we perceive to be available to us. Through our behavior, we invite other people to interact with us in a manner that perpetuates our stories about who we are as persons.

---

[1]We want to express our sincere appreciation to Krystal and her mother for allowing us to share their experiences. Names and other details have been changed to protect the family's confidentiality.

Children and adolescents who have been victims of child sexual assault have lived experiences that include violation and exploitation. The experience of sexual assault is one of profound powerlessness and helplessness that can affect young people in a variety of ways. For many young people, this experience of being overpowered and controlled by another invites them to feel out of control of their own feelings or behaviors (Durrant & Kowalski, 1990). They may be overcome by problems such as fear, anger, sexual urges, restrictive or binge eating, running away, misuse of drugs and alcohol, or the like. They may react in ways to try to regain some sense of control in their lives, such as withdrawing from friends or family, "spacing out," or excelling in some area (academics, athletics, or art).

The way in which a young person interprets the experience of abuse can have a profound impact on her story about herself.[2] Children and adolescents who have experienced sexual assault are at risk for developing negative stories about themselves that are dominated by the experience of abuse and its effects (Durrant, 1987; Durrant & Kowalski, 1990; White, 1995). Many of the young people we have met in our work developed disqualifying stories. These stories prevented them from noticing examples of their competence, talents, or accomplishments, and invited them to explain away experiences of being treated by other people in a caring, worthwhile, or respectful manner (Adams-Westcott, Dafforn, & Sterne, 1993).

A narrative approach does not assume that all children who experience sexual assault begin to interpret their lived experiences through an abuse-dominated lens (Durrant & Kowalski, 1990). We have worked with some young people who experienced victimization but did not begin to story themselves as "victims." These children and adolescents had supportive people in their lives who treated them with compassion and helped them punctuate their courage in challenging secrecy and disclosing the abuse. These people helped the young persons understand that they were not responsible for what happened to them. Any changes in emotions or behavior the young persons might be experiencing were perceived as temporary and understandable reactions to such a negative experience.

In addition to the confusing and painful experience of being touched in a sexual way, some young people are subjected to disempowering stories imposed on them by the perpetrators. A perpetrator may invalidate a child's experience by denying that the abuse ever occurred

---

[2]We choose to use feminine pronouns because the majority of young people who have consulted us are girls. We recognize that from 10% to 13% of adult men were abused as children (Finkelhor, 1994).

(Hoke, Sykes, & Winn, 1989). The young person may be told that she is responsible for or deserving of the abuse. She may be encouraged to experience self-blame and self-hate and to engage in self-punishing behaviors. We have worked with young people who were further disqualified by the perpetrators' use of power tactics, such as withdrawal of affection, surveillance, intimidation, threats, or torture (see Stewart, 1991, for a discussion of overpowering practices). Children who have had meaning imposed on them in these ways often have difficulty trusting their own experiences.

Abuse-dominated stories may be reinforced by the ways in which other people react to the effects of abuse. The young person who is experiencing her emotions or behavior as out of control may be responded to in negative ways by important people in her life. A vicious cycle may develop that inadvertently perpetuates the experience of powerlessness and self-hate (Durrant & Kowalski, 1990). For example, I (JAW) worked with an 8-year-old girl who had been removed from her foster home and placed in a children's shelter after her foster parents discovered she was touching herself in a sexual way. The foster parents believed that masturbation was sinful and used corporal punishment to discourage the behavior. The girl had difficulty stopping the behavior and began to see herself as "a bad person" who must have deserved to be abused by her stepfather. The foster parents reinforced this view by interpreting any transgression (e.g., forgetting to feed the dog) as more evidence that she was "bad."

Reactions to disclosure also often have a significant impact on a young person's understanding of abuse and its effects (Adams-Westcott & Isenbart, 1990). Children's attempts to tell adults about their experiences of abuse are often tentative. A child may interpret an adult's failure to understand in ways that reinforce the abuse-dominated story. When the perpetrator is a family member, the reactions of the nonoffending parent(s) appear to be particularly important. Unfortunately, some parents are too overwhelmed by the discovery that a trusted relative has assaulted their child to be able to help the young person make sense of the experience in a way that challenges the abuse-dominated story. They experience themselves as helpless and powerless, and do not see themselves as able to help the child experience some sense of mastery over her emotions and behaviors. We have worked with some parents who were themselves so influenced by the perpetrator's story that they refused to acknowledge the authenticity of their child's disclosure or to validate her experience. Other parents believe that the child has experienced abuse, but do not believe that the family member identified by the child as the perpetrator committed the offense.

Popular literature about child sexual abuse and the traditional psychiatric models on which much of this literature is based have the potential to reinforce a negative story about the self. These models assume that children who experience abuse inevitably suffer long-term emotional and interpersonal difficulties, and prescribe a specific set of steps that are necessary to help the children recover. Important people in a child's life who understand abuse within this framework may begin to look for "problems" and inadvertently invite their development. They may interpret the young person's reactions to life transitions as evidence of "psychopathology." Over time, the young person may begin to pathologize herself (Durrant & Kowalski, 1990).

Cultural expectations also influence the story the young person develops about herself (Freedman & Combs, 1996a). How the young person makes sense out of the abuse and its effects is influenced by the ideas she has been exposed to about what it means to be male or female in our society. Like many other young women in our culture, the girls we have worked with who have experienced abuse are influenced by the belief that they should give up their own voices and value the preferences of others (Jordan, Kaplan, Miller, Stiver, & Surrey, 1991; Taylor, Gilligan, & Sullivan, 1995). Young women in Western culture are constantly subjected to sexualized images of what they are supposed to look like in order to be attractive to men. Attempts by young women to measure up to this unrealistic ideal have contributed to the culture's current preoccupation with physical appearance, weight, and eating (Madigan & Epston, 1995; Zimmerman & Dickerson, 1994).

These gender stories can have profound effects on young people who have experienced sexual assault. Their lack of entitlement puts them at risk for exploitation in other relationships. Some adolescents begin to seek connection through sexualized behavior. To try to achieve cultural ideals of attractiveness, they may subject themselves to power tactics such as surveillance and comparison that were used by their perpetrators. It is not surprising that young people who have experienced sexual assault are overrepresented among those presenting for treatment for anorexia nervosa and bulimia nervosa (Wonderlich et al., 1996).

The personal story that a young person who has experienced abuse develops about herself is influenced by cultural stories that confuse intimacy, sex, and violence. One of the dominant discourses about sexuality in Western culture is that the male sexual drive is intense and compelling. This view legitimizes the use by men of certain power tactics to satisfy these urges. Many explanations for incest are situated within this discourse. For example, some theorists have argued that a father who feels inadequate "naturally" turns to his daughter if his wife is sexually unavailable. Such explanations have been challenged by feminist and social constructionist writers (e.g., Hare-Mustin, 1991). Sanders (1988;

see also Liske, 1993) has argued that what we call "sexual abuse" is not a sexual experience at all, but a form of violence. He points out that we do not refer to being assaulted with a bat as "baseball." He believes that the term "genital assault" reflects the experience of the person who has been victimized.

The cultural perception that the experience of assault is a "sexual" experience influences the story the young person develops about herself. Many children and adolescents who have been sexually assaulted begin to experience themselves as "dirty." They feel culpable for having participated in such reprehensible behavior. Many young people blame themselves because their bodies responded with pleasure or because they believe they should have been able to stop the abuse. This self-blame can invite a young person to isolate herself or to engage in self-injurious behaviors. Interpreting their experience within a cultural story that perceives abuse as violence rather than as sex might allow these young people to experience more understanding and less blame from both themselves and others (Adams-Westcott & Isenbart, 1996).

Intervention by the child abuse system can have either a positive or a negative impact on the child's story about herself. Too often, the impact is negative. Although there has been some accommodation for children, the court system (at least in the United States) uses adversarial processes that were designed for adults. The past decade has witnessed the development of children's advocacy centers for the purpose of minimizing the "secondary victimization" experienced by children and adolescents who have already experienced abuse and neglect. These centers utilize specially trained medical and law enforcement personnel to talk to children about their experiences of abuse and to prepare them for possible participation in the legal process. Practices designed to serve the "best interest of the child" have been developed to help young people experience a sense of mastery and support.[3] Despite these developments, many of the children with whom we have worked described feeling even more powerless after repeatedly discussing the details of the abuse, submitting to a gynecological exam, and testifying in court.

DEVELOPING MORE VALIDATING STORIES

Our work with young people who have experienced child sexual abuse is influenced by the narrative approach developed by Michael White, David Epston, and their colleagues (see, e.g., Freedman & Combs,

[3]Most often, the "best interest of the child" is determined by adults, without consultation from the children these practices were designed to assist. We are interested in developing practices that are more accountable to young people.

1996b; White, 1995; White & Epston, 1990; Zimmerman & Dickerson, 1996). Though much of our work as narrative therapists takes place in conversation, intervention takes place in the world of experience. As narrative therapists, we are interested in helping people create lived experiences in their everyday lives that support more preferred stories about who they are as persons.

The focus on lived experience makes narrative therapy particularly effective for children who have not yet developed the skills to use language to describe their experiences. Narrative therapists use many expressive arts (painting, drawing, sculpture, mask and puppet making, sandtray drama, puppet theater, storytelling, music, dance, etc.) to help children (1) express their experiences, (2) separate from problem stories, and (3) perform more preferred stories (see Barragar-Dunne, 1992, and Freeman & Lobovits, 1993).

Abuse-dominated stories rob young people of the experience of competence, agency, or compassion for themselves. Interventions that invite a young person to separate herself from such a disqualifying story allow her to begin to identify more validating experiences in the past and present.

The first meeting with the young person provides an important opportunity to help her begin to separate from the abuse-dominated story.[4] White and Epston (1990) discuss the importance of joining with people as unique individuals before talking to them about the problems that bring them into therapy. When meeting a young person for the first time, we make a special effort to learn what she values in life. We ask about her friends, teachers, interests, pets, favorite subjects in school, and the like. We are interested in beginning to discover those aspects of her everyday life that are not dominated by abuse and its effects. We also listen for experiences she might describe of people whose view of her is not influenced by the abuse-dominated story.

The process of separating the young person from the abuse-dominated story is facilitated by experiences that externalize the effects of abuse. "Externalizing conversations" use language or activities to locate the problem outside the person (Epston & White, 1990). In work with young children, the problem may be personified by giving it a name and representing it visually through a drawing or some other nonverbal ex-

---

[4]Our work is influenced by the rites-of-passage analogy. This model views change as a cycle of separating from old ways of being that no longer fit the person, experimenting with new ways of being, and incorporating these new ways of being into the person's story about the self. Within the context of this analogy, we assume that a young person had moments prior to her coming to therapy that were not completely defined by the abuse-dominant story. We ask questions to identify the changes that created a context for the abuse to be disclosed.

pression. The particular description externalized is selected from the young person's language or nonverbal expression of her experience. Externalized descriptions often evolve over the course of therapy. We may externalize the problem; the effects of the problem; problem stories; or beliefs, patterns of interaction, cultural expectations, and practices that support problem stories.

We are interested in helping young people experience mastery and competence. As such, our work is sensitive to practices that might invite experiences of powerlessness or helplessness. As a result, we do not ask children to recount the details of how they were assaulted. We agree with Durrant (1987) and White (1995) that approaches to therapy that require people to relive their experiences of being assaulted replicate the experience of powerlessless and have the potential to be retraumatizing. We might tell a young person we are meeting for the first time:

> "Your mother told me that your stepfather touched you in a confusing and hurtful way. I'm really sorry that he hurt you. I understand that you told the police detective, the social worker, and the doctor how he touched you. I'm not going to ask you to tell me what happened. I've talked to a lot of kids who have been touched by adults in confusing and hurtful ways. Even after they get to know me, a lot of the kids I work with never talk to me about how they were assaulted. Some of the kids I work with do decide that it's helpful to talk to someone about what happened to them. Those kids may decide to talk to me or to another person they trust."

Although we are careful to avoid interventions that might invite the young person to re-experience trauma, we are equally careful to provide opportunities to validate the young person's experience. During the first meeting we begin to talk about abuse as an experience that happened in the *past,* and that may continue to have effects in the *present,* but that does not have to continue to affect the young person in the *future.* We explain that we are curious about whether what happened to her in the past still "bugs" her today. We begin to externalize the effects of abuse by inviting the young person to either talk about these effects or communicate her experience in nonverbal ways. One 8-year-old drew a picture of a little girl with a tear in her eye. She wrote the words "mad," "sad," "scared," and "weird" in cartoon-like balloons to illustrate the girl's experience. Other children have used puppets, a dollhouse, or a sandtray to act out the effects of abuse. Adolescents have created collages with concentric circles that represent the abuse-dominated story, how the abuse continues to affect them today, and what their future will look like when they have escaped the effects of abuse.

Once we have developed an externalized verbal or nonverbal description of the way the abuse has affected the young person and her family, we begin to ask questions that locate examples of times in the past and present when she resisted the effects of abuse. We might discover times when she overcame fear and secrecy and told someone about the abuse; times when she was invited by the perpetrator to blame herself for the abuse, but recognized that he was responsible; times when she overcame the idea that girls should give up their voices, and shared her thoughts and feelings; times when she refused to be taken advantage of in a relationship; times when she recognized an accomplishment; or times when she was treated as a person of worth by someone she admired and respected.

Locating experiences that contradict the abuse-dominated story invites the young person to begin to access her own self-knowledge. Through questions, play, or drama, we invite young people to show us (and themselves) how they were able to accomplish these achievements. In contrast to the externalized language we use when we speak about problems, we use "internalizing language" that locates the qualities and skills that support these accomplishments inside the young person (Zimmerman et al., 1995).

We have found that children who have been severely abused often have difficulty internalizing positive developments. From the time of our first meeting, we are always listening for examples of experiences they have had with people who recognize these developments. Inviting a young person to take the perspective of a supportive teacher, Scout leader, foster parent, or friend helps her begin to recognize these positive qualities in herself. Acting out the experience of these supportive people through play allows the young person to see herself through their eyes and to experience herself as a person of worth (White, 1988c, 1995).

White (1995; White & Epston, 1990) refers to this process of externalizing the problem and internalizing positive qualities and developments as "re-authoring." With young people who have experienced abuse, we are interested in helping them appreciate unique outcomes as examples of courage and resistance to continued exploitation. With children, externalizing the effects of abuse is often sufficient to begin the re-authoring process. With many of the adolescents we have seen, the re-authoring process is facilitated by questions and activities that externalize the abuse-dominated story. We ask questions about how a young person got recruited into believing such a negative story about herself. As part of this process, we may externalize the story that was told by the offender about the young person, or the power tactics he used to keep her from challenging his view. We may externalize cultural expectations that support the abuse-dominated story. We may ask an adolescent to consider via conversation or artwork those beliefs about gender, sexuality, appearance, and eating that are influencing her story about herself. The process of separating these beliefs allows the young person to evaluate their effects and decide if they fit her preferences.

SUPPORTING PREFERRED STORIES

As the young person begins to re-author her story, therapy becomes a context to help her add to her lived experiences, both inside and outside the consultation room, in ways that support the more validating story. Sharing the changes she is making with important people in her life helps her challenge secrecy and isolation, and invites them to interact with her in ways that support the emerging story.

Whenever possible, we involve supportive parents in therapy sessions with their children.[5] Participating in activities that externalize the effects of abuse invites a parent to interpret problems experienced by a child as a temporary effect of the experience of abuse. The parent can then identify interactions that support the abuse-dominated story and can choose to interact with the child in more validating ways. In responding to questions about past successes or positive developments the parent has witnessed, the parent helps the child discover examples of courage and competence in her everyday life.

When parents are not supportive, young persons can identify significant people to invite to therapy sessions, team meetings, or celebrations. Some children we work with invite foster parents to participate in ongoing therapy sessions. Other children invite people to serve on a "nurturing team" (White, 1995). Members of this team meet one or more times to develop a plan to help the young person challenge the effects of abuse. Other children invite significant people to attend celebrations of positive developments in their lives. Including child abuse professionals assigned to a child in team meetings or celebrations catches them up with the child's challenges and accomplishments, and helps them make recommendations that support her preferences.

Therapy groups can provide a powerful context to help young people escape isolation and rediscover their competence (Adams-Westcott & Isenbart, 1995). Group members share their expertise by consulting with each other about how they were able to overcome secrecy and escape the effects of abuse (Epston & White, 1990). One group of 10- to 12-year-old girls decided to make a video about their experiences, using

---

[5]We choose to work with nonoffending parents and children separately when the parents are themselves so influenced by the effects of abuse that they are interacting with the children in disqualifying ways. We invite these parents to consider how abuse is affecting them as people, partners, and parents. We resume family sessions when the parents begin to challenge the way the abuse affects their interactions with their children.

a television talk show format. Prior to the taping, they listed questions they were interested in discussing. For example, one girl suggested that they discuss how they decided to tell someone about the abuse. The therapist (CD) suggested questions that were chosen to extend the story and punctuate each young person's agency in escaping abuse. Questions group members decided they were interested in discussing were added to the list:

> What did you say to yourself to help you overcome secrecy?
> How did you decide to listen to yourself and trust yourself?
> What does it mean about who you are as a person that you were able to tell someone about the abuse?
> Who do you know who would be least surprised to discover that you stood up for yourself in this way?

Over time, this talk show format evolved into a ritual that helped members document their strengths and talents. When a member was approaching "graduation" from the group, other members would spend time preparing interview questions. One member would assume the role of host and interview the girl who was leaving about what she did to escape the effects of abuse. Other members of the group served as the audience who witnessed her discussing these victories. This conversation was taped and given to the girl who was graduating to share with significant people in her life. The tape provided a reminder of her accomplishments that could be reviewed during any difficult times she might experience in the future. Group members observing the interview learned from the graduate's experience. The observing position helped them reflect back on their own stories and re-experience the courage and strength they demonstrated in challenging abuse and its effects.

KRYSTAL'S STORY: LISTENING WITH YOUR "HEART EARS"

When I (Cheryl) met 9-year-old Krystal for the first time, she and her family appeared overwhelmed by worry. Her family had moved in with friends while her parents worked on completing a house they were building in a nearby community. A month after the move, the two young girls living in the home disclosed that Krystal's 14-year-old half-brother was molesting them.[6] In response to questions from child protective services investigators, Krystal revealed that he had been abusing

---

[6]Krystal's half-brother and parents participated in a program for adolescent boys who have molested younger children.

her for some time prior to the move. Following the discovery of the abuse, the family moved to a motel until their house was habitable. Krystal's brother was sent to live with grandparents.

Krystal's mother began sharing her worries from the moment we were first introduced. Given that her car was always breaking down, how was she going to get her children to school and counseling? Would protective services disapprove of the fact that Krystal and her brother rode to school in the same car? Could her son spend time with the family during the upcoming holidays? Would Krystal suffer any long-term damage as a result of the abuse? How could she help her son? What should she do about her husband's fury toward him?

After listening to her mom's worries, I began to ask questions to get to know Krystal as a person. Her mother described Krystal as a good student and talented artist. She stated that before the abuse Krystal sang and laughed all the time. Krystal interjected a little song that made everybody laugh. She admitted that she had not felt like singing for some time, and that no one in the family was laughing very much because they were worried about all this stuff. The mother shared her concern that Krystal worried about everybody else's feelings and didn't pay attention to her own. She suggested that it might be best for Krystal to talk to me alone.

After her mom left, Krystal started drawing a picture, and I asked if I could ask her some questions while she was drawing. She agreed, and I began to ask questions that externalized worry as one effect of abuse. "What is worry getting the people in your family to do? What is worry keeping people from doing? How is worry keeping you from having fun and singing?"

In the second appointment, I continued to ask questions to externalize worry. Mom commented that Krystal often tried to worry for her parents about things like money and their living arrangements. She let Krystal know that they could handle worry by themselves and did not need her help. Krystal shared a "big worry" with her mother. She explained that she had overheard her mother telling someone that her dad was so mad at her brother that he could kill him. Her mother reassured Krystal that although her father was very angry with her brother for molesting Krystal and her friends, he would never really hurt her brother.

After her mother left the room, Krystal asked to play with the sandtray. She buried a treasure chest in the sand. Next she arranged some furniture in the sand and surrounded it with a fence and some trees. She explained, "This is like my family before. We had a happy little family, and then the sexual abuse was like a tornado." She then knocked over the furniture and trees, scattered them around, and announced, "This is what our family is like now." Next she got three dolls and explained, "This is my mom and dad and me, and we are unburying the hidden treasure." The conversation then turned to how she could create a map to guide her in uncovering these treasures.

We continued our work together, meeting for a total of eight times over the course of a year. Krystal also attended five sessions of a 12-week therapy group for preadolescent girls who had experienced abuse. The family's tenuous economic situation, unstable living arrangements, and unreliable automobile precluded her regular attendance.

I had not heard from the family for several weeks when Krystal's mother called to schedule an appointment. Her mother explained that she had received a call from the counselor at school, informing her that during the past few weeks Krystal had been talking to her on a regular basis. During these conversations, Krystal had told her school counselor how much she missed going to therapy. Her mother was surprised to hear this, given that Krystal appeared to be doing well, her sense of humor was back, and she was singing all the time. When she talked to Krystal about the telephone call from the counselor, her mother was even more surprised to discover that Krystal did not think it was fair that her brother got to continue going to counseling and she did not. The following conversation is an excerpt from the fifth session. The session began with Cheryl and Krystal having a long discussion about their pets:

CHERYL: I'm wondering: Do you think worry bothers dogs?

KRYSTAL: Yeah.

CHERYL: Do you have any dogs that are bothered by worry?

KRYSTAL: Babe, he worries that we are going to get rid of him. He's an inside dog and he chews up a lot of stuff. We yell at him, like, "No, don't do that, Babe!" And he gets in the trash and we yell at him for doing that. He probably worries he's gonna get kicked out.

CHERYL: I understand that you are beginning to be the kind of person who notices when worry bothers people too.

KRYSTAL: My friend Sheila is worried.

CHERYL: Worry is bothering Sheila? I bet you remember some of the things that helped you get rid of worry.

KRYSTAL: A lot of my friends, they could tell when I was worried. I didn't really tell them why. I told them it was family problems and that was it. They played with me, and it made me feel better because I had someone to do something with. They ate lunch by me and stuff.

CHERYL: So they just spent time with you?

KRYSTAL: That's what I do with Sheila, play with her a lot. Her and her boyfriend are getting ready to break up, and I'm trying to help her with that.

CHERYL: One thing I've learned about you is that you're the kind of person who likes to help others. Can you see why I might think that about you?

We then had a conversation about calling Janet (JAW) on the phone and inviting her to join us. I had previously informed Krystal and her mother of my plan to move out of state, and they agreed to continue consulting with Janet. The conversation continued, following introductions:

CHERYL: Krystal was telling me how she's helping a friend of hers who's got really kind of a big worry. So Krystal has started to notice a whole lot of things about worry.

JANET: You've learned some things about worry by helping your friend?

KRYSTAL: (Nods "yes")

CHERYL: The last time I saw Krystal was in the summer.

KRYSTAL: I was 9 then. Now I'm 10.

CHERYL: So one of the big things we talked about at that time was how sometimes worry really just got so big that it took over Krystal's life. (To Krystal) Worry and sadness went together?

KRYSTAL: (Nods "yes")

CHERYL: Sometimes those two things would work together so it seemed like they took over her whole life, but other times the worry wasn't quite so big any more.

JANET: What helped shrink worry?

KRYSTAL: I pushed it away.

JANET: How did you do that?

KRYSTAL: With my magic wand that Cheryl gave me. [We had made a magic wand in an earlier session.]

JANET: How did you use the wand to push it away?

KRYSTAL: I just picked up the wand one day and said, "Go away!"

JANET: Did it go away?

KRYSTAL: About a week later. It started trying to sneak back in . . . [I said,] "I told you to go away." . . . And then about a week later it went away, just gradually.

CHERYL: So it sounds like it wasn't just the magic wand. There were some words you said to worry, and you had to say the words over and over.

KRYSTAL: "Go away! Go away! I told you to go away!"

CHERYL: So sometimes with magic, you have to use a magic spell?

KRYSTAL: "Alakazoom! Now go away! I told you to go to your room!" (*Giggles*)

CHERYL: So that was your magic spell—"You go away! You go away! You go away!" And it worked?

KRYSTAL: (*Nods*)

CHERYL: So I have a feeling that Krystal knows a lot more about escaping worry—maybe even more that she can tell us about today.

JANET: Very possibly. You have a friend who was troubled by worry too?

KRYSTAL: Her dad has cancer. I hang out with her and I play with her, like she did with me when I had troubles and stuff. Like a best friend does, just tries to help.

JANET: So you hang out with her, and when worry starts bugging her, do you do something?

KRYSTAL: Kind of . . . she calls me a lot and stuff. I don't really know how I do it, I just do.

CHERYL: Do you think that talking helps? You know, you were saying you've been going to your school counselor and really just talking . . . about your animals . . . maybe not talking about how worry was bugging you. . . .

KRYSTAL: Yeah.

CHERYL: So you think talking is a big thing?

KRYSTAL: That's what helps. Unless you talk about things, a big brick wall will build up in your brain, and pretty soon it will just explode. And you might tell someone you don't even know, and they could go blurt it out to a lot of other people, and then it will come back around to you and really hurt your feelings. So I think you should talk about it with someone you know will be okay and won't blurt out the stuff. (*To Cheryl*) And you're one of those people.

CHERYL: Thank you. I appreciate your vote of confidence.

JANET: So you keep this brick wall from building up?

KRYSTAL: Uh-huh.

JANET: How do you do that?

KRYSTAL: If you keep worry inside, when you get a worry and don't talk to someone about it, one worry will gradually start building up. So if you talk about it, one brick will start gradually falling down, and pretty soon if you get all your worries out, you won't have a brick wall and you'll be happy.

JANET: How do you decide who to tell about worry? You said Cheryl's one of the people that you talk to, and you talk to your school counselor.

KRYSTAL: First, you've got to talk to them and find out what kind of people they are and stuff. That's how you'll know if you want to talk to them or not. That's what I do.

JANET: How do you know they're the kind of people you want to talk to? What lets you know that?

KRYSTAL: You could ask a little bit about them. If you want to talk to them, you can. If you don't feel comfortable about it, you don't have to.

JANET: So you pay attention to what goes on inside.

KRYSTAL: If you have butterflies in your stomach and you don't feel like they're that good of a person, you don't have to talk to them. You can find someone else.

JANET: That's interesting. . . .

CHERYL: When I told you about Krystal, I told you she was an interesting person, and how much she thought about what's going on inside her and has paid attention to how to help herself. So it doesn't surprise me that she's able to notice butterflies; that's a good way to notice her inside feelings.

KRYSTAL: They're all flying around, and they poke your stomach and stuff and say, "I don't feel good about this person." So maybe I don't have to see her if I don't want to. I don't feel butterflies with you (*points to Cheryl*) or with you (*points to Janet*).

JANET: (*To Cheryl*) If I were to talk to Krystal's friend and ask her what Krystal did to help her shrink worry, I wonder what she would say?

CHERYL: (*Thinking*) Hmm . . .

JANET: *(To Krystal)* Do you have any ideas about what she would say if we asked her that question?

KRYSTAL: She might say ... probably ... she goes to the hospital a lot and talks to her dad, and she probably knows that he's going to be okay because he's under chemo and stuff, and he'll probably survive. She talks to her mom about it. She's seen the school counselor too.

JANET: So what do you think Sheila would say helps her to keep worry away when she talks to you?

KRYSTAL: She talks to me about how her dad looks and how sad she is that he might die. I told her that it would probably be okay and hugged her, and she started crying.

JANET: So would she say that you listen?

KRYSTAL: Sometimes.

JANET: Sometimes ... what do you do other times?

KRYSTAL: I play games with her a lot and just hang around her like a real friend does.

JANET: So you spend time with her and talk to her about other stuff?

KRYSTAL: Not just about her troubles. We talk about school, because we both really like school and stuff. So we talk about school lunches *(makes a face)* ...

CHERYL and JANET: *(Laugh)*

KRYSTAL: ... and how they're disgusting and everything, and how we really like our moms' food. And we like to compare stuff a lot.

JANET: You like to see ways that you're alike and ways that you're different?

KRYSTAL: She's got short hair and a bunch of freckles. She doesn't like her freckles, but I always tell her, "They're just beauty marks." And she says, "That's a good way to look at it."

JANET: So part of what you did when you helped Sheila send worry away was to help her look at things in a different way?

CHERYL: Sounds like that might be part of it. I wonder how Krystal learned to do that?

KRYSTAL: Your heart tells you to.

JANET: Your heart tells you to?

KRYSTAL: I don't know. Maybe you can ask God how to do it or something. A lot of times I pray and ask how to do it, and he always talks to me back. You may not hear it, but you can feel it. It's kind of like a tinge in your heart. You can tell that he's [listening] to you and stuff, and that's probably where I found out.

CHERYL: (*Puzzling*) It's almost like you have "inside ears" or "heart ears." Do you have "heart ears"?

KRYSTAL: Thanks a lot! (*Laughs*)

CHERYL: Somehow you learned to listen to what your heart is telling you. Then you used your heart to listen to your friend when she was talking to you.

KRYSTAL: (*Nods "yes"*)

CHERYL: So there are different kinds of listening that you can use. How did you learn to listen with your heart? She said God talks to her in her heart, but how did she learn to do that kind of listening?

KRYSTAL: I don't know. (*Laughs and shrugs her shoulders*)

CHERYL: Have you talked to anybody else about this kind of listening that you do?

KRYSTAL: No, not really. I am a talker and I do talk about my feelings, but not much about how I got them or something—see, because I don't really know how I got them, so I can't really talk about it.

CHERYL: But it's an interesting thing to wonder about: Where do these things come from? I have a friend, and we have long conversations sometimes about that kind of thing. It helps me to talk to my friend about it, because talking about it helps me pay more attention to it, so it seems more real.

JANET: So when you pay attention to it, what difference does that make?

CHERYL: It's like . . . for instance, like listening with your "heart ears." Just because we've talked about it today, I'll probably think about it from time to time during the day. Paying more attention to it will help me do it more.

During this session, we were interested in helping Krystal develop self-knowledge and learn to trust her own experience. We asked questions that helped her rediscover the steps she had taken in the past to push worry out of her life. Next, we invited her to take the perspective of her friend Sheila. By explaining how she was able to help her friend, Krystal described the inner conversations that allowed her to take those steps to help herself. She discovered that she could "listen with her 'heart ears',", and pay attention to the "tinge in her heart" and the "butterflies in her stomach." These "inside feelings" helped her choose supportive people she could talk to about her worries. These discoveries added to her growing sense of competence and mastery.

During the next two sessions, I (*JAW*) invited Krystal to internalize a more validating story about herself. We introduced a distinction between "worry" and "caring." We continued to discuss worry, using externalized language. Krystal decided that she was able to "pay attention to the tinge in her heart" because she cared about other people. We began to talk about caring, using internalized language. As Krystal discussed examples of her standing up for others, we discovered that she was a person who had "strong ideas." For example, she told me about her decision to befriend a girl at school who was often taunted by classmates because they "thought she was retarded." Krystal explained that she did not like the way the girl was being treated and challenged her friends to include the girl in their activities. When asked what strong idea had influenced her decision, she explained that she believed that everyone should be treated with respect.

The next session provided an opportunity for Krystal to use her caring and strong ideas to stand up for herself. Her mother called for an appointment when she noticed that Krystal was not laughing and singing as much. Her mother discussed her own worries about Krystal's safety. Her brother was sleeping in a travel trailer parked in the family's yard. Although her mother never left them alone, he spent time in the house during the day. He was refusing to attend counseling sessions and was becoming increasingly aggressive in his interactions with all family members. Krystal explained to her mother that she cared about her brother, but did not like the way he was treating her. He was acting like a bully and was not treating her with respect. When I asked if it would be helpful to schedule a family session, Krystal became tearful and explained that she did not want to talk to her brother in therapy. She believed that this would bring up all of the sad feelings she had experienced when he was abusing her.

I talked with her mother about how impressed I was that Krystal was able to pay attention to her inside feelings and stand up for herself by letting us know that she did not want to talk to her brother in a therapy session. I explained that some therapists believe that it's important for kids who were molested to talk to the persons who molested them in therapy sessions, but that I trusted Krystal's strong ideas about what was best for her right now. I was curious how talking to her brother might be different after she had more practice standing up for herself. Did she think she might be able to talk to him without feeling sadness? I wondered what her mother had noticed about Krystal at a younger age that would have led her to predict that she would be able to use her caring and strong ideas to escape worry and stand up for herself in this way. After answering this question, Krystal's mother reassured her that she would take steps to deal with her son's behavior. She requested information about placing him in a group home where he could continue to participate in treatment.

Our last session took place several weeks later. Although her brother was still living at home, Krystal reported that she felt much safer. Her brother was now reinvolved with therapy and was treating her with more respect. She was really excited because her mother had arranged to spend special time with her each week. She explained that worry had not been bothering her, and she shared three examples of times when she stood up for herself. Because her grandfather had died earlier that month, she described feeling sad from time to time; however, she experienced this sadness as different from the sadness she experienced because of the abuse. We talked at length about how her grandfather knew she was a person with a big heart and strong ideas who could stand up for herself and for people she cared about. At the end of the session, Krystal decided to catch Cheryl up on her progress and faxed her the following note:

> Dear Cheryl,
>
> I'm doing just fine. How are you doing?
> *Guess what?* I got some contacts. And a new job
> (doing dishes!). I get paid $3.00 every other week.
> It's boring but it's money!!!!!!!!!!!!!!!!!!!!!!!!!!!!!!!!!!!!!
> Guess what else, my hair is long. WORRY DOES
> NOT BOTHER ME ANY MORE!!!!!!!!!!!!!!!!!!!!!!!!!!!
> I stood up for myself the other day!!!!!!!!!!!!!!!!!!!!!!!
>
> YOUR FRIEND ALWAYS,
> *Krystal*

CHANGING OUR STORY ABOUT THERAPY

Our work has evolved in the 10 years since we were first introduced to narrative ideas. Prior to adopting this approach, we viewed the therapist as the primary agent of change and assumed that the most important changes took place in the consultation room. We practiced traditional ideas about "recovery" from child sexual abuse, which required a confrontation with the offender and charged the therapist with responsibility for insuring the ongoing safety of the child who had been victimized.

When we began learning the narrative model, we spent hours reviewing videotapes and generating carefully worded candidate questions. As we adopted narrative ideas as ways of thinking, we became more focused on privileging the person's experience and less concerned with getting the language just right. We began to privilege those experiences that challenged the effects of abuse and the abuse-dominated "victim" story.

We view therapy sessions as an opportunity to create more validating lived experiences. We are most interested in helping young people and their parents create validating interactions in their everyday lives.[7] We work with young people to develop connections with supportive others. Interacting with other people who recognize their competence and worth helps them begin to recognize these qualities in themselves.

Supportive people can also serve as a resource to help a child stay safe from further victimization. Many of the families with whom we have worked face challenges similar to those of Krystal and her parents. Unreliable cars, uncertain housing, and no gas money prevent them from regularly attending therapy sessions. Even parents who make it to sessions on an ongoing basis can themselves be overwhelmed by the effects of abuse. Supportive others can help young people learn to listen to their own experiences and develop more validating solutions to problems that occur in their daily interactions.

We were encouraged that Krystal chose to develop a relationship with her school counselor. We viewed this as a sign that she was determined to find resources and get help in solving problems. We were also encouraged by Krystal's report that most of her conversations with the counselor were not about worries, but about topics (like her pets) that were important to her. In the past we might have viewed this as evidence of "denial." Instead, we viewed these conversations as adding to those lived experiences that support a more validating story. Krystal advised us that good friends don't just talk about troubles; they play and hang out together.

In the past, we would have been especially concerned that Krystal did not want to talk to her brother in therapy. We were pleased that she was able to listen to her experience and stand up for herself. We respected her statement that she did not want to re-experience the sadness she had experienced during the abuse. We asked questions to punctuate this unique outcome and identify other situations where she was able to use her strong ideas about respect and fairness to stand up for herself.

Traditional views would have invited us to pathologize Krystal's mother. Instead, we recognized her efforts to get treatment for her chil-

---

[7]Kathy Weingarten's (1992) ideas about intimacy have had a major influence on our thinking. She conceptualizes intimacy from a social constructionist and feminist perspective, which considers the ways in which people coordinate their actions to co-create meaning. We are interested in helping people discover how to take an active role in co-creating interactions that support preferred stories.

dren, despite the challenges the family was facing. She recognized that Krystal might pay more attention to her mother's feelings than her own, and suggested that Cheryl meet with Krystal individually. She assured Krystal that she and her husband could handle the family's worries without Krystal's help. She managed to get Krystal's brother to treatment most of the time. She became sensitive to signs that worry was starting to bother Krystal again. Within the family's limited resources, she developed a plan to keep her son from molesting Krystal or her friends. Finally, she intervened when he began to intimidate family members.

Our work with Krystal and her mother invited us to continue to evaluate the influence of traditional ideas about the treatment of child sexual abuse on our work. We are most likely to take an expert stance and impose our views in situations where we are concerned about the safety of a child. When we turn down invitations to think in traditional ways and maintain a collaborative stance, we find that parents are able to access their own expertise and take responsibility for the safety of their children. We share the excitement young people experience as they overcome the effects of abuse, discover a sense of personal agency, and create more validating stories about themselves.

EDITORIAL QUESTIONS

Q: *I (CS) like the way you have portrayed the everyday, spontaneous quality of your work with Krystal. You've also managed to let us see her as a human being with some difficult struggles, rather than as a permanently damaged "victim."*

One question for me was how you thought about Krystal's mom's concerns that Krystal "worried about everybody else's feelings and didn't pay attention to her own." Cheryl made a comment about Krystal's being "the kind of person who likes to help others." Later, the three of you talked about her helping a friend who had worries, and this led to some re-authoring conversations and creative new ways of dealing with her worries. If Krystal successfully developed ways to worry less, but was still concerned about others and liked helping them, would her mom still perhaps have had concerns? Are there other events that might help us understand her mom's view of how therapy proceeded? How might you have dealt with this concern of her mom's if in fact she had continued to have this reaction?

A: Our thinking is influenced by the writers (see Jordan et al., 1991) who have suggested that the metaphor of "connection" is a better fit for women's experience than the metaphor of "separation/individuation."

As such, we place a positive value on caring and concern for others. We believe that this caring becomes problematic when young women are influenced by the belief that they are valuable only to the extent that they are concerned for others. So we shared her mother's concerns and asked questions to help Krystal learn to pay attention to and privilege her own feelings. We maintained an open invitation to Krystal's mother to participate in therapy sessions, but recognized that her regular attendance at sessions was precluded by the realities of locating child care for her younger children and supervision for her son. If Krystal's mother had continued to have concerns, we would have more actively sought her ongoing participation in sessions through the use of letters. We would have been interested in her mother's ideas about ways to overcome worry while caring for other people. Indeed, we suspect that the events of the past year had given Krystal's mother considerable experience with this dilemma. We might have used artwork or stories to catch her mother up with Krystal's progress in listening with her "heart ears" and using her strong ideas to stand up for herself.

Q: *(CS) Second, you mention toward the end of the chapter that as your work has evolved, you "became more focused on privileging the person's experience and less concerned with getting the language just right." Could you say more about this? What happened when you tried to get the language right? What or whose language were you trying to get right? What sorts of things are different for you and/or for the client when you privilege the person's experience instead?*
A: Both of us have well-worn copies of Michael White's articles (1988a, 1988b, 1988c) that provide examples of various categories of re-authoring questions. I (JAW) recently reviewed my notes about my work with a woman who consulted with me in 1988 and 1989. These notes were taken on a form with column headings labeled with these categories: "unique outcome," "account," "redescription," "possibility," and "circulation." My notes from 1988 are replete with questions—candidate questions I generated prior to the sessions, questions I asked during the sessions, questions I wished I had thought to ask, and so on. My notes in 1989 focus on the person's description of her experiences, and much less on the questions I asked to inquire about their experiences.

The positive effects of privileging each person's experience are most apparent in our work with families who have experienced child sexual abuse. When we reflect back on our work using models that impose meaning, we experience our work using narrative approaches as more effective, more fun, and more meaningful. We used to spend the first 6 months of therapy "challenging denial and confronting resistance." The families we worked with felt judged and pathologized.

When we privilege each person's experience, our work is much more collaborative. We experience a sense of generativity as meaning is co-created in the interaction. The families we work with today are surprised when we ask them about their experiences and invite them to evaluate for themselves whether or not these experiences support their preferred directions. They describe these interactions as extremely validating. We are truly honored to witness the people we work with experience a sense of developing agency, as problems are externalized and steps are taken in the development of more preferred stories. We have found that this work affects who we are as people, sometimes in very profound ways.

REFERENCES

Adams-Westcott, J., Dafforn, T., & Sterne, P. (1993). Escaping victim life stories and co-creating personal agency. In S. Gilligan & R. Price (Eds.), *Therapeutic conversations* (pp. 258–276). New York: Norton.

Adams-Westcott, J., & Isenbart, D. (1990). Using rituals to empower family members who have experienced child sexual abuse. In M. Durrant & C. White (Eds.), *Ideas for therapy with sexual abuse* (pp. 37–64). Adelaide, South Australia: Dulwich Centre Publications.

Adams-Westcott, J., & Isenbart, D. (1995). A journey of change through connection. In S. Friedman (Ed.), *The reflecting team in action: Collaborative practice in family therapy* (pp. 331–352). New York: Guilford Press.

Adams-Westcott, J., & Isenbart, D. (1996). Creating preferred relationships: The politics of recovery from child sexual abuse. *Journal of Systemic Therapies, 15,* 13–30.

Barragar-Dunne, P. (1992). *The narrative therapist and the arts.* Los Angeles: Possibility Press (Drama Therapy Institute of Los Angeles).

Durrant, M. (1987). Therapy with young people who have been the victims of sexual assault. *Family Therapy Case Studies, 2*(1), 57–63.

Durrant, M., & Kowalski, K. (1990). Overcoming the effects of sexual abuse: Developing a self-perception of competence. In M. Durrant & C. White (Eds.), *Ideas for therapy with sexual abuse* (pp. 65–110). Adelaide, South Australia: Dulwich Centre Publications.

Epston, D., & White, M. (1990). Consulting your consultants: The documentation of alternative knowledges. *Dulwich Centre Newsletter,* No. 4, 25–35.

Finkelhor, D. (1994). Current information on the scope and nature of child sexual abuse. *The Future of Children: Sexual Abuse of Children, 4,* 31–53.

Flaskas, C., & Humphreys, C. (1993). Theorizing about power: Intersecting the ideas of Foucault with the "problem" of power in family therapy. *Family Process, 32,* 35–47.

Freedman, J., & Combs, G. (1996a). Gender stories. *Journal of Systemic Therapies, 15,* 31–46.

Freedman, J., & Combs, G. (1996b). *Narrative therapy: The social construction of preferred realities.* New York: Norton.

Freeman, J., & Lobovits, D. (1993). The turtle with wings. In S. Friedman (Ed.), *The new language of change: Constructive collaboration in psychotherapy* (pp. 188–225). New York: Guilford Press.

Hare-Mustin, R. (1991). Sex, lies and headaches: The problem is power. In T. Goodrich (Ed.), *Women and power: Perspectives for family therapy* (pp. 63–85). New York: Norton.

Hokes, S., Sykes, C., & Winn, M. (1989). Systemic/strategic interventions targeting denial in the incestuous family. *Journal of Strategic and Systemic Therapies, 8,* 44–51.

Jenkins, A. (1990). *Invitations to responsibility: The therapeutic engagement of men who are violent and abusive.* Adelaide, South Australia: Dulwich Centre Publications.

Jordan, J., Kaplan, A., Miller, J. B., Stiver, I., & Surrey, J. (1991). *Women's growth in connection: Writings from the Stone Center.* New York: Guilford Press.

Liske, C. (1993). Gary Sanders on sexuality and loving intimacy: A *Participator* profile interview with Dr. Gary Sanders. *The Calgary Participator, 3,* 22–31.

Madigan, S., & Epston, D. (1995). From "spy-chiatric gaze" to communities of concern: From professional monologue to dialogue. In S. Friedman (Ed.), *The reflecting team in action: Collaborative practice in family therapy* (pp. 257–276). New York: Guilford Press.

Sanders, G. (1988). An invitation to escape sexual tyranny. *Journal of Strategic and Systemic Therapies, 7,* 23–34.

Stewart, K. (1991). Three stances on a theme of power, certainty and intimacy. *Dulwich Centre Newsletter,* No. 2, 51–55.

Taylor, J., Gilligan, C., & Sullivan, A. (1995). *Between voice and silence: Women and girls, race and relationship.* Cambridge, MA: Harvard University Press.

Weingarten, K. (1992). A consideration of intimate and non-intimate interactions in therapy. *Family Process, 31,* 45–59.

White, M. (1988–1989). The externalizing of the problem and the re-authoring of relationships. *Dulwich Centre Newsletter,* No. 4, 3–21.

White, M. (1988a). The process of questioning: A therapy of literary merit? *Dulwich Centre Newsletter,* No. 2, 8–14.

White, M. (1988b). Saying hullo again: The incorporation of the lost relationship in the resolution of grief. *Dulwich Centre Newsletter,* No. 3, 14–21.

White, M. (1995). *Re-authoring lives: Interviews and essays.* Adelaide, South Australia: Dulwich Centre Publications.

White, M., & Epston, D. (1990). *Narrative means to therapeutic ends.* New York: Norton.

Wonderlich, S., Donaldson, M., Carson, D., Staton, D., Gertz, L., Leach, L., & Johnson, M. (1996). Eating disturbance and incest. *Journal of Interpersonal Violence, 11,* 195–207.

Zimmerman, J., & Dickerson, V. (1994). Tales of the body thief: Externalizing and deconstructing eating problems. In M. Hoyt (Ed.), *Constructive therapies* (pp. 295–318). New York: Guilford Press.

Zimmerman, J., & Dickerson, V. (1996). *If problems talked: Narrative therapy in action.* New York: Guilford Press.

Zimmerman, J., Dickerson, V., Combs, G., Adams-Westcott, J., Freedman, J., & Madigan, S. (1995, November). *Narrative therapy: Myths, misconceptions and politics.* Symposium presented at the annual conference of the American Association for Marriage and Family Therapy, Baltimore.

9

From Imposition to Collaboration

GENERATING STORIES OF COMPETENCE

KATHLEEN STACEY

Many young people who attend community mental health or family therapy services, often on the recommendation of educators who are concerned about their behavior, experience language-based learning difficulties (LBLDs).[1] However, the existence or significance of the learning difficulties is not always recognized by teachers or therapists. Conversely, many young people receiving learning support are not referred for family therapy, despite the significant impact the learning difficulties are having on their lives. A more desirable approach would be a "both–and" situation, in which young people and their families and teachers have access to both learning and therapy support services.

Another desirable approach, which this chapter specifically addresses, would be for the people involved in the lives of these young people to engage in practices of language that generate stories of learn-

---

[1]This is the term I prefer to the more commonly used "language disorders," as it is less pathologized language, but is also inclusive of literacy difficulties whose connections to speech–language skills have often been disregarded until more recently.

ing, success, and competence, rather than stories of deficit, failure, and incompetence. Externalizing language that facilitates stories of competence is offered and grounded in my work with Matthew. As the LBLDs these young people experience cannot be completely separated from the young people themselves, the work is couched more appropriately in a collaborative rather than a protest metaphor (Stacey, 1997). A brief description of different metaphors in narrative work is also provided.

THE DISCOURSES OF LANGUAGE-BASED LEARNING DIFFICULTIES

The stories or descriptions dominating the lives of young people living with LBLDs have often been imposed by others as outcomes of educational and developmental assessments. Because language is a place of struggle for these young people, they are extremely vulnerable to internalizing descriptions by others in forming their self-narratives.[2] These descriptions usually involve deficit-based terms that implicate their whole persons and encourage young people to develop a hopeless, defeatist lifestyle. They shape the dominant discourses in the speech–language pathology, education, and psychology professions (Stacey, 1992, 1995a, 1995c). As these descriptions seem compelling, or at least the authority of those who speak them seems daunting, the influence of existing alternative knowledges about abilities known to the young people, their families, their peers, or educators is diminished.

In contrast, externalizing conversations serve to identify young people's competence in learning and solving problems, despite the interference of LBLDs in their lives. When professional descriptions from educational and developmental assessments are combined with young people's self-knowledges and externalizing conversations, more self-embracing rather than rejecting stories can emerge. This alternative discourse has some roots in the literature on early intervention and special needs, which has adopted more family-focused and competence-based approaches (Stacey, 1994b).

---

[2]Bruner and Haste (1987) have suggested that "'making sense' is a social process; it is an activity that is always situated within a cultural and historical framework" (p. 1). Through their social interactions with adults, "children create narrative accounts of their lives, accounts that are represented as a world view, as social maps of the world" (Garbarino, 1993, p. 8). When adults bring attention to children's failures and the ways in which they don't measure up to educational or behavioral expectations, children enter into a worldview and self-narrative of incompetence.

"EARS THINKING" AND "EYES THINKING": A DIFFERENT WAY OF TALKING

Exposure to the ideas of narrative family therapies led me to develop and apply the concepts of "ears thinking" and "eyes thinking" when talking with young people about the difficulties they have encountered in their learning (Stacey, 1992, 1994a, 1995a). Introducing these concepts requires careful and paced explanation supported by visual cues to insure that young people with LBLDs connect with these ideas.

I usually draw a simplistic picture of a head and explain to young people that there are two sides of the brain, which do all their thinking. I show and explain how the information they hear through their ears is sent to one side of the brain, and the information they see through their eyes is sent to the other side. I show how the information crosses from one side of the brain to the other to reach the special "ears thinking" and "eyes thinking" places. Because either "ears thinking" or "eyes thinking" may have trouble doing its job, I emphasize that the two sides of the brain need to talk to each other to best help young people with their learning.

I explain further that "ears thinking" is about *words* that we speak, listen to, read, and write.[3] "Eyes thinking" is about *pictures and actions* that we see or do/make. I then discuss with the young people which sort of thinking is easier for them: "Working out things you see with your eyes, or working out words you hear with your ears?" Young people with LBLDs often quickly decide that "ears thinking" is harder than "eyes thinking."

Another useful aspect of the "ears thinking" and "eyes thinking" externalizing conversation is to assign ages to the two components (White, 1991a). Young people are usually well aware of their own ages and can use these as a point of comparison for judging where their "ears thinking" and "eyes thinking" are at. I suggest that since they are clearly very good at "eyes thinking," it may even be older than they are. They are _____ years old; how old do they think "eyes thinking" is? Invariably, young people name an age older than themselves, and I usually accept whatever age they nominate. Then I ask how old "ears thinking" is. I may suggest that it probably hasn't caught up to them because it is

---

[3]Because reading and writing involve "eyes thinking" skills, some may find this distinction confusing. Reading (*decoding* sounds/words) and writing (*encoding* sounds/words) are linguistic processes that involve understanding a complex sound–symbol code. Those who try to read by relying on visually memorizing words and sound combinations, as some young people with LBLDs do, find that they cannot "crack the code" sufficiently to read and write novel language in the way they understand and generate novel oral language.

having trouble doing its job. Invariably, young people nominate a younger age. We also assign ages to how "ears thinking" manages listening, speaking, reading, spelling, and writing tasks, as "ears thinking" often does better in some areas than others.

Next, I tell young people that one way to get "ears thinking" to do its job is for "eyes thinking" to help it out, and that I (or someone else who is supporting the young persons' learning) will help them teach "eyes thinking" to help "ears thinking" do its job. If "ears thinking" does its job, life will be easier for them (in whatever way their lives are being troubled by the problem). Not only is the assigning of ages a useful concrete tool; it suggests there will be growth in ability over time, since young people know they get older. Although it does not promise that "ears thinking" will catch up and surpass their age (because it may not), it does suggest a way forward.[4] It is another sign of hope for the young persons, their families, or significant others. Finally, it acknowledges the competence already achieved by young people in helping their "ears thinking" do its job.

"EARS THINKING" AND "EYES THINKING": USING A COLLABORATIVE METAPHOR

The protest metaphor has become the best-known and most popular metaphor for situating externalizing conversations. However, it is not the only one used or the most appropriate one in many instances. Externalizations can be divided into at least two basic categories—outer and inner externalizations (see Stacey, 1997, for a detailed discussion). Both can operate from the frame of wanting less influence of a problematic feature, or wanting more influence of a nonproblematic feature (e.g., strengthening one's relationship with trust, playfulness, hope, or confidence). Outer externalizations are used when a problem is viewed predominantly as a negative and removable feature of a person's life. Three metaphors available for outer externalizations are as follows:

---

[4]I am not suggesting that LBLDs are simply delays in the "normal" developmental pattern of language and literacy acquisition (this has been debated in the field, but most people have agreed that LBLDs are more complex than this). In most instances, young people have not developed, or are struggling to use, specific language abilities that do not show growth with maturation. The assigning of ages makes conceptual sense, as it forms an analogy with a known description of how one attains more complex or advanced abilities.

1. Protesting the existence and effects of the problem and wishing to banish it from one's life. An example of such a problem might be temper, trouble, worry, or fears.

2. Readiness for growth/evolution/transition from the current situation to a preferred situation in which the problem is no longer present (or not present in the same way). Such a problem can have a developmental nature (e.g., soiling, bedwetting, worry, or fears).

3. Surpassing or transcending the problem through a reconstruction of the meaning system surrounding the nature of the problem. If an alternative meaning system informs the problem, including the history of that meaning system, then the problem is no longer fed by the belief system on which it depends. This can enable people to refuse submitting to the definition of self the problem requires for its existence. An example of such a problem might be shyness, incompetence, guilt, abuse, homophobia, sexism, or racism.

Inner externalizations are used when the problem is not necessarily viewed as a negative and removable feature. Some problems cannot be viewed in this way when there are physiological or neuropsychological difficulties present. Three metaphors available for inner externalizations are the following:

1. Collaboration by working with the problem so as to minimize its negative effects and to open space for preferred possibilities (in a case where protesting by ignoring the demands the problem places on a person usually serves to make it worse). Examples of such problems might be chronic health problems or learning difficulties.

2. Balancing by confining the problem to the positive part that it may play in the person's life, rather than letting the problem dictate the person's life. An example of such a problem might be altruism/being for others, overresponsibility, worry, or overcommitment to work/study.

3. Embodiment of particular qualities or skills that act to minimize the effects of problems (e.g., strengthening one's relationship with and internalizing inner strength, self-respect, or hope). This metaphor is usually coupled with other metaphors that focus more on diminishing or eliminating a problem.

Externalizing conversations for "ears thinking" and "eyes thinking" are situated in a collaborative metaphor. Most of us would not wish to protest the presence of "ears thinking"; it is vital to our language-saturated lives. However, when it is not doing its job and lets us down, it pays to collaborate with "ears thinking" so that it works for rather than against us.

GETTING TO KNOW MATTHEW[5]

Matthew was given a "language disorder" label when he entered school at age 5 and attended a special learning unit for a year. He received four to eight visits a year from an education department speech–language pathologist, as well as teacher assistant time to follow up his speech–language program on a more regular basis. In the fourth grade, he was considered to be functioning well enough academically for this support to be stopped, although this was not Sharon's (his mother's) preference. In fifth grade, he moved from the city to a rural area with Sharon, his stepfather, and four teenage siblings. As Sharon received little support from the new school in appreciating Matthew's learning struggles and their effects on his life, she sought alternative sources. This led her to Child and Adolescent Mental Health Services (CAMHS), a community-based mental health service in South Australia for young people aged 0–18 years, for which I work.

I first met Matthew in late 1994; he was aged 12 and at the end of sixth grade. The CAMHS psychologist had completed an assessment on his general learning abilities and referred him for family therapy. Because I was a speech–language consultant[6] by initial profession, I was able to perform a dual role and completed a review of Matthew's speech–language skills. This indicated that significant LBLDs were still present. It was at this point that the language of "ears thinking" and "eyes thinking" was introduced.

When I asked Matthew and Sharon about the impact the learning difficulties (or "ears thinking" not doing its job) were having on his life, they said it was quite significant. He was having great difficulty with peer relationships, was excluded by many of his peers, and found it difficult to connect with their interests. He struggled to be organized in regard to his schoolwork, homework, and many home responsibilities. He had great difficulty keeping up with writing tasks, often forgot verbal instructions, and struggled to extract rich meanings from fiction texts. He often forgot to use eye contact, and his attention frequently drifted out of conversations. His descriptions or responses were often nonspecific or vague, as he frequently did not understand questions, vocabulary, or the situation, although he tried to act as if he did in the hope that he would work it out.

[5]This is Matthew's chosen pseudonym, and his story is used here with his written permission. Indeed, he is quite excited at being even more famous, having had a brief version of his story appear in a previous paper (Stacey, 1995a) and a videotape of an interview with him shown in New Zealand and Australia.

[6]As I have chosen to move away from pathological language as much as possible, I prefer to use "speech–language consultant" to refer to my first profession.

Sharon found much of her time taken up with trying to convince people that Matthew had difficulty with his learning and was not just lazy or unmotivated. Furthermore, she found herself consistently invited into being an advocate for Matthew's best interests, the main support for his learning, a confidant for his worries, a motivator when he felt low, and an interpreter for others who tried to converse with Matthew but overestimated or otherwise misjudged his comprehension. In fact, she was the person who most strongly believed in his abilities. Her experiences were very similar to those of other parents who live with young people's learning difficulties (Stacey, 1995b; Stewart & Nodrick, 1990).

Matthew enjoyed reading, particularly science texts where he could memorize specific facts. He loved computers, was particularly good at math, liked to entertain himself with a rich fantasy life, and enjoyed playing archery. Although we would never have predicted this, he had an aptitude for learning other languages at school, such as French and German. Matthew had one friend at school and some older friends at archery. Matthew's best friend, Wipeout (an imaginary friend), had recently been packed off to another state, as he was "getting bored" and had started to interfere with Matthew's development of other friends.

TALKING WITH MATTHEW: LANGUAGE AND METAPHORS

Before presenting some of my work with Matthew "*in vivo,*" I explain more about the specific language and metaphors present in the conversations. In addition to the language of "ears thinking" and "eyes thinking," situated in the collaborative metaphor, we considered how Matthew was entering himself more strongly into a Problem-Solving career in contrast to a Giving-Up career,[7] which was the direction "ears thinking" had previously taken. The idea of different careers was situated in the outer-externalization metaphor of readiness for growth/evolution/transition, as we collected evidence of the Problem-Solving Career's growing strength and Matthew's transition from a self-narrative of failure to one of competence. A transcendence metaphor could also have been used, as Matthew increasingly refused to submit to the definition

---

[7]The other name for the Problem-Solving career was the Problem-Solver career, and that for the Giving-Up career was the Giver-Upper career. These names were used interchangeably in our conversations.

of himself required by the Giver-Upper career and identified with one that fitted with the Problem-Solver career.

In our early work, Matthew identified those areas where "ears thinking" did its job the best, as well as those areas in which it struggled. By drawing on these and other resources, such as "eyes thinking," Matthew collaborated with "ears thinking" by training it to do successively more difficult tasks with words/language (i.e., listening, speaking, reading, and writing). In this way, he minimized the negative effects of "ears thinking"'s struggles, and opened space for "ears thinking" to grow in competence and to assist him in managing situations that drew heavily on language and literacy skills. As our work progressed, we collected evidence of Matthew's acting in concert with a Problem-Solving career and believing in his competence when the Giving-Up career would have encouraged him to act differently. The dialogues presented in this chapter demonstrate how the Giving-Up career diminished in strength as the Problem-Solving career became increasingly influential over his life.

In the dialogues, notice that I chunked my information into shorter sections, even pausing in the middle of an idea or sentence to check that Matthew was with me with a "Yeah" or "Mmm" (the equivalent of the North American "Uh-huh" in Australian English) as confirmation. I rarely went into an extended talking turn or monologue. I often revisited ideas, in a more pedantic way than I would with a young person who did not struggle with learning, to insure that Matthew had understood and that my conversation with him was meaningful and helpful. I frequently rephrased a question, having given him extra time to respond, by acknowledging that I didn't ask it in a helpful way or responding to his request for a repeat, or when his answer indicated that he missed the point of the question or responded as if it were a different question. The latter problem usually occurred with "How?" questions. Matthew often found explanations, particularly extended ones, extremely difficult to provide without prompting or cueing from his listener.

I also took general questions and broke them down into their specific contexts, so that the questions were more fully grounded in the realities of his life. Also, note how I often repeated back what he had just said. This insured that I understood him and offered him a chance to confirm or change his response if he accidentally said the wrong thing. This was important, as one of "ears thinking"'s tendencies in not working hard enough for Matthew was to give "on-the-surface answers" (e.g., to choose one of the options offered in a choice question, without checking whether that was the answer that best fitted with his experience). Ways of using language in inclusive ways with young people like Matthew are discussed in more detail elsewhere (Stacey, 1995a).

RELINQUISHING THE GIVING-UP CAREER: IDENTIFYING COMPETENCE IN LEARNING AND PROBLEM-SOLVING

During this conversation, we drew a picture to depict the two previously identified careers of Problem-Solver and Giver-Upper, and to map the degree of influence they had over Matthew's life at that time. We then proceeded to identify how he had strengthened the Problem-Solver career. You will notice that at times I didn't go slowly enough; I got ahead of him and had to back up and recheck things.

KATHLEEN: Do you remember how we were talking about learning to be a Problem-Solver? How you can have a career as a Problem-Solver?

MATTHEW: Mmm.

KATHLEEN: Do you remember what we meant by that?

MATTHEW: Yeah.

KATHLEEN: What did we mean?

MATTHEW: Well, like, helping other people, umm . . .

KATHLEEN: (*pause*) What does it mean to have a career?

MATTHEW: Oh, sort of like a job.

KATHLEEN: Yeah, it is, or you could have a career as a Giver-Upper.

MATTHEW: Mmm.

KATHLEEN: Do you remember that?

MATTHEW: Yes.

KATHLEEN: And one thing that Mum was saying was that although you wanted to have a career as a Problem-Solver, sometimes you feel really bad about things . . .

MATTHEW: Yeah.

KATHLEEN: . . . and you were developing a bit of a career as a Giver-Upper.

MATTHEW: Uh-huh.

KATHLEEN: What do you think Mum meant?

MATTHEW: Like giving real easily, like succu . . . succumb.

KATHLEEN: Succumb! That's a good word. I didn't know you knew that word!

MATTHEW: It means to give up (*said proudly*).

KATHLEEN: It means to give up—very clever. So you thought at that time you were giving up a little bit too easily?

MATTHEW: Yeah (*slowly*).

KATHLEEN: You were succumbing to things that were tough for you. Were they "eyes thinking" things, or were they "ears thinking" things?

MATTHEW: "Ears thinking" (*said at the same time as I say it in the question*).

KATHLEEN: They were "ears thinking" things?

MATTHEW: Mmm.

KATHLEEN: So did you think that you were getting enough practice with Problem-Solving to have a career, or did you need more practice?

MATTHEW: Well (*slowly*), just a little bit more practice—like that should have done the trick.

MATTHEW: So which career was stronger last year? Which career was stronger, the Giver-Upper career or the Problem-Solver career?

MATTHEW: It was sort of like an in-between.

KATHLEEN: So it was about half and half.

MATTHEW: Yeah, in between.

KATHLEEN: So last year, it was sort of half and half (*speaking slowly and writing on picture*)—career as a Problem-Solver, career as a Giver-Upper.

MATTHEW: Yeah.

KATHLEEN: Now, was that okay with you . . .

MATTHEW: Yeah.

KATHLEEN: . . . to have both careers?

MATTHEW: Yeah.

KATHLEEN: Do you want a career as a Giver-Upper?

MATTHEW: Well . . . not really—no.

KATHLEEN: Oh, you don't! So is it okay to have it half and half, or should one be stronger?

MATTHEW: Well, half and half . . . probably . . . probably . . . umm . . . ahh . . . I'd say half and half, because sometimes I'm good, sometimes bad, sometimes good, sometimes bad.

KATHLEEN: All right. But even if it's good or bad, do you want to have a career as a Giver-Upper where you just give in . . .

MATTHEW: No.

KATHLEEN: . . . or would you like to have it, even when it's bad—have a career as a Problem-Solver and find a way to sort it out?

MATTHEW: (*Points to the Problem-Solver part of the picture*)

KATHLEEN: You want this one.

MATTHEW: Yeah.

KATHLEEN: So having half of this career and half of that career, that's no good to you?

MATTHEW: Yeah . . . that's no good to me.

KATHLEEN: So instead of it being half and half, sort of like 50/50—you know percentages, don't you?

MATTHEW: Yeah.

KATHLEEN: What would you like this percentage to look like?

MATTHEW: Sort of like . . . 90 . . . 10 [i.e., Problem-Solver/Giver-Upper].[8]

KATHLEEN: 90/10—so that's what you are aiming for. So here, this is 1994 [the year before this conversation], and this is what you want it to be.

MATTHEW: Yes.

KATHLEEN: So now where is it? This is sort of like the future over here (*pointing to the 90/10 goal*). So let's do 1995. How much has your career as a Problem-Solver got bigger?

MATTHEW: By 40, and reduced for the bottom, 40.

KATHLEEN: Oh, that's in the . . . is it 90/10 now, or is it only part way there?

MATTHEW: Probably part way there. I'd say probably 85.

KATHLEEN: Right now it's about 85, is it?

MATTHEW: Yeah.

KATHLEEN: So that makes that down there . . .

---

[8]You will note that Matthew determined the percentage of influence of each of these careers so that they added up to 100%. This was how *he* made sense of the careers; it was not a requirement. I would have readily accepted percentages for the *strength of influence* of each career in his life that added up to more than or less than 100%, as this would have been a different but equally viable way of looking at the relationship of the careers to his life.

MATTHEW: Ahh . . . (*thinking for a while*).

KATHLEEN: That's 85 out of 100. What is left?

MATTHEW: Fifteen, I think.

KATHLEEN: Fifteen—all right. So at the moment you are 85 and 15, and what you are aiming for is even better, 90 and 10. So you have made . . . 35%.

MATTHEW: As a Problem Solver!

KATHLEEN: Yeah, and this has got smaller—35% has gone away of your Giver-Upper career. What do you think of that?

MATTHEW: That's pretty cool!

KATHLEEN: That's pretty cool! Now, how have you done it? . . . How have you started to become a Problem-Solver, an even stronger one?

[Below is an example of his difficulty with answering a "how" question: He often answers "Really good," as if it were a "What do you think of using your . . . ?" or "How do you feel about using your . . . ?" question. Here I ask how he has used his "eyes thinking" more. When he replies, "Yeah, really good," I repeat the "how" question.]

KATHLEEN: How have you used your "eyes thinking" more?

MATTHEW: Yeah, really good.

KATHLEEN: But how have you used it? . . . What have you had to do?

The conversation turned to identifying specific evidence for the unique outcome of using his "eyes thinking" as a resource for his "ears thinking." Matthew indicated that he had been doing the following:

- Picturing what he read in his head.
- *Seeing* the tactics to use when he played a sport.
- Brainstorming ideas before writing a story by picturing what the story could be about.
- Looking at people when they talked and telling his "ears thinking" to concentrate on what they said.
- Finding a way for "eyes thinking" ideas to get through the storm[9] in the middle of his brain and talk to his "ears thinking."

---

[9]The "storm" was an analogy (almost a metaphor, which is notable, as metaphors are difficult for young people struggling with LBLDs to understand) that Matthew invented when we discussed how "ears thinking" and "eyes thinking" did not always talk across

- Building up his "nerves of steel" by doing things that he usually found scary (e.g., by balancing on water pipes laid across the river).

Several of these examples showed that he was using the speech–language strategies I had introduced to him—in particular, the picturing/visualizing of ideas or actions. After talking about visualizing the tactics he used in sports, Matthew referred to a joke between us when he said, "Looks like I'm turning out to have psychic powers!" When we talked more about how he was working out how to get through the storm in the middle of his brain, the following exchange occurred:

KATHLEEN: Do you think there is still a storm in your brain, or has it quietened down?

MATTHEW: Sort of quietened down; it's only part clouds.

KATHLEEN: Oh, it's only part clouds, so it only gets in the way a little bit.

At this point, I suggested he apply for membership in the Problem-Solvers Club (a league invented for therapeutic purposes in which young people complete an "application form" and receive a certificate of membership). Matthew thought this was pretty cool, as he was the first South Australian member from a rural area. He said, "I'll be a star—bonus!!" Also, he was very excited that he could "tutor" other young people in the future who might need his ideas about Problem-Solving.

PERFORMING THE PROBLEM-SOLVING CAREER

I have found that grounding discussion in real-life experience for young people with LBLDs increases the chances that they will understand what I am talking about, make concrete connections to their everyday experiences, and enjoy the experience of therapy (despite its tendency to be highly verbal). I often do this by role-playing real or possible events in a young person's life. For Matthew, this was also an opportunity to bear

---

the brain. He suggested that there could be a storm in the middle of his brain. We discussed how a storm would stop you from reaching a place you wanted to go, or make it harder to get there without being changed in some way. We were trying to find ways to create a clear path through the storm so that "ears thinking" and "eyes thinking" could communicate more directly and help each other out.

direct witness to the strength of competence in his life, and to draw comparisons with his mother as to how he might have handled situations when the Giving-Up career was much stronger in his life. Matthew and I developed the following role play. As we became loud and boisterous, we didn't realize we had gathered a secret audience, as Sharon and one of Matthew's brothers peered around the door to see what we were doing! (I usually visited Matthew at his house.)

The role-play scenario was an important soccer match, where I (playing Matthew's soccer coach, Don) and Matthew simulated the opposition's scoring a goal against Don and Matthew's team. As Don, I stormed over to Matthew and began yelling at him in front of the other players. This was meant to show how this situation would usually go for Matthew (i.e., before his Problem-Solving career had reached his preferred strength for it).

DON: Bloody hell, Matthew, where the hell were you looking? I mean, why didn't you stop the goal?

MATTHEW: (*Walks away*)

DON: Look, don't bloody walk away from me, where in the hell are you? This is a really important game. What do you think you are doing?

MATTHEW: (*Pacing around, giving no eye contact*)

DON: Do you realize that we might lose? We're tied now. . . .

MATTHEW: It's only a game, Don! (*Yells it back at Don and looks at him*)

DON: But it's really important, Matthew! I mean, this is the final!

MATTHEW: (*Still pacing and not looking*)

DON: Bloody hell, Matthew, who are you? Gee, you give me the shits.

We then discussed the role play. Matthew indicated that he was not taking me too seriously, as he knew this was pretend; this helped his Problem-Solver career to emerge more strongly in this first try, although he would like it to be stronger. If he had taken me really seriously, he would have walked off the field, been very upset, and tried to call his mother—similar to when the Giver-Upper career was much stronger in his life. Sharon later informed me that Matthew had great difficulty with such situations, and that until recently the Giver-Upper career had most influence over him at these times. We noted the elements of a Problem-Solver career that he was beginning to use:

- Not taking the situation too seriously.
- Not accepting negative descriptions of himself.
- Having a response so he could answer back.
- Offering his (Matthew's) perspective on the issue.
- Assuming that Don would eventually stop going on about it.
- Walking away and not arguing or fighting back.

We then role-played a future unique outcome for the same situation, when Don had become more of an audience to the alternative story of Matthew's having a Problem-Solving career (we assumed that Matthew would have persisted with and improved his use of the strategies above). Matthew played Don, and I played Matthew. This allowed Matthew, as Don, to demonstrate further Problem-Solving abilities as he provided the ideas to prevent a goal from being scored again.

ENCOURAGING SELF-REFLECTIONS ON THE MEANING OF A PROBLEM-SOLVING CAREER

I used several questions and comments in reflecting on the role play with Matthew. They could be considered "landscape-of-consciousness" questions, which

Encourage persons to review the developments as they unfold through the alternative landscape of action[10] and to determine what these might reveal about:

a) the nature of their preferences and desires,
b) the character of various personal and relationship qualities,
c) the constitution of their intentional states,
d) the composition of their preferred beliefs, and lastly,
e) the nature of their commitments. (White, 1991b, p. 31)

Therapists are often under the illusion that such questions need to be complex and eloquent; however, such questions tune out "ears think-

---

[10]"According to Bruner (1986), the 'landscape of action is constituted of (a) events that are linked together in (b) particular sequences through the (c) temporal dimension—through past, present, and future—according to (d) specific plots'" (White, 1991b, p. 28). The landscape of action can be elicited through such questions as these: "How/when/where did this happen?", "Who was there?", "What did you/they notice you doing?", "What did you tell yourself or think at this time?", "How did you get ready to take this step", and so forth.

ing" for young people with LBLDs. In the following excerpt, I offered alternative questions or comments that still referred to personal qualities, preferences, and commitments:

KATHLEEN: If you thought that you always made mistakes and were no good at things, would it keep you doing your work, or would it make you want to stop doing your work?

MATTHEW: I'd keep trying—everybody learns from their mistakes.

KATHLEEN: That's a Problem-Solver's answer!

MATTHEW: Yeah!

KATHLEEN: What would be the Giver-Upper's answer?

MATTHEW: Just don't do it, just give up . . .

KATHLEEN: And don't even try?

MATTHEW: Yeah.

KATHLEEN: It sounds like it is almost hard for you to give me a Giver-Upper's answer.

MATTHEW: I think I am turning out to be a real Problem-Solver (*spoken with some surprise*).

KATHLEEN: I think there is a distinct possibility you are, because if it is now 85%, that's the stronger one—that's the one that wants to answer. The Giver-Upper doesn't want to answer. Because every time I ask you a question about the Giver-Upper career, you turn it into a Problem-Solving answer.

MATTHEW: I think I am turning it into a future-type answer (*again with surprise*).

KATHLEEN: You think so?

MATTHEW: Yeah.

KATHLEEN: You're making your future stronger?

MATTHEW: Yeah.

In the remainder of this and subsequent visits, Matthew increasingly made self-reflective comments about his small achievements in the strengthening of his Problem-Solver career and what this meant about him as a person. For example, he would say things like "I'm doing this really fast," "I think I'm becoming a Problem-Solver," or "Hey, I worked that out!" As you can gather, the idea of becoming a Problem-Solver in life was extremely appealing to Matthew, given the many experiences of failure he had survived.

INTEGRATING "EYES THINKING" AND "EARS THINKING" LANGUAGE INTO LANGUAGE-BASED ACTIVITIES

The following dialogue offers a taste of how "ears thinking" and "eyes thinking" language was embedded in language/literacy tasks from a speech–language therapy perspective.

KATHLEEN: Now we are going to write about this story [the one we have just acted out in the role play]. What is the first part of your writing plan?

MATTHEW: *(Reflectively and slowly)* Umm, what is it?

KATHLEEN: What do you do with your "eyes thinking" first?

MATTHEW: Convert it into a picture, then interpret it—what it's trying to say.

KATHLEEN: Do you need to do that first?

MATTHEW: No, I think I've got it, I've got the picture in my head. Now convert it—no, interpret it about what it's trying to say.

KATHLEEN: Do you need to do a brainstorm first, where you just write down quick ideas?

MATTHEW: Mmm, yes. That's what Mr. Z [his teacher] does—brainstorm.

KATHLEEN: Do you want to do that with your writing plan with the big words [used as cues], or can you just, like, do it quickly?

MATTHEW: With my—probably with my writing plan.

Matthew went on to brainstorm words and ideas for each of the "big" cue words, which are drawn from Nanci Bell's (1991) work and include "what," "where," "size," "color," "number," "shape," "background," "movement," "perspective," "mood," "when," and "sound." In doing this, he used his "ears thinking" to find the words that matched the picture his "eyes thinking" had created in his head. He then wrote a first draft of the story (predominantly by himself!). Lastly, we began a revising and editing process: revising for meaning, then editing for grammar, spelling, and punctuation. The revising process included returning to his brainstormed notes and checking whether those words and ideas were included in the story, then finding places to include those ideas to create a richer account. Although this process is tedious at first, it allows "ears thinking" to deal with one layer at a time. It also helps a young person to avoid becoming overwhelmed by the task or being encouraged to give up.

Unsurprisingly, this was a long process when first introduced, and much scaffolding was needed to assist Matthew to develop better "listener or audience awareness skills" (i.e., skills for identifying and satisfying a listener's or audience's needs for information, in order to facilitate their understanding of the speaker/writer's context and intended meaning). This concept was explained as follows: "Although your 'eyes thinking' can see the picture really well, it is only through your 'ears thinking' finding lots of words to describe all the parts of the picture that your listeners can get their 'ears thinking' to send it to their 'eyes thinking' and see it the same way as you." In addition, I drew a picture to help this reflexive idea make more sense.

NOTICING PERSONAL AGENCY AND DEVELOPING AN AUDIENCE FOR A SELF-NARRATIVE OF COMPETENCE

The following conversation with Matthew and his mother, Sharon, was about a story that Matthew had written as practice between visits. Story writing, or any written work that required maintaining a topic over more than a short paragraph, had been extremely difficult for him. His "ears thinking" was very reluctant to persevere with this work, as the Giving-Up career had talked Matthew out of his competence and stolen his confidence. To be able to write longer narratives would be evidence of the Giver-Upper career's further diminishing its influence over his life, and of the increasing strength of the Problem-Solver career. Several landscape-of-action questions were used in this conversation with Matthew and Sharon, along with a persistent endeavor to notice his personal agency.[11]

KATHLEEN: So this story was written over 2 days, and at one point Matthew thought he was at the end; then you gave him some en-

---

[11]Much discussion among narratively influenced therapists centers on the place of intentionality in practice. Given that such intentionality has often been at the service of predetermined and usually negative, pathological descriptions of clients, and of therapists' preferred outcomes or answers, caution about intentionality is well placed. I think it is impossible to be completely nonintentional, just as I believe it is impossible not to communicate, so I prefer to be accountable for my intentionality when it occurs. Furthermore, I prefer it to be apparent rather than hidden, so that I can be more transparent about my practice. When it comes to noticing the ways in which young people act on their own behalf and what this might mean about them, I have no difficulty admitting that intentionality pulls at me quite strongly to pursue such a conversation.

couragement, and he wrote a bit more and he thought he was at the end. Then you gave him some more encouragement, and then it was *positively* the end.

SHARON: That's right.

KATHLEEN: Now, Matthew, you've just told me that this is the *longest* story that you have probably ever written.

MATTHEW: Yeah.

KATHLEEN: And you know that for sure?

MATTHEW: Yeah (*very definitely*).

KATHLEEN: How did you manage to get it so long?

MATTHEW: Hmmm ... I don't know, it's quite hard to say (*small chuckle*). Just with some, well, just with a little bit of help, well, some encouragement.

KATHLEEN: Encouragement from ...

MATTHEW: From Mum.

KATHLEEN: Because you know, last year if we were doing this ... [I realize I may make assumptions here, so I decide to check it from his point of view by asking questions.] Well, you know how we have talked about your career in Giving-Up and your career in Problem-Solving?

MATTHEW: Yeah.

KATHLEEN: And I think you told me a little while ago what the percentages are, and I think the Problem-Solver career is up to 80% or something pretty high like that—in fact, it was 85%.

MATTHEW: Yep.

KATHLEEN: And only 15% of the Giver-Upper career is left. Now when you got to here, one and a half pages, and you thought this might be the end ...

MATTHEW: Mmm.

KATHLEEN: ... and Mum gave you some encouragement and said, "You can do some more," which career took over here?

MATTHEW: Problem-Solving.

KATHLEEN: The Problem-Solver career took over here. All right, what did it have to do to get you writing again?

MATTHEW: Umm, oh ... well ... umm ... (*Looks away at something else going on in the kitchen*)

KATHLEEN: What did the Problem-Solving career have to do to get you writing again? What did it do to convince you to write again (*spoken more slowly and with emphasis*)?

MATTHEW: Well, keep going 'till you get to that limit.

KATHLEEN: Yeah . . . but how did you get the message to keep going?

MATTHEW: Uh . . . mmm.

KATHLEEN: Which career . . . let me start again. Which career did you listen to at this point? What career did you listen to, the Giver-Upper career or the Problem-Solver career?

MATTHEW: Problem-Solver career.

KATHLEEN: And you said that Mum gave you some encouragement. If Mum didn't give you that encouragement, what do you think would have happened?

MATTHEW: Well, I would have just stopped there.

KATHLEEN: You would have just stopped there. All right, so that would be where that 15% of that Giver-Upper career would have . . .

[The conversation is interrupted here by a phone call. After the call, I reiterate an earlier point and then continue with the line of questioning.]

KATHLEEN: What made you stop here? Which career made you stop?

MATTHEW: Probably the Giver-Upper. Then Mum said, "Well, do more."

KATHLEEN: And you did. But what if the Giver-Upper career was really strong? [What if] Mum said, "Do some more," but the Giver-Upper career was really strong—what would you have done?

MATTHEW: Well, uh . . . I wouldn't be able to do it.

KATHLEEN: So, Mum gave you some encouragement. Was that the only thing that helped you to do it. . . .

MATTHEW: Yeah.

KATHLEEN: . . . or was your strong Problem-Solver career helping as well?

MATTHEW: Well, Mum as well . . . a bit of both.

KATHLEEN: I'm just wondering, Sharon, if Matthew's Giver-Upper career was really strong, whether he would have still been able to do it, even with your encouragement?

SHARON: He wouldn't have been able to do it if I hadn't kept on saying to him, "No, Matthew. I won't accept that from you because I *know* you can do it. Go back in your room, sit down, and do it, because I want it done." And he just went back and he did it.

KATHLEEN: I'm just wondering now because his Problem-Solver career is now at 85% strength, and it has convinced him that he can solve problems most of the time. Before, when his Giver-Upper career was strong and said, "No, it's not worth it. No, you can't do it. No, don't bother," do you think he would have responded in the same way to you?

SHARON: No.

KATHLEEN: What would have been different?

SHARON: I would have only gotten maybe a half a page out of him. He would have just given up, and even if I had sat with him and kept him going a little bit, with my own ideas as well as his own, he would have only have written that half a page.

KATHLEEN: Right . . . So his ability to go back and do some more *by himself*—you gave him some encouragement, but he actually did it by himself—that's actually quite a new development.

SHARON: Oh, yeah—well, that's a first. This is a first.

KATHLEEN: A first—this is unique?

SHARON: This is *a* first.

KATHLEEN: All right! So there should be a few cheers then, shouldn't there?!

SHARON: Oh, yes.

MATTHEW: (*With some excitement*) Yeah, a celebration!!

KATHLEEN: A celebration! And what's more, you went back not just once . . .

MATTHEW: . . . but twice!!

KATHLEEN: So what did you prove to yourself?

MATTHEW: That I'm a really good Problem-Solver.

KATHLEEN: Yeah, and that you can do something even when you don't think you can do any more.

MATTHEW: That's right.

KATHLEEN: So where were these ideas hiding? You got to the end, you thought it was the end—where were these ideas hiding? (*Pointing back to the story where he continued it on two occasions*)

MATTHEW: Umm . . . hmm.

KATHLEEN: That you hadn't yet used. These were new ideas, you hadn't used them. Where were they hiding?

MATTHEW: Well, basically, up in my head.

KATHLEEN: In your head—in your "ears thinking" or in your "eyes thinking," were they hiding?

MATTHEW: "Ears thinking" . . . well, in my brain.

KATHLEEN: In your brain—but were the ideas hiding in your "eyes thinking," like your picture of what happened, or were they hiding in your "ears thinking," in the words to go with it?

MATTHEW: Well, hiding in the . . . well, basically, in the "ears thinking."

KATHLEEN: They were in the "ears thinking." How did you get them out of your "ears thinking"?

MATTHEW: Well, I just thought until . . . how can I put it?

KATHLEEN: Did you say you thought it or you saw it?

MATTHEW: I thought it.

KATHLEEN: And did you think of it by seeing it, or did you think of it by hearing it?

MATTHEW: By hearing it.

KATHLEEN: You were hearing it (*surprised*)? Did you need to use your "eyes thinking" to come up with these ideas?

MATTHEW: Well, a little bit of it.

KATHLEEN: So you saw it a little bit with your "eyes thinking." So how did your "eyes thinking" get the words out of hiding?

MATTHEW: I just wrote them down.

KATHLEEN: So, by seeing it with your "eyes thinking," that helped pull the words out of where they were hiding, and then you wrote them down?

MATTHEW: Yep.

KATHLEEN: Then they weren't hiding any more, were they?

MATTHEW: That's right.

KATHLEEN: They were right out there on the page. . . . So do you think this is another step in your Problem-Solver career?

MATTHEW: Yeah, definitely.

KATHLEEN: Is this a step that you like to see?

MATTHEW: Yep, I love to.

KATHLEEN: So what would happen if you saw more of these steps, where you keep doing work when you didn't even think you could do any more?

MATTHEW: Well, I'd just keep going and going and going.

KATHLEEN: You think you will.

MATTHEW: Yeah.

KATHLEEN: All right, you're convinced that you will now.

MATTHEW: Yeah.

KATHLEEN: So, is this Problem-Solving career—you said it was at 85%—has it crept up a little bit at all?

MATTHEW: I think so, yeah, a little bit, yeah.

KATHLEEN: What would it have crept up to if it's crept up just a little bit?

MATTHEW: If I had that little bit of extra help, I could get that little bit done.

KATHLEEN: Yeah.

MATTHEW: And get the rest of my ideas in my . . . out, get the rest of the, my ideas out.

KATHLEEN: So getting that encouragement from Mum was very helpful.

MATTHEW: Yeah, and we're doing this major project . . .

Matthew went off on what looked like a tangent, but it ended up being a comparison between the encouragement Sharon had given him and the "tips" his teacher had given him to do a project. We then decided that the Problem-Solver career had crept up to 86%.

COMPETENCE AND THE PROBLEM-SOLVING CAREER AS A WAY OF LIFE

Future conversations with Matthew identified new developments in his strengthening Problem-Solver career. Thinking in terms of his personal competence and Problem-Solving abilities began to capture Matthew's enthusiasm, and he needed less encouragement to consider thinking in such terms. We spent time deconstructing the practices, beliefs, and "talk" of the Giver-Upper career, considering how Matthew's life might have turned out if it had maintained a strong influence, and tracking the early beginnings of the Problem-Solving career. Some of the questions used were these:

- What would have happened if the Giver-Upper career had kept on being strong?
- How would you be feeling?
- What would people see you doing?
- What would they say about you?
- Would they start believing that you couldn't do anything?
- What made you think that giving up was what you had to do?
- What do you have to give in to, to make the Giver-Upper career strong?
- What would the Giver-Upper career say to you?
- Did it even talk you out of things you knew you could do?

In all of this work, the use of visualization to enable Matthew to make direct connections with past experiences was vital to his engagement with the therapy process. He then began spontaneously to visualize himself solving problems or using his competence in the past and to use these visualizations to assist him in the present (see Stacey, 1995a, for further discussion on using visualization).

REVIEWING THE HISTORY OF THE PROBLEM-SOLVING CAREER

This conversation reviewed the steps Matthew had taken to strengthen the influence of the Problem-Solver career in his life. It also shows how Matthew was being a consultant to others younger than himself who were having trouble with learning.

KATHLEEN: This last couple of weeks, how many steps do you think you've been making, because you told me about remembering how to delete on the computer?

MATTHEW: Yeah, that's one.

KATHLEEN: And then you told me about . . .

MATTHEW: Finger power on the computer.

KATHLEEN: Using all your fingers so you have finger power on the computer.

MATTHEW: Umm . . . and sometimes, helping other people.

KATHLEEN: Helping other people?

MATTHEW: Yeah, so that's a third step.

KATHLEEN: What sort of helping have you been doing?

MATTHEW: Like giving another person who's having problems with their learning that extra step up.

KATHLEEN: Uh-huh. Can you give me an example, something you've done?

MATTHEW: Let's say someone couldn't do a multiplication sum. I'd say, "Just times that by this. When you've finished the first line, add the placement zero, then you go on to that, then add it up, then you've got your answer!" (*Very pleased with himself at this explanation*)

KATHLEEN: Uh-huh, and how did they find that helpful?

MATTHEW: Yeah, pretty helpful indeed.

KATHLEEN: They found that helpful. All right. And how old are these people?

MATTHEW: Sometimes, well . . . they are usually fifth or sixth . . . no, not sixth-graders but fifth-graders. And sometimes we're doing reception, tutoring receptions. [This is equivalent to the kindergarten year in North American schools.]

KATHLEEN: And what do you like about doing that?

MATTHEW: Well . . . it gives them the experience . . . it gives, like, them to boost up their help . . . it gives them help . . .

KATHLEEN: It gives them help. And does it boost . . . go on (*we speak at the same time*).

MATTHEW: Yeah . . . well, not really boost up, well, just help them and . . .

KATHLEEN: Do you think it might boost up their confidence?

MATTHEW: Yeah, boost up their confidence, that's it!

KATHLEEN: Yeah. Why do you think that's important?

MATTHEW: Er . . . well it actually teaches them self-confidence . . . and, like, well . . . well, it teaches them, well, it teaches them confidence and like, so they don't like, so they don't, like, take . . . so they don't, like, give up sort of thing.

KATHLEEN: So they don't give up? So they don't develop a Giving-Up career?

MATTHEW: That's right!

KATHLEEN: Now, why did you decide . . . what made you decide . . .

MATTHEW: Oh, and the other seventh-graders were doing that as well.

KATHLEEN: What made *you* decide that people boosting their confidence was important?

MATTHEW: Yeah, that was really important.

KATHLEEN: But what made you *decide* it was important?

MATTHEW: Phew.

KATHLEEN: What makes you think that's important?

MATTHEW: So they, like, if they don't . . . if they don't know what it is, they can just ask anyone and they can help them. So they don't, like, give up all the time.

KATHLEEN: So they can get help if they need it.

MATTHEW: Yeah, that's right.

KATHLEEN: Could it also mean if they don't get it the first time, they could try a second time?

MATTHEW: Yep.

KATHLEEN: And that would stop the Giving-Up career too, wouldn't it?

MATTHEW: Correct.

KATHLEEN: Because if you try a second time, you're not practicing giving up, you're practicing . . .

MATTHEW: Problem-Solving! Was . . . is that . . . was that a fourth step?

KATHLEEN: Well, I think that was three steps—well, it might be four steps. So it was . . . learning how to delete, using your finger power with all of your fingers, helping the younger students . . .

MATTHEW: Helping the receptions.

KATHLEEN: Yeah, so that's a step in Problem-Solving.

MATTHEW: And teaching other people that they're confide . . . and teaching confidence.

KATHLEEN: And teaching confidence! Yes.

MATTHEW: So that's four things . . . I've boosted up!! (*Very excited about this*)

KATHLEEN: You're right, it is a fourth step. So you've been taking lots of steps in your Problem-Solving career! I wonder what it has got to right now.

We decided that the Problem-Solver career had grown to be 87%, the Giver-Upper career was 12%, and 1% was undecided. Matthew guessed that this 1% would probably decide that the Problem-Solver career was a better career, as it would make him happier in life. Later that session, we discovered that remembering things he had to do was a fifth step, and Matthew volunteered that enthusiasm could be a sixth step. We agreed that although he had been practicing enthusiasm for a long time, with lots of encouragement from his mum, he had been giving it extra practice lately. He then suggested that "once I get to 20 steps, I'll be passing with flying colors!"

Later that visit, when questioned about how the Giving-Up career undermined his confidence, Matthew suggested that it would tell him things or get him to say to himself things such as these:

- "Why do it? Don't bother, you're not good at this."
- "Why bother? I can't do this."
- "No, they'll laugh at me for trying—even easy things."

Furthermore, he said that the Giver-Upper career took his ideas away from him so he couldn't use them for Problem-Solving.[12]

CATCHING UP ON SPECIAL ABILITIES: GOING FROM STRENGTH TO STRENGTH

When I caught up with Matthew after he had started high school, he wanted to demonstrate his special abilities with speaking German (a new subject), which were quite stunning. This led to us realizing that his "ears thinking" had some special abilities that we had not really talked enough about before. These special abilities included showing different voice characteristics when performing other people's roles or during everyday conversation, speaking German and French with good accents, and learning to talk and read these languages. Discussion with Sharon indicated that Matthew had had trouble learning her first language,

[12]This conversation occurred close to the end of the seventh grade. In the last 6 months of seventh grade, before going on to high school, Matthew had also practiced Problem-Solving with me by writing to the Regional Special Educational Consultant, who was available to provide support to the school for students with special learning needs. Because Matthew's teacher was convinced that he was lazy and unmotivated rather than struggling with LBLDs, the teacher had declined any offers for direct communication. By communicating with the Regional Special Education Consultant, we were able to influence the teacher indirectly to accept some of the "ears thinking" strategies Matthew and I had developed, as he was prepared to respect the consultant's input. Matthew authored most of these documents, with my support—they were also opportunities to use his "ears thinking" strategies for writing tasks. Due to space limitations, more details and copies of the documents exchanged between Matthew and the consultant could not be included.

Maltese. It became clear to us that in learning German and French, he was using "ears thinking" and "eyes thinking" skills together more consistently, and that this led to easier learning.

A review of Matthew's careers indicated that the Problem-Solver was 89%, the Giver-Upper was 10%, and 1% was still undecided. Matthew decided that there was a pattern: Any undecided percentage point that came out of the Giver-Upper career eventually went into the Problem-Solver career, but stayed there—it never returned. He then gave evidence of the strengthening of the Problem-Solver career with his better marks in his first high school report, compared to his primary school reports.

KATHLEEN: What else tells you your Problem-Solver career is getting stronger?

MATTHEW: Well, I've been helping. I have one friend who has trouble with his work in maths, so I, like, help him.

KATHLEEN: So, helping a friend with maths.

MATTHEW: You should see this one—outstanding, outstanding (*showing me his report*).

KATHLEEN: Oh, these are your other areas (*reading from his report*): Responsibility in care group is outstanding; uniform, neatness, appearance is outstanding; and punctuality is just right.

MATTHEW: Just right in the middle. That's overdone, that's underdone, and that's just right (*pointing to the different columns*).

KATHLEEN: So you've got nothing that's underdone!

MATTHEW: So it's just right. (*Lots of giggles by us both*)

The conversation turned to uncovering several unique outcomes that fitted with the Problem-Solver's career. We reviewed Matthew's friends at school—he had several, including boys and girls whom he hadn't known before going to high school. Furthermore, he was quite tuned in to one of his friend's experiences of breaking up with a girlfriend; he said that the friend was feeling, "terrible, just terrible. He hasn't been his normal self since!" We also contemplated whether it should be how it "usually is," according to Matthew, that the boy dumps the girl, because in this case the girl dumped his friend. Matthew believed it was understandable, as "she didn't get any attention." He also thought that either person could choose to end the relationship. This was an example of Matthew's being able to talk about other people's experiences with an awareness of how the events might have felt for them—something he had found very difficult to articulate for himself or others previously. Matthew wasn't interested in talking about his own special new female friend at school, whom his brother mentioned as he walked through the room. He seemed embarrassed and insisted that it was none of his brother's business; it was just between "me and my brain!" This was an example of Matthew's being able to stand up for himself and cope with some friendly teasing without feeling demoralized or unable to respond.

Matthew and I developed an idea to write to a listserv through the Internet for a group of narrative or solution-focused therapists. Matthew wanted to see whether any therapists worked with young people who might want to become his pen pals. (He also, very benevolently, suggested that therapists were "nature's own problem solvers"!) Matthew received two responses to his request and planned to write to these young people. He and I had now worked together for 19 months; we agreed at this point, together with his family, that we would drop back from visits every 3–4 weeks to checking in every 3 months. With his Problem-Solver's career only 4 points away from his goal of 95%, he felt confident that he could take these steps by himself and was getting the support he needed at school for continuing to help his "ears thinking."[13]

EDITORIAL QUESTIONS

Q: *(DN) In your work with young persons, you must interface with speech pathologists and/or special educators who are informed by conventional, modernist notions of LBLDs. How do you communicate with professionals who subscribe to pathologizing stories in a way that maintains your own integrity and does not disqualify young persons? Do you have any advice from your own personal experience that you could pass on? I ask this question because it is a challenge for me to interface with colleagues/professionals who operate from a very different paradigm.*

A: Let me first state that such people are acting in ways they believe are helpful and often prove to be helpful to young people. They would not

---

[13]The move to high school proved to be very positive, once Matthew had worked through some initial trepidation. Most importantly, there was no difficulty recruiting an audience to understanding the effects of LBLDs on his life, the importance of supporting strategies to assist his "ears thinking" to do its job more effectively for him, and his strengthening Problem-Solver career, as his special education support teacher's perception of Matthew was similar to ours. In fact, he was quite astounded at Matthew's achievements.

be in their work unless they had a commitment to supporting young people who live with learning disabilities. I find that most people are intrigued by or at least respectful of the style of language I use, regardless of whether they are interested in the theoretical ideas that inform it. Furthermore, they find it useful to be oriented toward other aspects of the young person as "person," as this usually generates more hope. The most difficult situations to negotiate are the times when the behavior in which a young person is engaging speaks more loudly to educators/professionals than the learning difficulties the young person is experiencing. It is at these times that pathologizing versions have a stronger influence and invite the phrase of which a colleague and I have become increasingly wary: "Gary needs to learn that . . ."

Until the young person learns whatever has been stated, the young person is disqualified from receiving compassion, appreciation, and support. I usually take this as an expression of the adults' frustration in the face of learning difficulties. I believe, especially for regular class teachers, that learning difficulties can be a threat to their sense of professional competence. As teachers have few supportive environments in which to speak about these perceived threats to competence without facing blame and failure, the invitation to see incompetence as residing with young persons themselves is more compelling. Furthermore, it fits with the prevailing notions about ownership of problems.

Thus, I try to orient conversations toward the effects of learning difficulties on young persons' lives, relationships, sense of competence, communication efforts, feelings, and behavior. I try to acknowledge how this interferes with classroom management, home–school communication, and peer relationships, and to note how it results in the young persons' waiting for offers rather than initiating requests for help from educators. I try to explore whether, in trying to manage their learning difficulties, young people have developed habits that have outlived their usefulness or are not as appreciated by other people, especially adults. If so, these can be named—and, ideally, the adults most affected by these habits can join forces with the young persons in putting an end to the habits or limiting where they can be practiced.

In essence, I endeavor to create space for a different way of talking about the issues that the adults are raising, in which problems continue to be externalized and "loss of face" is minimized. I am often steadfast in these endeavors, so I also have to be aware of how leaning toward "missionary zeal" can get in the way of my relationships with other professionals. So, some selective ignoring is often useful here, as is initiating a conversation about the effects of trying to support young persons with learning difficulties on the adults' work. I hope the adults will find out that I am also interested in supporting them, not just the young persons.

Finally, acknowledging the successful efforts the adults have made to support the young persons' learning is also vital to conveying respect for them and their own knowledge.

Q: *(CS) Kathleen, your transcript demonstrates for me a wonderful combination of faith, patience, persistence, humor, flexibility, and respect. I'm amazed at how you so successfully combine teaching/coaching skills with therapist curiosity and other narrative talents! You have creatively originated a whole new language of "eyes thinking" and "ears thinking," which is a unique way of extending White's and Epston's ideas about externalizing conversations. Simultaneously, you draw from your rich speech and language background in simplifying, scaffolding, and structuring your questions to make them understood.*

Since you bring a unique background in speech and language to this book, I would like to focus on this. Could you say a few words about particular traditional speech and language research, or developmental research/assessment in general, that has proven helpful to your work? Are there specific traditional concepts or ways of working with visual and auditory difficulties that have been central to your work?

Conversely, what aspects of traditional ways of working with LBLDs are least useful for you? You briefly mentioned a conventional focus on deficits and totalizing. Could you give us a couple of concrete examples of questions that might be asked or interventions that might be done from a more traditional mindset, so we can get a clearer idea of both the differences and the similarities between your work and other approaches to LBLDs?

A: I think that Lev Vygotsky, Jerome Bruner, and Michael Halliday, to name a few, are examples of people whose work has influenced mainstream speech–language work in ways that I find helpful—although I now interpret their work through a different lens than the one I was originally taught. I have difficulty with collapsing mainstream speech–language work into a traditional box, as it has gone through a number of transformations since the 1960s. It has moved from a focus on grammatical forms and articulation of sounds, to including semantics or meaning in language in context, systemic understandings of speech sound production, and narrative and/or discourse structure and use. Like psychology, it has also expanded its behavioral and sociobehavioral knowledges and practices to include cognitive, psychosocial, and (very recently) discourse knowledge and practice, although its research base is still heavily dominated by logical–empiricist research, with some case studies and ethnographic studies sprinkled around.

Concepts that have been helpful to my work are that language is made up of grammatical, semantic, and pragmatic knowledges, and that there are both distinctions and interconnections between visual and auditory processing of information, which need to be addressed for young people struggling with language learning (see Stacey, 1992, 1994a, 1995a). Approaches to LBLDs that I find less helpful are those that, despite a cursory acknowledgment of the relationship between socioemotional and linguistic development, ignore the socioemotional effects of living with LBLDs and focus predominantly on language and academic issues for these young persons; minimize the need for behavioral issues in connection with language issues; focus on specific language skills without putting them in the context of a child's language and literacy needs in everyday living; ignore cultural and/or sociopolitical contexts that influence a child's style of learning and the standards to which the child is compared; and those that engage in (often subtle) parent blaming, either for the presence of the learning difficulty or for a perceived lack of support for the therapy program. I think these issues are fairly familiar to therapists, although situated within different problem descriptions. I find it difficult to encapsulate all this in a couple of concrete examples, however, see Stacey (1995b, 1995c) for further discussion.

Q: *(CS) As you are well aware, some narratively oriented questions are reflexive and involve a high level of abstraction and complexity. Do you have any concrete advice for therapists wishing to work narratively with young children in general? Are there some common features in your work with children with and without LBLDs?*
A: My advice would be to become less enraptured with the frequent eloquence of narratively oriented language and more connected with the language that makes sense to a child, and to break questions down into component parts. Drawings, puppets, and play can also be useful. These are common features in my work with children (see Stacey [1995a]). The differences are often more patience on my part and a willingness to go slower in order to end up going quite fast with young people with LBLDs in therapy. The other difference is to work in partnership with someone with speech–language knowledge who can support these young people in this area of their lives.

Q: *(CS) I have appreciated your emphasis on how children's voices are often undervalued in our adult-centered world. You have pointed out how this general trend is even more pronounced for those with LBLDs and/or from minority cultures. Could you say a few words for those readers who might be unfamiliar with your and Cathy Loptson's ideas on this (Stacey & Loptson, 1995)?*
A: To draw on the words of bell hooks (1989), for these young people in a Western and more Anglo- and Celtic-dominated culture, "language

is a place of struggle" (p. 28). Young people are not able to engage in the complexity and nuances of language that adults engage in, mainly because of their more limited experience and cumulative knowledge of language and operations of the world. If the language on which young people need to rely is further alienated from them by their having difficulties in the manipulation, generation, and use of language, or by their being born outside of the language of power, their voices are silenced in an adult-dominated world. Adults make the rules; set the standards; determine priorities and criteria; judge value, appropriateness, and relevance; control resources; and administer consequences. Language is one of the most valued ways of having influence over these activities. There are other ways, but they are usually not valued or understood. When language is a place of struggle, then the struggles are multiplied.

REFERENCES

Bell, N. (1991). *Visualizing and verbalizing for language comprehension and thinking*. Paso Robles, California: Academy of Reading Publications.

Bruner, J. (1986). *Actual minds, possible worlds*. Cambridge, MA: Harvard University Press.

Bruner, J., & Haste, H. (1987). *Making sense: The child's construction of the world*. London: Methuen.

Garbarino, J. (1993). Childhood: What do we need to know? *Childhood, 1,* 3–10.

Goolishian, H., & Anderson, H. (1990). Understanding the therapeutic process: From individuals and families to systems in language. In F. W. Kaslow (Ed.), *Voices in family therapy* (Vol. 1). Newbury Park, CA: Sage.

hooks, b. (1989). *Talking back: Thinking feminist, thinking black*. Boston: South End Press.

Stacey, K. (1992). Language: A point of convergence: Integrating family therapy and speech pathology. *Family Therapy Case Studies, 7*(2), 3–19.

Stacey, K. (1994a). "Ears thinking" and "eyes thinking": Language as a point of convergence: Mark revisited. *Family Therapy Case Studies, 8*(1), 37–45.

Stacey, K. (1994b). *Family-focused and systemic approaches with children experiencing language based learning difficulties: Influences on service provider knowledge and practice*. Unpublished master's thesis, Pacific Oaks College, Pasadena, CA.

Stacey, K. (1995a). Language as an exclusive or inclusive concept: Reaching beyond the verbal. *Australian and New Zealand Journal of Family Therapy, 16*(3), 123–132.

Stacey, K. (1995b). The impact of learning difficulties on families' lives in terms of loss and change. *Proceedings of Understanding Loss and Managing Change: A National Multidisciplinary Conference*. Adelaide, South Australia: Royal College of Nursing.

Stacey, K. (1995c, May). *Interfaces between language, social-emotional development and social competence from a systemic perspective: An introductory paper.* Paper presented at the National Conference of the Australian Association of Speech and Hearing, Brisbane, Queensland.

Stacey, K. (1997). Alternative metaphors for externalizing conversations. *Gecko: A Journal of Deconstruction and Narrative Ideas in Therapeutic Practice, 1,* 29–51.

Stacey, K., & Loptson, C. (1995). Children should be seen and not heard?: Questioning the unquestioned. *Journal of Systemic Therapies, 14*(4), 16–32.

Stewart, B., & Nodrick, B. (1990). The learning disabled lifestyle: From reification to liberation. *Family Therapy Case Studies, 2*(1), 61–73.

White, M. (1991a). *Introduction to re-authoring and narrative therapy.* Intensive course presented at the Dulwich Centre, Adelaide, South Australia.

White, M. (1991b). Deconstruction and therapy. *Dulwich Centre Newsletter,* No. 3, 21–40.

10

Collaborative Conversations with Children

COUNTRY CLOTHES AND CITY CLOTHES

HARLENE ANDERSON
SUE LEVIN

We all know we are unique individuals, but we
tend to see others as representative of groups. It's a
natural tendency, since we must see the world in
patterns in order to make sense of it; we wouldn't
be able to deal with the daily onslaught of people
and objects if we couldn't predict a lot about them
and feel that we know who and what they are. But
this natural and useful ability to see patterns of
similarity has unfortunate consequences. It is
offensive to reduce an individual to a category, and
it is also misleading.
—TANNEN (1990, p. 16)

This chapter reflects our excitement and enjoyment in writing about our
work with children. We find working with children as interesting, enriching, and successful as our work with people of any age. A delightful

255

yet emotional interview[1] in which one of us (Harlene), four children, and their parents take part, forms the basis of this chapter, and creates a vehicle for our discussion of a collaborative approach to therapy (Anderson, 1995, 1997; Anderson & Goolishian, 1988). The children in this interview are 4, 6, 8, and 11 years old, and are engaged with Harlene in a first meeting that has coalesced around their parents' expressed concerns. This interview portrays our belief, shared with a portion of our larger community, that children are valuable; they deserve respect and an opportunity to have a voice.

The idea to meet with Mindy[2] and Charles and their four children evolved out of a conversation that Mindy, Charles, and Harlene had the day before. In that conversation, they talked about the difficulties Mindy and Charles were having in negotiating their recent "arrangement." Mindy had recently rented an apartment in town, about an hour's drive away from the family home in the country. Mindy and Charles had considered this arrangement for several months and felt they had finally worked out a plan that both could live with. The children lived with Dad in the country and visited Mom in the city or in the country. What happened, however, was not what either imagined, as Mindy's need for "space" created "pulls" with the children. Mindy's words reflected the inner pull she felt from herself and the outer pull she felt from the children:

> "And there's a part of me that even wants more disconnectedness than there is right now. I've been talking with Charles about—the pull is the kids. I have devoted my life to these children. I have given them every ounce—I'll go to tears again—I've given them every ounce of everything that I've had. And so it's like he said, that he's [Charles] a big boy and that we'll work it between us, but the *kids*—I can't—the disconnection—they stay connected to me with the heartstrings. They want to pick up the phone and they want to call me, and they want me at home, and whatever they want, but they want that connectedness. And so I've been talking in terms of—I want to tell them that I'm going on a 2-week vacation, or some amount of time that they can register in their mind or mark

---

[1]This interview is available on videotape from Master'sWork Productions, 1315 Westwood Blvd., Los Angeles, CA 90024; (800) 476-1619. We thank Masters' Work for permission to use the interview dialogue. The entire interview was 50 minutes; the excerpts used in this chapter are in chronological order.

[2]Names have been changed to protect confidentiality, though all clients mentioned in this chapter (including Achelra, who is discussed briefly later) have consented to have their stories told.

off on the calendar or do whatever they want to. But I need that disconnection, because they're pulling me hard."

Charles reported his concern for the children since the collapse of the back-and-forth nature of the plan:

"What I'm saying is it's fine for me, that I can deal with it. She can go be separate. She can go to her place in the city and stay for as long as she needs to stay. I can pull back off of that and be okay, but the kids cannot. The kids are in real distress. . . . Because when we talked about having a place in town, it was—the deal was we could spend a couple of days in town [this referred to Charles and the childrens' staying at a grandfather's house], and she could spend a couple of days in the house in the country. That way, the majority of time, they'd have access to Mindy. . . . But it's turned into something different."

Mindy, Charles, and Harlene talked about the arrangement and how Mindy and Charles were handling it with each other and with the children. Questions that emerged about the children included the following: How did they think the children were understanding and making sense of the arrangement? What did they each say when the children asked questions about the arrangement? What did Mindy say to them when they called her on the phone? Finally, what were their worst fears for the children? At the end of the hour, Mindy, Charles, and Harlene agreed that the next step seemed to be a meeting with the children. The meeting was arranged for the next day. Harlene had met the children previously because they always came with their parents, playing and reading inside when the weather was bad, and outside when the weather was good. Her contact with the children was usually a brief social exchange, except for one meeting with the mother and the 8-year-old daughter, at the mother's request.

For the curious reader, Mindy and Charles (who are in their mid 30s) and their four children have orchestrated their lives in various unusual ways, in addition to the current country–city arrangement. In Mindy's words, "We do things nontraditionally." Married for 19 years, Mindy and Charles were high school sweethearts who shared a dream. They worked hard, saved their money, bought a piece of land in the country, and built their own home step by step. Charles describes it as a "back-to-the-land homestead lifestyle." They are very self-sufficient and they live modestly, since Charles retired early so that he *and* Mindy could be full-time parents. The children were born at home and are home-schooled.

INCLUDING CHILDREN?: A MODERNIST QUESTION

The field of family therapy has recognized its tendency not to include children in therapy sessions, and some practitioners are making efforts to change this (Combrinck-Graham, 1991; Dowling, 1993; Villeneuve & LaRoche, 1993). Other mental health professionals have also discussed the question of when, and when not, to include children (Wachtel, 1994). Recommendations about inclusion seem to revolve around three types of concerns: concern for each child, based on the child's age, developmental level, and psychological/emotional needs; concern for the family, based on family structure, the issues in the family, and, the family's developmental stage; and concern for the therapist, based on the expertise and comfort level of the therapist. For example, when a family with children is facing divorce, most therapists agree that the children need attention. There is disparity, however, regarding whether the children should participate in psychotherapy to satisfy their emotional needs, or whether therapy should focus on teaching the parents how to attend to their children's emotional needs during this transition (Campbell, 1992; Wallerstein, 1991; Wallerstein & Kelly, 1977).

In our view, whether to include children in therapy or not is a modernist question. Modernism is an epistemological tradition related to empiricism and the natural sciences that posits reality as something knowable, and subsequently implies that there are *answers* to questions such as the ones above. People living within this tradition bear the responsibility of *knowing* the answers, or looking to experts to find them. Therapists practicing within this tradition, for instance, make decisions about whom to include in therapy, based on their "knowledge" and "expertise." Therapies based on postmodern philosophies, such as social constructionism, have developed in response to discomfort with modernism (see, e.g., Berger & Luckman, 1967; Gergen, 1985; Anderson & Goolishian, 1992; McNamee & Gergen, 1992; Shotter & Gergen, 1993; Anderson, 1997). From a social constructionist position, the decision of inclusion would not be left to a therapist.

Culture affects perceptions and expectations of children (Ariés, 1962). Children have been treated differently among cultures, and within cultures from century to century. Modernists use cultural information to make judgments about good and bad child-rearing practices, and believe that empirical study is helping us develop better ways to understand, raise, and protect children. Social constructionists question the assumptions in such evolutionary explanations that civilizations are constantly moving forward on a linear path.

Social constructionism considers that we, as humans, construct what we know. Knowing occurs in a shared, social exchange, in language. From this viewpoint, individuals operate in an intersubjective and *shared* meaning system (Levin, 1992). Therapy from a social constructionist perspective does not follow predetermined maps or formats. Maps and formats are created collaboratively, and are unique and specific to the particular client(s) and therapist at a certain point in time.

CHILDREN ARE PEOPLE TOO: OR, IS LABELING NECESSARY?

A respect for clients and their concerns, and a curiosity and openness about who should participate in therapy conversations, are hallmarks of a collaborative approach to therapy, as developed by Anderson and Goolishian (1988, 1992). Other hallmarks to be illustrated here include following a client's lead, maintaining coherence, generating meaning, entertaining new and contradictory ideas, and keeping multiple conversational directions open. Respect, concern, curiosity, and openness may seem simple and straightforward concepts that are reportedly shared by therapists who operate out of other theoretical orientations, but they begin to crumble when therapists view clients as members of "special populations."

Once clients are defined as members of "special populations," they are labeled as different. They become known by the characteristics or behaviors associated with this categorization, and the rest of their *selves* get lost and out of focus (Levin, 1992). Once a therapist diagnoses and therefore labels a client, he/she then *knows* what to do. This modernist "knowledge" directs a therapist's thoughts and actions and leaves little room for alternatives. Labeling a child, for instance, carries implications that limit the kind of interactions most therapists would have with her/him.

We do not believe that therapy relationships require using labels and categories, nor do we approach therapy that way. We do not think of our work with children as any different from work with any other age group. The word "child" may come up in conversation with clients or colleagues, as it is a commonly used shortcut, but it does not carry any special predeterminations for us about that person or how we will work with him/her. We want to learn about persons from themselves and from the others who are involved in their lives, whether these include biological family members, child protective services workers, school counselors, or best friends.

Though we do not find it helpful for therapy, there are occasions when categorization or labeling is necessary and pragmatic. For example, how would school funding be allocated if children in a given geographic area were not identified and counted? Assessing the needs of underprivileged children has led to the development of important programs such as Head Start and Aid to Families with Dependent Children. Many children would not get adequate health care or nutrition if it were not for community interventions based on statistical categories. Despite the utility of many of these programs, there are at least an equal number of instances where professionals believe that identification or categorization of children has done more harm than good. Overdiagnosis in the area of attention deficit disorder is one of the most glaring examples of this problem (see Law, Chapter 11, this volume).

We believe that our responsibility as therapists is to talk with clients in ways that are respectful and generative. Labels and the stereotypes by "outsiders" are neither respectful nor generative. How persons are labeled is not all there is to know about them. Self-identity is fostered in this type of therapy by going beyond labels, beyond stereotypes, beyond our biases and predetermined ideas about people. This frees and allows for multiple, contradicting, and simultaneously existing selves.

GETTING STARTED

A therapist using a collaborative approach follows a client's lead. This position, of staying "one step behind" a client, grants prominence to the client's views, concerns, and constructions of the problem. In this way, the client determines what is important to talk about. Taking this position also leads a therapist to become a learner (Anderson, 1997; Anderson & Goolishian, 1992), as a therapist takes each person's comment(s) as an opportunity to learn more about the person, what she/he considers important, and how she/he sees the world. Children often are not afforded this level of interest by adults; their ideas are minimized and discounted (Stacey & Loptson, 1995).

Each session, its participants, and its focus are informed by the previous conversation. Clients and therapists are equally engaged in the process of deciding who should be in therapy—or, as Andersen (1991) asks, "Who should be talking to whom, about what?" During the session with Mindy, Charles, and Harlene, for example, the idea for the next day's meeting and for including the children evolved within the conversation. The idea was not therapist-driven, but what Mindy and Charles thought best at that point in time (Anderson & Goolishian, 1992).

It is hard to describe the uniqueness of Denise, Melissa, Sylvia, and Joel, the children you will meet in the following excerpts. Transcriptions of dialogue do not portray all that occurs in an interaction. You do not see Denise's tears as she talks about being scared that Mom and Dad will divorce; neither do you know when Joel crawls up into Dad's lap, or when Mom attempts to comfort Denise with a hug.[3] These children are compellingly articulate, engaging, and well behaved in this 50-minute interview, and reportedly are so as a general rule. Four-year-old Joel is as attentive, and as forthcoming with his own contributions to the session, as his older siblings.

At the beginning, and throughout the interview, Harlene is intensely involved in following each child's[4] comment closely, learning more about each comment, finding and maintaining coherence with each child and his/her stories, and not directing the conversation. This involvement displays her respect, concern, curiosity, and openness toward each child and his/her ideas. Though the interchange may appear tedious and slow, painstaking attention to their ideas and language engages them in a shared, collaborative effort. They and their thoughts and worries are the focus of therapy, not the therapist. Let us now turn to Harlene's opening words.

HARLENE: So I guess I would like to say, first of all, thank you for coming again today. I think our meeting today, in a way, is really an example of the way I work, because one of the things that I talk about in my work is that each conversation informs the next, so the idea about all of us getting together and talking today came out of the talking that the three of us did yesterday. Normally we might have scheduled the session next week or in 2 weeks . . . we did it today so that we could videotape it in conjunction with yesterday's. So why don't we introduce the two of you, Mindy and Charles, and let people know who you are. So (*to the children*) would you say your name one more time and maybe how old you are?[5]

DENISE: Okay, my name's Denise, I'm 8 years old.

HARLENE: Welcome.

MELISSA: My name is Melissa, and I'm 6 years old.

HARLENE: Welcome.

SYLVIA: My name is Sylvia, and I'm 11 years old.

---

[3]Those who would like to have a multidimensional "picture" of this session are referred to the videotape available from Master'sWork.

[4]You are invited to substitute the word "client" here. As discussed earlier, we do not use the term "child" or "children" to imply that young clients are being treated differently from any other clients.

[5]As this session is being videotaped to be a teaching tool, Harlene's comments keep the imagined audience in mind.

JOEL: I'm Joel, and I'm 4 years old.

HARLENE: Hi, Joel, and good morning. Thank you guys for coming. What did your mom or dad tell you about coming today, because this is a little different than what we usually do? Usually when I talk with Mom and Dad or with your mom, you're playing on the porch, or in the yard, or doing something like that, so usually we don't talk this way, do we?

DENISE: No.

HARLENE: Did you know I was going to be talking to you?

DENISE: Mom and Dad told me when we were waiting.

HARLENE: When you were waiting, okay. What did they tell you?

DENISE: They told me that you probably would be videotaping, and that we were going to come in too. They might ask us a few questions, answer them as well as we could, that's pretty much all. Anyone else have any comments?

HARLENE: So you're kind of wondering what kind of questions I'm going to ask you?

DENISE: Yeah.

HARLENE: Yeah, I guess I would be too if I thought somebody was going to ask me some questions. Well, let me tell you why I wanted to talk to you. Because when your mom and dad and I were talking yesterday, one of the things we were talking about was some of the changes in your family over the last few weeks—the change meaning the new apartment in town and your mom being, it sounds like, more at the apartment than at home? Is that accurate?

DENISE: Yes.

HARLENE: Okay, and your Dad being kind of like—did you see the movie *Mr. Mom*? Okay, your dad kind of being like Mom. Even though I know that your mom and dad are usually home with you a lot, and people who heard us talking yesterday know that you're in a home school program, so that you are schooled at home and not in a regular school, and that your dad works kind of differently than most dads do, so people know a *little* bit about you already. But we wanted to talk about some of these new arrangements, and I guess I also wanted to know what kind of questions that you might have, or what kind of worries or concerns you might have, because your mom and dad think that you are worried about them.

DENISE: In a way I am.

HARLENE: In a way you are, okay.

DENISE: 'Cause sometimes when they have a big argument, I get kind of scared they're going to get divorced.

HARLENE: Get scared that they're going to get divorced. Okay. Really scary, huh? Yeah. What about the rest of you? Are there some things you're scared of with Mom and Dad, or some questions you have?

MELISSA: Not particularly.

HARLENE: Not particularly. Okay. Do you share the same fear that Mom and Dad might get divorced?

MELISSA: Yes.

HARLENE: Okay. And sometimes you say that out loud to them?

DENISE: I've told Mom . . . I think I've told Dad, have I?

CHARLES: Told me what, honey?

DENISE: Fear.

CHARLES: Yeah.

DENISE: Well, I think that I expressed to you—at least, like yesterday morning, remember?

CHARLES: Yes.

HARLENE: And you were shaking your head yes, Sylvia, that you've expressed this fear also, out loud?

SYLVIA: Yes.

HARLENE: Okay, and you have, Melissa? And Joel, you have too? Okay. And when you say you're scared that they are going to get divorced, what do they say to you?

DENISE: Well, I forgot.

HARLENE: You forgot.

DENISE: They tell us that they don't think they're going to get divorced, that they don't plan on it.

HARLENE: They tell you they don't think they're going to get divorced and they don't plan on it.

DENISE: That they hope they don't, at least.

HARLENE: Oh, that they *hope* that they don't, at least. Do you want to say something, Mindy?

MINDY: I remember telling you that we're working as hard as we can to work through a difficult time.

HARLENE: So it sounds like though, when they try to reassure you, that maybe it's not very reassuring—you're still worried.

DENISE: Well, sometimes when you're worried, it's kind of hard to stop, you know.

HARLENE: Yeah, Sometimes when you have a worry, it's kind of hard to let go of that worry.

DENISE: Yeah.

HARLENE: Okay, so [you've] worried about divorce. Are there some other things that you're worried about that's kind of hard to stop?

DENISE: Well, I don't know. There's sometimes I'm worried that Mom–instead of getting a divorce, Mom just stays in town all the time, or something, or just stays in one place all the time and they hardly see each other, and we have to—not have to, but we go back and forth from one house to the other house.

HARLENE: Uh-huh, and that's something that you don't like? Going back and forth and . . . ?

DENISE: Well, I've been doing it a lot, at Grampa's house, but they're usually both with me when I do that, and there'd only be one.

HARLENE: So that's the real difference, then, in terms of with the apartment—that it's usually one person there or one person at home, whereas at Grampa's house it might be that more of the time your mom and your dad were both with you.

DENISE: Except for when Mom goes off to meetings or Dad goes off to work.

HARLENE: Yeah, okay. So, Sylvia, Melissa, or Joel, do you have any more worries?

JOEL: I do!

HARLENE: You do? Okay, what's your worry?

JOEL: Well, you know what?

HARLENE: What?

JOEL: Our electricity went out. (*Laughs*)

HARLENE: Oh, your electricity went out? That is a big worry, isn't it. That is a big worry. Yes. I guess people watching this tape don't know that we're having a very unusual couple of winter days, and so there was ice on the electrical lines.

JOEL: And the trees.

HARLENE: And the trees, yeah.

JOEL: On the way, we got an icicle.

HARLENE: Oh, you got an icicle. So, you're kind of a very practical man like your dad.

DENISE: He'd rather talk about things that have been going—things that we're doing rather than feeling.

HARLENE: Oh, he'd rather talk about things that you're doing rather than feelings, okay.

DENISE: I'd rather talk about my feelings, of course.

HARLENE: Your feelings, of course. You're laughing, Sylvia—what do you think?

SYLVIA: I think she's being silly.

HARLENE: You think she's being silly.

MINDY: I think she's being accurate.

HARLENE: Oh, you think she's being accurate, okay. (*Mindy laughs*) Okay, so when Mom and Dad try to reassure you that they're working on things and that they're not going to get a divorce— that's what they say? They're not going to get a divorce?

DENISE: No.

HARLENE: No, they don't say it that way.

DENISE: They *plan* that they won't.

HARLENE: They *plan* that they won't. Okay. So, is it the way that they word it that makes you doubt, as well as that Mom is gone a lot now?

DENISE: I think yes. Kind of both.

Harlene takes care to use each response to inform her next comment or question, in a generative process. Meaning is generated in conversation, *in the moment,* and not from her interpretations or predetermined assumptions. Harlene explores each child's worries. She talks respectfully with Denise about her worries about divorce. She also respects Joel's worry about losing electricity, following his concerns with talk about icicles, until another voice comes in to change the course of the conversation. Each person's story takes center stage for that moment, while Harlene creates and safeguards room for the development of new meaning. This is provided through Harlene's careful attention to each person, and her curiosity about their stories and ideas. Each person's story is given the chance to develop.

In the conversation above and throughout the interview, Harlene keeps conversational directions open. She asks each of the children if they have comments they would like to share, thus offering an opportunity to participate without requiring it. Entering the conversation does not commit one to a particular path, but is more like an invitation to test the water: Each person has the opportunity to go deeper, or to back out if it does not feel comfortable. The therapist does not choose the depth or direction of the therapeutic conversation for the participants.

MULTIPLE, COEXISTING STORIES

Therapists and clients, children and adults, all are active and equal contributors to therapy conversations in a collaborative approach. A therapist working from this perspective must be able to inquire about, and respond to, multiple stories, descriptions, and explanations. Each person must feel that his/her view is heard and respected, and that one view is not favored over another. Clashing voices, competitive views, and defensive postures dissolve in this joint participation. This does not mean that there is not room for discrepant and contradictory stories, but that the differences are not problematic tensions; instead, they are food for thought, for inquiry, and for exploration. When this occurs, the conversation becomes symphonic, as all contribute their stories within the story, ultimately creating a new story for each. New meaning occurs as thoughts are expressed, clarified, and expanded. As each person talks, others listen: Outer and inner dialogues occur simultaneously and overlap.

Even one-person therapy centers around a client's multiple, coexisting stories, which shift in prominence from moment to moment and from interaction to interaction. For example, in another therapy situation, 11-year-old Achelra, who was referred to therapy with one of us (Sue) by her child protective services caseworkers, had "mixed feelings" about therapy. Though Achelra's frustration at "having to talk"[6] about her past sexual abuse by her father was the dominant story she told about the referral to therapy. Achelra also reported wanting to find out if she could trust other people with her past. Achelra's biggest concern was finding out if she could trust her foster parents, with whom she had been living for 2 months at the time of referral. Prior to this placement,

---

[6]Though Sue never took a position that Achelra "had to talk," her caseworker did. Much time was given to discussing this situation, as everyone's position (including the caseworker's) was included in the conversation.

Achelra had spent a year in another foster home, and had been moved at the foster parents' request.

Sue and Achelra explored these contradictory but coexisting interests of hers; this led eventually to Achelra's decision to experiment with telling her foster parents about her past abuse. This "telling" was done in many small steps designed by Achelra, and was done for *her* purposes (e.g., in order to find out how her foster parents would respond) rather than the caseworker's purposes (because it would be "therapeutic"). Achelra considered this experiment successful, and reported that she was glad that she had been referred to therapy (Levin, 1997).

Attending to the multiple participants (even if they are not all in the therapy room, such as the caseworker in the example above) and their stories requires—as illustrated in the following section of the interview—continued attention to concerns raised, while also demonstrating mindfulness of other perspectives and directions unexplored. Aware that the parents have been listening and having their own internal thoughts as the children have talked, and curious about their thoughts, Harlene turns to the parents and asks. There are many reasons and potential interpretations for why Harlene would choose to do this. Talking with one person, then another, continues to enlarge the conversation.

Each therapy conversation is a multiplicity of criss-crossing, overlapping, and sequential dialogues (internal and external) within the conversation. As some talk, others silently listen and think. We always want to access each listener's silent thoughts, and add her/his piece to the story.

DENISE: . . . then Dad retired and they began to fight, pretty much. But now they've lowered down, since Mom has been in town.

HARLENE: Oh, since Mom has been in town, the fights have lowered down.

DENISE: Yeah, because they haven't had time, or they just haven't been doing it. Sometimes they still argue. I try to let them know when I'm feeling sad, though.

HARLENE: Well, let me hear from [Mom and Dad] for a moment, because I'll bet that while y'all are talking that they've been having lots of things going on in their heads . . . lots of thoughts. What kinds of thoughts are you having?

CHARLES: I'm just really pleased that y'all are sharing within so well, but I want to hear that you're expressing what you really are feeling, and I hope that if you're holding back anything, or if you have anything else that you'd like to share with it, that you've noticed, anything you want to say is okay with me. Anything that's really going on with you is okay to share. I just want to reinforce that I'm real concerned about y'all's feelings and that I want you to have a good and happy and full life, and I'm just doing the best I can with trying to make that happen.

MINDY: Okay, we've been talking for a long time. I try to keep y'all aware of what's going on as much as I can. Daddy and I started, I think, yesterday, arguing a little bit in the morning . . . disagreeing on something . . . I wanted to catch a quick lunch before we had to do . . .

DENISE: Before you had to drop us off at Cathy's.

MINDY: . . . and Daddy didn't want to, Daddy wanted me to fix it there, and so Mother went into an uptight mode and Daddy had a reaction to it, and I watched both of your faces, and both of your faces saddened a bit, and were ready for . . . it's okay . . . it is *okay*, I think, for Mommy and Daddy to disagree. I want you to think about the times that you as sisters argue. And then make up with each other. What happened yesterday morning was . . . it was quick.

HARLENE: It was quick.

MINDY: It was *quick*. . . .

SYLVIA: What it was just because I was asking you, "Could you drop us off at Cathy's or something?" But it was quick.

MINDY: It was quick, but I saw the look on your faces and I know that upset you, but you and I aren't always agreeing on everything, and *Daddy* and I aren't going to always agree on everything. And we're still working it out. We still try every day. I am far from perfect, but I keep trying to learn and learn about things, and Sylvia, the other day when I was at home and started taking my sewing machine with me? And I watched you, and I saw a reaction in you about me taking my sewing machine? Can you tell me what you were feeling when you crawled down underneath the desk?

SYLVIA: Well, for one thing, I found something.

MINDY: Okay. Were you sad? And why were you sad?

SYLVIA: I don't know, I'm just sad for you taking your *machine*.

HARLENE: 'Cause that was kind of like she was really going, if her machine was going, because we know how much she loves her machine?

SYLVIA: Yes.

HARLENE: Yes.

MINDY: I took the machine . . . I want to tell you that I took my machine so that I could have a connection with y'all, while I'm doing the work that I need to do. I took my machine so I could make you some clothes or somehow be connected with you without being at home . . . all the time. Doesn't mean I'm not coming back, it doesn't mean that I don't love you, because if love you *desperately.* I love you *desperately.* . . .

Here the conversation expands from Harlene and the children to include Mindy, as Harlene, Mindy, and Sylvia discuss Sylvia's concerns about her mother's moving her sewing machine from the family's house to the mother's apartment. As there are no predetermined rules for therapy conversations, this three-way interchange is considered just as useful as any other, and there is no attempt to stop or change it.

HARLENE: So, if I guessed when Mommy and Daddy argue now, since Mommy is in the apartment in the city a lot, that that makes you even more worried and more upset than when they argue when they're at home? Oh—it's kind of like it shines a spotlight on it or something, is that right?

MELISSA: See, because they argue at home, well, they've been . . . our mom moving somewhere out there, but they should have had to find a place. We've had a little bit more time with her, and him too. But now since she's got that place already, she wouldn't have to look. It's hard.

HARLENE: Let me ask you something else. I'm wondering, do you have any friends whose parents argue? Do you see any friends' parents argue, or do you have any friends whose mommy or daddy is gone a lot?

MELISSA: Yes.

HARLENE: You do?

MELISSA: Uh-huh.

DENISE: Cathy and her husband has been . . .

SYLVIA: Not husband, father. He's at work. That's about the most I've seen anybody's father gone.

MINDY: Do Bob and Sharon fight?

SYLVIA: Uh-huh.

JOEL: I don't know.

MELISSA: Uh-huh.

HARLENE: Like your mom and dad, or just like . . .

DENISE: I don't know . . . Sharon gets up and *screams* at him.

HARLENE: *Louder* fights, huh?

DENISE: But see, we don't know what they're about.

HARLENE: Oh, you don't know what those fights are about?

DENISE: Sometimes we know what Mom and Dad's fights are about because we *overhear*. Like the other day with the—that Mom was talking about—when Mom wanted to eat out and Dad didn't want to . . . we knew what that was about . . . eating there or eating out.

HARLENE: Let me ask you this. Let's say that Mom and Dad *are* going to have some arguments or some fights, or at least that's what your mom said. (*To Charles*) Would you agree or disagree with that?

CHARLES: Yeah, I would agree with that. . . .

HARLENE: Okay. There are going to be some [fights]. And given that, is there anything that they could do or say that would help you? In terms of not being so worried?

As this exchange continues, Harlene explores the children's worries about the parents' arguing and the mother's leaving from another angle. She wonders if the children think that Mindy and Charles will probably continue fighting and arguing. The children agree, and she then asks if there is anything that would help them with their worries. Harlene's curiosity is broken down into small pieces and introduced tentatively, in such a way that it can be included in or discarded from the conversation. This form of interjection keeps a therapist's choices about the conversation on equal ground with those of the other participants—no more or less important to consider.

The conversation takes multiple directions, none of which are considered ultimate or permanent. Harlene, an active member of the conversation, asks questions that grow from what has been talked about, and also introduces a few questions that come from her own thoughts and reflections that have been formed by the conversation. Denise responds to Harlene's question at the end of the exchange above by reporting that she "does not worry as much when her parents fuss" now. Harlene asks her to clarify, saying that she has been under the impression that Denise is very worried indeed. Denise goes on to explain that she does not see her parents fuss or argue too much, since her mother has moved into an apartment. This changes the direction of the conversation toward a discussion of some of the positive changes that have occurred with Mom's move. Harlene's curiosities and questions about the children's worries and their perceptions and experiences of their parents triggers a new direction of conversation, providing an opportunity for a new story to emerge.

ORDINARY PEOPLE

Most people come to therapy with concerns about everyday, ordinary dilemmas. The process and content of therapy, therefore, are not always dramatic and flashy. To an observer, a conversation in therapy might seem mundane or even boring. To the participants involved, however, it is serious business and often exciting. When a therapist works from a position in which he/she is not determining the direction or content of what happens in therapy, clients feel free to talk about whatever is bothering them, no matter how trivial it may seem to others. Some people may find children difficult to listen to, since their conversational styles are usually different from those of adults, and may seem simplistic (Faber & Mazlish, 1980; Stacey & Loptson, 1995). It is important, however, to consider the implications when a therapist communicates lack of interest in children's conversations. Children, like adults, feel devalued and discounted when they are not heard (Levin, 1992). Respecting children and exploring their concerns, ideas, and interests (even if they seem ordinary to adults) creates a relationship in which children feel supported and important. We believe that all clients should have the opportunity to feel this way in therapy, and that all people should have the opportunity to feel this way in relationships.

In the next segment, the children describe wearing different clothes when they are in the city (where Mom's new apartment is) and in the country (where they live with Dad in the family house). Multiple, overlapping, and connecting conversations illustrate the importance of hearing and responding to children in their own terms. This exchange creates an opening for the children to report their confusion and struggle to clarify the rules and expectations of their parents.

HARLENE: So where do you think we should go from here? Is there some more of this you'd like to talk about in here today, or . . .

JOEL: Yes.

HARLENE: Yes, okay?

JOEL: Well . . .

HARLENE: What?

JOEL: Well, I'm scared that Mom and Dad are going off.

HARLENE: You're afraid they're going off. You keep saying that.

SYLVIA: I feel that sometimes what brings the fights back is because we try to come to town in decent clothes, but sometimes we ask that we come in clothes that have the knees that have holes in them, or the sleeves, or something.

HARLENE: Oh, so you have country clothes and city clothes?

SYLVIA: Yeah.

HARLENE: Okay, so how does that bring on a fight?

SYLVIA: Well, because Mom gets ticked off.

HARLENE: Oh, ticked off at . . . ?

SYLVIA: Because we aren't dressed nicely and she . . .

MINDY: Because . . . you know who I'm ticked off at.

SYLVIA: Well, umm . . .

MINDY: Generally, who am I ticked off at?

SYLVIA: Daddy.

MINDY: Because he hasn't learned the difference between city clothes and country clothes.

HARLENE: Oh . . .

MINDY: So that brings on a fight, is what she's saying.

SYLVIA: Not a fight, but a disagreement.

HARLENE: Disagreement, okay.

DENISE: It does.

SYLVIA: This morning Daddy said not to wear these, but then Mother wanted to talk to me, and she told me *to* wear these.

HARLENE: Yeah, how did Daddy do today? That's right, because you went back to the country with Daddy last night and came in this morning. Are these [referring to the clothes the children are wearing] in the category of city clothes, or country clothes, or what?

SYLVIA: These are city clothes.

HARLENE: These are city clothes.

MINDY: Well . . .

SYLVIA: The jeans . . .

HARLENE: I don't see any holes.

SYLVIA: Well, they've got faded knees, see, you can tell. . . .

As the conversation continues, the children share more of their experiences since the parents' separation. The discussion includes talk about whether the toilet lids can be left up or not, who does the cooking, who does the dishes, and who makes chocolate chip cookies, now that Mom is not at home with the children. The children seem proud to report their new activities; for example, they are making pancakes, toast, and coffee, and serving breakfast in bed on Sunday mornings. A strong sense of accomplishment is established, as the children eagerly tell another story—one that positions them anew. Here they have the opportunity to be heard as competent, independent, and functional, very much in contrast to sad, worried victims of their parents' struggles.

NEVER-ENDINGS AND NEW BEGINNINGS

Just as each question is not known ahead of time, but is informed by the previous response, so each session closes in a new and unpredictable way. We hope that at its conclusion, each session has created some new possibilities, highlighted stories and voices that have been previously unaccessed, opened new doors where there have been none, answered old questions, and raised new ones. We do not think of sessions, or therapy, as ending. Each conversation *in the room* is influenced by and influences the conversations that each participant, including the therapist, is involved in *outside the room*. We believe that the generative process that is created in a therapy room goes with clients and therapist as they leave. Sessions, therefore, do not have to conclude with a grand intervention or interpretation—actions that fit with hierarchical practice, not collaboration.

People do not stop thinking when they leave a therapist's office. Clients report changes evolving from multitudinous events in their lives; the connections are sometimes related and sometimes not related to therapy conversations. The dialogue below represents the final exchanges of this therapy session, as Harlene shares her hope that the session may have helped a little bit. This triggers Joel's suggestion of another thing that may help (Dad's getting an alarm clock), while Denise describes the session as helping her to "express without . . . fear." Harlene's statement of hoping the session has helped a bit is not a solicitation for a reply. She does not have an expectation that anyone will respond, yet two of the children do. This illustrates the participatory freedom created when a therapist behaves in a collaborative manner. It also reflects the constant introduction of new story lines into the conversation.

The "end" of this session, an artificial construct dependent on time, stops Harlene from talking more with Joel about his ideas about Dad's oversleeping. Likewise, there is little time to talk with Denise about her experience of "being able to express without having a fear." Both of these expressions, like any others during this session, could have generated meaningful discussion. To reiterate, we believe that these "endings" create new beginnings—for internal conversations, for external conversations, for therapy conversations, and for nontherapy conversations.

HARLENE: Okay, so maybe we've talked about your worries and your fears and your concerns, and we've talked about some of the things you're going to get to do . . .

DENISE: That helps you feel better.

HARLENE: Yeah, it'll make you feel better, yeah. And I hope that all of us talking about it today maybe has helped a little bit.

JOEL: I have another idea.

HARLENE: You have another idea! Oh, why am I not surprised? What's your other idea?

JOEL: Well, my idea is, well Dad stays in bed for a lot of time.

MINDY: Daddy stays in bed . . .

CHARLES: Dad stays in bed for a lot of time?

DENISE: Well, what he means is you sleep late. You're sleeping late . . .

JOEL: I have another idea.

HARLENE: Okay, one last idea.

JOEL: Get an alarm clock to wake him up.

DENISE: See, that's what I was going to say! This session has helped me a lot by being able to express without having a fear.

HARLENE: Without having a fear. Okay, this has helped you. We hope that we can find some other ways to help all of you, because I know your mommy and daddy are very worried about all of you, and I know that they love you very, very, very much. You're very, very special to them. They don't want to do anything to worry you, and they don't want to do anything to hurt you. So do you have anything you want to ask me, or do you have any advice for me in terms of the next time your mom and dad are going to talk with me?

DENISE: No.

HARLENE: No, okay. Well, I'll look forward to hearing what you've come [up] with for family day this Sunday.

DENISE: Uh-huh.

HARLENE: You have one more day to play it, huh? I thank you so much for coming.

DENISE: Thank you for letting us.

HARLENE: . . . Mindy and Charles, anything in particular you want to say, or . . .

CHARLES: No, I don't think so.

HARLENE: To me or the kids . . . ?

MINDY: Well, just for me, that I—that I never expected to be at this place [in my life]. I never expected to do a lot of work on me, and that it is very much a surprise to me, and it's very frightening for me. And you know how we talk about maps and maps telling us where we're going to go? I don't have a map . . .

DENISE: You lost it.

MINDY: I lost it.

HARLENE: Oh, she lost it.

MINDY: I don't have a map about this. I don't know where I'm going with it, and so I wait and I listen to inside, I listen to my heart. . . . And I try the very best that I can, and I make mistakes, and I try again. But I would never change anything about having y'all in my life.

A NON-SUMMARY

"Ending" this chapter with a summary would be inconsistent with our theory and practice. We do not believe that there is a single, correct understanding of this text that we want to highlight; nor could we predict, capture, or represent the multiple thoughts about these ideas that you, our readers, may have. Just as we do not finish sessions with a summary, intervention, or interpretation, we do not presume to do so in this chapter. Where we leave off, we hope, is the beginning of other conversations for you and for us.

EDITORIAL QUESTIONS

Q: *(CS) When most people think of "narrative therapy," they think of the creative contributions of Michael White and David Epston's re-authoring approach. In their writings, I've seen Harlene and Harry [Goolishian] speak of "client narratives" for at least 8 years or so.*

When Harlene and I had a recent conversation about the narrative metaphor, I believe she indicated that she thought all therapies influenced clients' narratives.

I know that Peggy Penn and Marilyn Frankfurt (1994) have spoken of working with "narrative multiplicity," and you speak of "keeping multiple conversational directions open." Could you say something about the ideas informing your notion of narratives, so the reader can better grasp relevant distinctions from or similarities to a re-authoring approach to narratives?

A: We are often asked questions about how our approach is similar to other approaches that use a narrative metaphor. We are curious to find in rereading our chapter that we do not use the term "narrative," although our tendency is not to refer to our work as narrative. "Narrative" was a useful term some years ago to differentiate a literary, hermeneutic approach to understanding people from a structural, scientific one. Today, however, the way that narrative is used in the field no longer fits for us. We do not think of ourselves as narrative experts.

This does not mean that we do not think that "narrative" or "storytelling" is not an appropriate term to describe how people organize, account for, and make sense of their experiences. It refers more to distinguishing the narrative metaphor as situated under a modern or postmodern therapy umbrella (Anderson, 1997).

We do not believe that people *have* narratives about themselves—selves that are separate and internal, and that operate independently of others. In our postmodern social constructionist view of selves, individuals are relational; they are continually constructing themselves in relationship with others, their history, and evolving context (Gergen, 1994). Any narrative, therefore, that may be attributed to someone is not that person's internal property, but rather a social, multiple-voiced, and dynamic product.

Q: *(CS) I am fascinated with how the flow of your chapter echoes how you prefer to be with clients—weaving in and out with transcript (even close to the beginning of the chapter) and explanations of your work, the flow of one section into the other, the lack of a comprehensive, tying-it-all-up-in-a-package-and-bow-conclusion, and so on!*

I'd like to ask you to talk a little more about problem "dissolution" as compared with problem "resolution," because I think many readers growing up in our modernist world often think in "resolution" terms. Thus, as they read this chapter, they continue to anticipate the "big" moments where they imagine Harlene will focus on "the central problems/dysfunctions/discourses" in this family so that these can be "resolved." I find that my experience of reading this transcript is radically altered when I loosen myself from this lens and instead look through a "dissolution"-through-dialogue frame!

For instance, I'm struck by these open-ended explorations—the way the presenting concerns evolve and change without a thematic or problem focus. In the couple session preceding the family one, the mother talks about needing some more time alone, whereas the kids still wish she was at home with them in the old arrangement. Dad says the kids are in distress about not having more access to their mom. When the family session begins, what starts out as the children's fear of their getting divorced and wanting reassurance that this won't happen shifts to the story of the kids going back and forth between houses. This story recedes as the focus is on whether arguing is normal, expected disagreement between people or an inevitable sign of incompatibility. This evolves into Mom's poignant voicing of her taking the sewing machine to be more, not less, connected with the kids; then Denise saying she isn't as worried about her parents arguing; and so forth.

At the end of the session, I am left feeling that a lot has happened in spite of no "problem resolution." Do you think that others hearing about your work look at your work through "problem resolution" glasses? Could you talk about some assumptions that inform your ideas about "dissolution" as well as about "resolution"?

A: The notions of language and knowledge as relational and generative are central to how we conceptualize human systems, the "problems" they present, and how we position ourselves in relationships with clients—how we talk and act with them in regard to their problems. In McNamee and Gergen's (in press) words, "Language [and knowledge created through it] is a resource that permits particular forms of action and suppresses others" (p. 4). If we accept the idea that problems are created and exist in language, they also become nonexistent or dissolve in it. What once seemed problematic is no longer experienced or thought of in the same way. In dialogue, people access a self-agency that allows them to think about and approach their once problematic situation in a manner that it becomes not so. To put it differently, hope and possibility can be seen where none seemed to exist before. We do not know how Mindy would explain her experience.

Often people who present in therapists' offices (and most therapists) use "problems-seeking-solutions" language; it is intrinsic to Western culture. When a person is concerned, alarmed, or miserable about something, he/she usually wants it solved or resolved. Also culturally intrinsic are the suggestions of external expertise and hierarchical relationship. Believing that a therapist has privileged expertise on how other people should live their lives relies on and engenders the traditional notions of individual responsibility and individual authorship.

We do not choose to focus or privilege problem, resolution, or solution talk. Because, in our experience, meeting other persons within their language has been effective, we use this language when clients, colleagues, or students choose to use it. This does not mean that we choose to accept or reject a person's definition of a problem; rather, it means that we are always learning about how each person thinks about and talks about her/his situation. Nor does it mean that talking about a problem concretizes it. We are not interested, however, in participating in the kinds of conversations that risk reifying a problem or privileging one theme, narrative, or viewpoint over another.

There is a difference between "talking about a *problem*" and in "*talking* about a problem." We think that people have series of experiences and conversations with themselves and others, which they sometimes organize into something they call a "problem." It is as though the problem is a shorthand through which people communicate about complicated issues. We are always curious to understand how particular meanings and explanations of a problem have been favored, and through this curiosity we find that a problem is talked about in a different way. In taking our learning position and inviting clients' expertise and authority, we find that they begin to experience problems not as static entities, but as dynamic and fluid. Since there is no such thing as a problem in a concrete sense, there can be no problem resolution in a traditional sense.

We hope that a reader will not think that we condone monstrosities defined by our cultural and moral views as problems—for instance, child abuse or suicide. In our practices, we meet with many people struggling with these life events. What we are interested in, however, is sincere and complete attention to the uniqueness, social context, and history of each person's concerns and ideas about what needs to be different. In our experiences, we have found that exploring and hearing about clients' situations from a learning, or not-knowing, position creates an environment in which their concerns are expressed and talked about in new ways that lead to new outcomes, including new views of themselves and their situations.

Harry Goolishian and I (Harlene) first chose to use "dissolve" when referring to our experiences and clients' reflections on what happens to problems in therapy. We wanted to distinguish our work from the meanings and therapist positions traditionally associated with the words "solution" and "resolution." We continue to use it in our attempt to capture the transformational essence of the kind of dialogic process and relationship that we refer to. We want to elucidate a concept; this is the importance, not the word itself. In addition, we also find that thinking in terms of resolution/solution risks tempting therapists to know ahead of time, to guide clients toward therapist knowing—neither of which, in our opinion, is in the spirit of collaboration.

Q: *(CS) It seems to me that Harlene is orienting toward how the conversation might enlarge and include more perspectives—toward the process of how the family members' stories are getting told, rather than focusing on specific aspects or the content of their stories. You allude to therapy conversations as a beginning catalyst for helping internal and external conversations evolve.*

From this perspective, it's almost as if the therapist helps people breathe more "dialogic oxygen" and this expanded breathing continues to happen after the session, leading to greater possibilities for dialogue and understanding. If I can play with this metaphor just a bit longer, this oxygen seems to permit a greater freedom for clients "not to know"—not to have to have a modernist "map" of exactly how to be in all situations. For example, my words for how Mom poignantly ends the transcript would be that perhaps these reflective therapy conversations have helped her realize she doesn't need to follow a script or "map" or a theme for how to be—that each moment can be responded to uniquely by tuning in to her "heart." Perhaps equally important is that Mom has a sense that her heart will be listened to, if not always agreed with—that dialogue can occur and misunderstandings dealt with. "Country and city oxygen"! How does this sit with the two of you? What reactions do you have? Have you gotten feedback from clients about subtle shifts in how they talk to themselves and others after sessions end?

A: Our intention is focused on the process of the conversation and the nature of the relationship, rather than the content of the conversation and the subjects of the relationship. We invite clients into conversations in which we listen, hear, and interact *with* them—in which clients and therapists mutually participate in clarifying, elaborating, extending, deepening, amplifying, and diminishing. In this shared inquiry—what Shotter calls "joint action" (Shotter & Gergen, 1993), this dialogic process—clients become curious about themselves in a way that they may not have been before. When conversations are dialogic, potential, possibility, and transformations are inherent in them. Similarly, inherent in new forms of dialogue are new forms of relationships; people position themselves differently with each other. That is, as space opens up, crystallized, polarized positions—blaming, judgmental, pejorative, disruptive, silencing—fade; problems dissolve and relationships transform.

Therapists often act as if there are boundaries between conversations—for instance, boundaries between conversations within and outside the therapy room, or between before- and after-therapy conversations. Conversations are dynamic and fluid. Each conversation is situated within other conversations, and each mutually influences the other—past, present, and future. A therapy conversation, like any other conversation, does not stand alone.

REFERENCES

Andersen, T. (1991). *The reflecting team: Dialogues and dialogues about the dialogues.* New York: Norton.

Anderson, H. (1995). Collaborative language systems: Toward a post-modern therapy. In R. Mikesell, D. D. Lusterman, & S. McDaniel (Eds.), *Integrating family therapy: Family psychology and systems theory.* Washington, DC: American Psychological Association.

Anderson, H. (1997). *Conversation, language, and possibilities: A postmodern approach to therapy.* New York: HarperCollins.

Anderson, H., & Goolishian, H. (1988). Human systems as linguistic systems: Preliminary and evolving ideas about the implications for clinical theory. *Family Process, 27,* 371–393.

Anderson, H., & Goolishian, H. (1992). The client is the expert: A not-knowing approach to therapy. In S. McNamee & K. Gergen (Eds.), *Therapy as social construction.* Newbury Park, CA: Sage.

Ariés, P. (1962). *Centuries of childhood: A social history of family life.* New York: Vintage Books.

Berger, P. L., & Luckman, T. (1967). *The social construction of reality: A treatise in the sociology of knowledge.* Garden City, NY: Doubleday.

Campbell, T. W. (1992). Psychotherapy with children of divorce: The pitfalls of triangulated relationships. *Psychotherapy, 29*(4), 646–652.

Combrinck-Graham, L. (1991). On technique with children in family therapy: How calculated should it be? *Journal of Marital and Family Therapy, 17*(4), 373–377.

Dowling, E. (1993). Are family therapists listening to the young?: A psychological perspective. *Journal of Family Therapy, 15*(4), 403–411.

Faber, A., & Mazlish, E. (1980). *How to talk so kids will listen and listen so kids will talk.* New York: Avon.

Gergen, K. J. (1985). The social constructionist movement in modern psychology. *American Psychologist, 40,* 266–275.

Gergen, K. J. (1991). Emerging challenges for theory and psychology. *1*(1), 13–35.

Gergen, K. (1994). *Realities and relationships: Soundings in social construction.* Cambridge, MA: Harvard University Press.

Levin, S. B. (1992). *Hearing the unheard: Stories of women who have been battered.* Unpublished doctoral dissertation, The Union Institute, Cincinnati, OH.

Levin, S. B. (1997). Achelra and the big experiment: A story of collaboration and connection with a scared eleven-year-old. In F. N. Thomas & T. S. Nelson (Eds.), *Tales from family therapy: Live-changing clinical experiences.* New York: Haworth Press.

McNamee, S., & Gergen, J. K. (Eds.). (1992). *Therapy as social construction.* Newbury Park, CA: Sage.

McNamee, S., & Gergen, K. (in press). *Relational responsibility.* Thousand Oaks, CA: Sage.

Penn, P., & Frankfurt, M. (1994). Creating a participant text: Writing, multiple voices, narrative multiplicity. *Family Process, 33,* 217–231.

Shotter, J., & Gergen, K. J. (1993). Social construction: Knowledge, self, others and continuing the conversation. In A. Deetz (Ed.), *Communication yearbook.* Thousand Oaks, CA: Sage.

Stacey, K., & Loptson, C. (1995). Children should be seen and not heard: Questioning the unquestioned. *Journal of Systemic Therapies, 14*(4), 16–32.

Tannen, D. (1990). *You just don't understand: Women and men in conversation.* New York: Morrow.

Villeneuve, C., & LaRoche, C. (1993). The child's participation in family therapy: A review and a model. *Contemporary Family Therapy, An International Journal, 15*(2), 105–119.

Wachtel, E. F. (1994). *Treating troubled children and their families.* New York: Guilford Press.

Wallerstein, J. S. (1991). Tailoring the intervention to the child in the separating and divorced family. *Family and Conciliation Courts Review, 29*(4), 448–459.

Wallerstein, J. S., & Kelly, J. B. (1977). Divorce counseling: A community service for families in the midst of divorce. *American Journal of Orthopsychiatry, 47*(1), 4–22.

11

Attention Deficit Disorder
THERAPY WITH A SHODDILY BUILT CONSTRUCT

IAN LAW

This chapter, through both a satirical view and an analysis of the medical evidence, critically evaluates the medical discourse's construction of the notion of "attention deficit disorder" (ADD) and outlines the way in which this construction is embedded in the cultural and social practices of the pathologizing of behavior, mother blaming, and the infantilization or "growing down" of children. These practices can have a disabling effect on those people whose experience of life is mediated by these constructions of meaning, and can blind us as therapists to contexts of violence, abuse, and the politics of gender. It is suggested, and illustrated with sections of a transcribed interview, that an approach to therapy that actively critiques (or at least refuses to be captured by) such social constructions and cultural practices can create a context in which there is greater opportunity for the discovery of strengths, competence, and success in overcoming problems of life, and for the discovery of meanings that have their eyes open to the dominance of sexist, ageist, and biological determinist ideologies in Westernized culture.

As a result of appearing in print, I am aware that, like a fly in amber, any author's thinking can be trapped in her/his writing to be stumbled across at a later date. Therefore, this chapter should be seen as an accurate reflection of some of my thinking on this issue at the time of its writing. Suffice is to say that this amber does not hold any of the developments that may have occurred in my thinking since then. It also should be known that this fly is still buzzing around the head of the body of psychiatric discourse and, at the time of this writing at least, has yet to be successfully swatted.

YOU CAN'T BE SERIOUS?!

There was a time when I would begin presentations, workshops, and discussions about the ADD construct by asking the group members to respond to a series of questions. I would ask them to think of any meetings and formal gatherings that they might have attended recently, and to raise their hands if they had observed the following behavior in either themselves or others:

- A lack of ability to attend
- Fidgeting
- Squirming
- Blurting out an answer before a question has been asked
- Difficulty in remaining seated when required to do so

You can imagine that with a bit of imagination and fun, such a gathering can become a little forest of hands, with people blurting out answers, jumping out of seats, and pointing out the squirming and fidgeting behavior of others. However, it may then seem sobering and/or ridiculous for those present to realize that in identifying their exhibition of these behaviors, they are rendering themselves vulnerable to a diagnosis of ADD.

And what, you may ask, is ADD? The American Psychiatric Association's (1994) definition of ADD—or "attention-deficit/hyperactivity disorder" (ADHD) as it is now formally known, even though ADD remains the preferred term in popular usage—rather cleverly subsumes the previous construct of hyperactivity that was fashionable in the 1970s. But the debate over the biological basis of children's behavior is not new to the current debate over ADD. An even earlier construct, "minimal brain damage," had to mutate to "minimal brain dysfunction" for the simple reason that despite much research, no evidence of brain damage was ever demonstrated. This mutation of constructs in order to maintain the "integrity" of biological theory got me thinking about the satirical application of the disease metaphor to the development of the ADD construct, because the assertion that ADD is neither viral nor bacterial is not supported by an everyday experience of this phenomenon. ADD seeps it way through a classroom like the latest strain of flu, and there are certain risk factors that make children vulnerable to the infection. For instance, having an older sibling with ADD appears to dramatically increase a child's risk of diagnosis, by the same doctor or psychologist, by the time the child has reached the older sibling's age. However, close proximity to a classmate with ADD seems only to be a risk when the caregivers of the respective children are good friends. Why is this? Is the sufferer infectious? Or is the caregiver an unwitting host, infecting children while remaining symptom-free? What about tracing the source of infection? If ADD gains a life in a host from the discourses of mainstream psychiatry and psychology, should we then be exercising disease control by quarantining and medicating the psychiatric and psychology profession?

Of course, we know that ADD sufferers may develop secondary complications such as the brilliantly named "oppositional defiant disorder" (ODD), which it left unchecked may lead to the chronic condition "conduct disorder" (CD). If we allow this construction of meaning to be totally free from an analysis of power and resistance, then who knows where it might end? Could we see a text entitled *Civil Disobedience: The Hidden Disorder*? Or a historical biography analyzing Gandhi's personal struggle with ODD? Is it possible that a national government could claim that its army of occupation is actually a convention of psychiatrists called in to treat a neighboring country's mass CD? Well, maybe not, but reaching a point so extreme that it becomes satirical is pretty hard when the reality is itself so extreme. Figures in history have already been identified and retrospectively diagnosed. An article in *Time* magazine (Wallis, 1994) has asserted that Benjamin Franklin, Winston Churchill, Isaac Newton, Leonardo da Vinci, and Albert Einstein all had ADD.

Not so long ago, it would have been comical to claim that we were about to make a quantum leap in the expansion to diagnose ADD *in utero*. Or to imagine a publication by reductionists claiming to have isolated the gene for ADD. Or to predict the discovery of ADD as a premorbid precursor or an early-onset syndrome for some adult pathologies. But, of course, we can now see that the reality has overtaken the ridiculous and traveled beyond—into the bizarre. On reading a local community paper (*Messenger*, 1994), I was confronted by the story of an infant being diagnosed with ADD at 18 months old. When I picked up a book on display on the counter of my local chemist (Nash, 1994), telling me how to recognize ADD in my children, it told me that the outcomes of twin studies have shown that ADD is hereditary. Parents and caregivers tell me that when they look at the violent, controlling behavior of their sons who have been diagnosed with ADD, it reminds them of the abusive behavior of their ex-partners. This then leads them to the conclusion that the ex-partners must have had ADD too and passed on the gene to their sons.

In a last-ditch attempt to highlight the ridiculousness of pathologizing behavior, I attempted to come up with some pathologies of my own, based on research I conducted on selected people using subjective and superficial observation. My first offering was

- "sheer bloody-mindedness disorder," but then I realized that to be taken seriously a medical condition has to have a basis in Latin. So I discovered
- "cantankerous obstreperous disorder," derived from the Latin root, *ob,* meaning "against," and *strepere,* "to roar." But the crowning glory of my research is
- "swine cranial syndrome," or to give it its common name, "pig-headedness disorder." (Abbreviated to PHD, the popularization of this condition may have some implications for postgraduate enrollments.)

Once more, though, my enthusiasm for pursuing this apparent silliness was dampened when I was yet again overtaken by the serious claims of pathologizers of behavior. A newspaper item (*Advertiser,* 1996) reported that a man had taken his own life because he could not face the onset of winter. His daughter called for more money to be made available for research into the little-known "illness" that had been "discovered" some 8 years earlier by a psychiatrist working in the United States. The acronym used as shorthand for this "illness," seasonal affective disorder (SAD) says far more about it than its full diagnostic title.

Perhaps the ridiculousness of biological theorists' inventing an increasing number of pathologies is not self-evident in the case of the ADD construct. If so, then let us take a look at the medical evidence.

THE DEBATE WITHIN MEDICINE

There appear to be two major claims in relation to ADD that proponents of pathology seek to justify on the basis of medical research: namely, (1) that ADD is a medically and scientifically proven fact, and (2) that there is therefore a need to establish a treatment program specifically for those persons diagnosed with ADD. The first claim—that ADD's existence as a psychiatric disorder is a medically established fact—is directly challenged by Reid, Maag, and Vasa (1994) in their critique of the "voluminous body of [ADD] literature." They systematically discredit the three assumptions that the ADD construct is based upon.

1. The assumption that the Fourth edition of the *Diagnostic and Statistical Manual of Mental Disorders* (DSM-IV; American Psychiatric Association, 1994)—the manual of taxonomy that the psychiatric profession uses to classify individual problems—can differentiate ADD (or ADHD) from other conditions is contradicted by the fact that ADD/ADHD is defined by a "constellation of behaviors that did not evolve from an empirical base [and] cannot be reliably differentiated from other disorders in terms of etiology, response to treatment, course, or relation to external referents other than the symptoms by which it is purported to be defined" (Reid et al., 1994, p. 200). In other words, the behaviors that have been grouped together to identity ADD/ADHD have no scientific basis for their choice and overlap with other existing conditions.

2. The assumption that behavior rating scales can be used to identify ADD accurately and reliably is contradicted by the fact that there is no empirical base to any cutoff point that would identify someone as having ADD. These descriptors typically lack objective anchors and are not operationally defined; both the behaviors indicative of an attribute and the quantity of behavior associated with any given rating are left to the subjective judgment of the rater. In other words, two people can observe exactly the same behavior, use exactly the same behavior rating scales, and reach entirely different conclusions.

3. The assumption that medical research has proved that ADD has an organic etiology—that it is caused by biology—does not stand up to examination. One particular study that Reid and his associates focus on is Zametkins et al.'s (1990) study of the differences in the rate of cerebral glucose metabolism between persons who were diagnosed with ADD and those who were not. It is often cited as proof of ADD's biological base, even though the researchers themselves qualified their findings. According to Reid et al., what Zametkin et al. have failed to demonstrate is a causal flow—that is, whether a change in biochemistry causes ADD or whether ADD causes a change in biochemistry. To use an analogy, if a person is startled, the ensuing release of adrenaline does not prove that "startled behavior" has a biological cause. The circularity of this argument, combined with the scientifically erroneous belief that a response to psychostimulants proves the diagnosis of ADD (persons who are not diagnosable as having ADD, such as those persons who were putting up their hands in the exercise described at the beginning of this chapter will also respond to psychostimulants), is summed up by Reid et al.: "Like its predecessor MBD [minimal brain damage],

you have ADHD because you exhibit the symptoms and you exhibit the symptoms because you have ADHD. Thus ADHD defines itself without the need for any external referent" (p. 203).

When it becomes clear that these three assumptions are based upon opinion and unproven hypothesis, and not on scientific fact, it also becomes clear that a belief in the psychiatric classification of ADD/ADHD is a leap of faith. As a result, not to take this leap of faith—in other words, to challenge the validity of the construct of ADD—is not to take a position against medicine. It is not by definition an antiscientific, antipsychiatry, antimedication stance. As Reid et al.'s review and critique amply demonstrates, this is a highly controversial issue within the medical profession itself. The medical profession is in fact airing the debate. For example, an issue of the *Australian Doctor* (1996) carried a piece titled "Debate: Attention Deficit Disorder—Controversies in Medicine," in which a pediatrician and psychiatrist put the case for and against the medically verifiable existence of ADD. In further highlighting the lack of medical consensus, the publication invited its readers (mostly doctors) to write with their views on the matter to a section called "Gut Feeling." So, by challenging the selective information and unfounded assertions of the ADD steamroller, I am not taking a view that contradicts the view of a united medical profession. I am, in fact, supporting a view that already exists within the medical profession.

When seen from this viewpoint, how then does the second claim begin to look? This claim is that those children who have been diagnosed as having ADD need a discrete medical and nonmedical treatment program, which is distinct from interventions that have already been widely applied to the areas of learning disability, emotional disturbance, the effects of child abuse, and other problems of childhood. It has become increasingly common for medical practitioners to refer children for various forms of counseling and nonmedical support when medication has failed to produce the desired change in behavior. The rationale given for this is that in severe cases medication may not be enough on its own and needs to be backed up with other interventions. It could be argued with equal if not greater validity that other interventions are necessary not because medication is not enough, but because it is entirely irrelevant to the situation in the first place. It is common practice within medicine that if a diagnosed condition does not respond to the appropriate medication, the validity of the original diagnosis should be questioned. However, in the case of ADD, faith in the diagnosis can become unshakable even when the situation is experienced as being no better or even worse after medication. If those children who are vulnerable to being diagnosed with ADD were to be responded to within our existing knowledge of screening for and addressing the effects of learning difficulties, neurological damage, and child abuse, what need would there be for a further pathological construction?

But I would like to make it clear that in holding this view, I am not disputing the fact that certain problems occur in the lives of some children and young people. These problems can involve not being able to engage in the classroom; being on the verge of exclusion, or already having been excluded, from school; aggression and noncooperation that isolate them from peers and siblings; and violence or temper that has them breaking objects, spitting, biting, kicking, hitting, and being verbally abusive. These are distressing and devastating events to all who suffer their effects, such as teachers, siblings, the children or young persons themselves, and parents (especially mothers, who will often accept the strong cultural/societal invitation to shoulder the responsibility for their children's behavior while at the same time feeling powerless to change or control it). That these events are facts, are actually occurring, is not in dispute here. Simply talking to the children and parents concerned makes it clear that these are unpleasant occurrences that are very unwelcome, and that everyone (including the children) feels powerless to control them. This much can be accepted. However, what is to be questioned is the interpretation of these events—the meaning that is attributed to them.

To start categorizing these children with a psychiatric diagnosis is to become blind to the fact that these same behaviors and problems are experienced by children and families in the context of child abuse, domestic violence (more accurately, male violence), and emotional trauma. This is not to say that all children who have been diagnosed with ADD have a history of being abused or are reproducing their experience of male violence. Many children have simply never been engaged in learning how to take charge of their lives from such problems. Some children just go at a million miles an hour because, in the vast diversity of the human species, that is how some children are. But these children are increasingly seen as a problem when child–teacher ratios are over 30:1, and when any sort of difference is increasingly seen as a problem and problems are pathologized. It is only when we become blind to the many different contexts of behavior perceived as problematic that we become available to seeing such behavior as a problem of biology, which is ADD. Moreover, we become available to the belief that treatment and interventions are required that are special to ADD, and we become blind to our long cultural history of expertise in parenting, teaching, social work, and counseling with children and families that have such problems. So how is it that the notion of ADD has thrived and spread through Western society? I would suggest that it is facilitated, if not aid-ed and abetted, by three cultural practices that are the products of biological determinist, sexist, and ageist ideology. These three cultural practices are the pathologizing of behavior, the infantilization or "growing down" of children, and mother blaming.

THREE CULTURAL PRACTICES

The Pathologizing of Behavior

The construction of any meaning is an expression of a certain discourse, and in the case of ADD the construction of meaning is a diagnostic category that is an expression of the dominant Western cultural discourses of traditional psychiatry and psychological testing. Foucault's (1965, 1979) analyses of the "history of madness," and of the objectification of persons through the process of classification, dividing practices, and subjectification, can lead us to believe that traditional psychiatry has reached its zenith in the achievement of its major piece of technology, the DSM-IV. Mainstream psychology is managing to keep pace, however, with an increasing battery of psychological tests and questionnaires that can categorize and compartmentalize events and experiences, free of any context. The power of this discursive practice is evidenced by the extent to which it is shaping of, and in turn shaped by, popular cultural experience. For many of us, the notion of self is inextricably linked with the option of personality. The notion of personality is seen as a configuration of attributes. The identification and measurement of these attributes are regular features of popular magazines. You can, of course, check off a series of boxes not only to find out what sort of person you are, but also to discover the configuration of characteristics of your significant relationships.

It would seem then that in Western culture there is now a frame of reference that is readily available to interpreting events, experiences, and dynamics as categorized, compartmentalized, fixed entities with a neurological/biological location. These entities are described in deficit-based language—the professional language of "less than." Meanings, understandings, and interpretations are reduced to a size that can be neatly located inside the person's brain, as pathology. As such, we are culturally primed to accept and perform a pathologizing interpretation of events that we experience as problematic. But this is not just an academic debate. These ideas have consequences; they have effects; they make some actions highly likely and prohibit other actions. They also shape our experience of ourselves, our relationships, and our world.

So what effects does the construction of ADD have on the families that are interpreted through this meaning system? A large number of the families I see in counseling are one-parent families. In most cases the sole parent is the mother, and the child who is identified as the problem is a boy. Upon exploration, some or all of the following is usually found. The mother may have a childhood history of physical/sexual abuse. She may have been subjected to domestic violence by her child(ren's) father or a subsequent partner. This may also have involved misogynistic verbal abuse aimed at denigrating and humiliating the mother. The child or children may have been a witness to this sexual/physical/emotional abuse, or may have been subjected to it themselves. In making a stand against violence and abuse by leaving the violent partner, the mother may then be dismayed to see abusive practices develop in her relationship with her male children. The child may become violent to people and objects and may be verbally abusive, often in a misogynistic manner. This may not occur in school, or even outside of the family home; it may only be directed at any siblings and at the mother. In effect, the child is repeating the practices of male violence perpetrated by the father *de facto*. Against her better judgment, the mother may be sucked into an escalating pattern of conflict that may get her yelling, shouting, being verbally abusive, and hitting or smacking.

Given the overwhelming statistics relating to the perpetration of violence and abuse by men on women, any critical analysis would require an emphasis on gender politics and the respective cultural discourses of masculinity and femininity—in particular, the culturally constructed and mediated sense of entitlement and righteousness that can enable men to feel justified in using practices of domination and control in relation to others. However, if the family is brought into contact with the ADD industry and the ideology of biological determinism, then the child is almost certain to be constructed as the problem, diagnosed with ADD, and prescribed Ritalin or Dexedrine. It will be understood that the child's behavior is the result of a chemical imbalance in the brain. Other factors may be recognized as contributors or issues that may need to be addressed, but ADD is not seen in the context of violence and abuse; rather, violence and abuse are seen in the context of ADD as a pathology.

The Infantilization or "Growing Down" of Children

As noted earlier, pathology uses a language that constitutes deficit. This deficit language is one of "less than," disability, incapacity, inadequacy, and incompetence; it is a labeling of damaged goods. It renders its subjects passive and mitigates against their taking action in their lives against a problem that is put down to physiology. The locus of control becomes a medication, not a person. The site of the problem becomes not the context but the child's brain. This intrinsically blames the child (or at least a physical part of the child) for the problem construction, but at the same time absolves the child of taking responsibility for acting against it, as the deficit-based discourse considers such responsibility to be beyond a child's ability. So instead of engaging children in taking on responsibility for taking control of their lives and discovering their own competence in employing alternatives to abusive practices that have a detrimental effect on their lives and on the lives of the people they care about—a process that many parents may associate with maturity and "growing up"—the ADD discourse engages them and their families in a process of "growing down." This process of infantilization places a diagnostic injunction on competence. It externalizes the locus of control and any sense of personal agency in attributing these functions to the medication. It thus separates and distances children from the experience of taking responsibility for their own lives and actions, and from the opportunity of discovering their own competence. Well, if this is the effect that these ideas can have on children, what effect can they have on parents?

Mother Blaming

To say that all fathers are absent would clearly not be true; however, in many families they are absent altogether, and in many others they are absent in the emotional and practical processes of caring for children. Even if there is a shared care arrangement, it is often the mother who takes on more responsibility and feels more distress in relation to the problems that arise with their children. This experience of distress has to do with gender politics and the cultural practice of mother blaming. This cultural practice is based upon the socially constructed invitation to women with children to see their identity as being primarily that of mother, with their self-worth and success as persons being dependent upon how well their children are constituted by, and constituting of, dominant cultural expectations. The judgment of the school and other mothers that a child is beyond control becomes a direct reflection on a mother's parenting. The mother may then experience a profound sense of self-blame, along with a sense of failure, guilt, helplessness, and perhaps anger or frustration with the child. When put in contact with the ADD industry, she is left to choose between resisting this culturally dominant construction of her context and accepting its definition. If she attempts to resist it and find another way, she will suffer the further judgment of others (such as other mothers, extended family members, the school, and doctors), who may blame her now for her irresponsibility in neglecting to get her child the medical help the child deserves. However, should she become defined by the ADD discourse, she will be freed from the mother blaming: She is no longer a failed mother, but a mother battling against the odds with a disabled child. Of course, once released from this torture, she may then become the instrument of the discourse in her attempt to liberate other mothers from their own private torture by introducing them to the ADD industry.

I would like to make it clear in saying this that I do not believe mothers are the problem, or are in some way weak. The construct of ADD is only one arena in which the cultural practice of mother blame flourishes; the responses to mothers whose children have been sexually abused constitute another (Freer, 1997). In the discursive construction of ADD, the child is not the problem. The mother or the parents are also not the problem. The problem is the dominant discourses of psychology, psychiatry, and patriarchy, which subjectify parent and child—rendering them passive and separate from their abilities, competence, and strengths, which would enable them to take action against the effects of violence, aggression, abuse, and boredom in their lives—that is the problem.

THERAPY IN THE PRESENCE OF
THE ADD CONSTRUCT

In order to follow the style of other chapters in this book, I have included a transcript of certain sections of a single interview. The interview was one in which I met with a 14-year-old boy called Paul; although that is not his real name, the conversation that appears here has been transcribed verbatim. Both Paul and his mother gave their permission for a number of our interviews to be recorded and included in some of my teaching and writing.

Paul's mother arranged for him to begin meeting with me where I work as a family therapist in independent practice. By that time, Paul was being seen by a general practitioner, a pediatrician, a psychiatrist, his school counselor, and a state social worker. All of this involvement was organized around the "diagnosis and treatment" of ADD(+H) (ADD with hyperactivity, as defined in the DSM-III-R, the immediate predecessor of DSM-IV). Paul's mother was willing to meet with me to inform me of her experience of Paul, which was one of guilt, anger, and resentment. Both she and her son had been subjected to severe and prolonged violence and emotional abuse by Paul's father and a subsequent partner.

Being given a diagnosis of ADD does not automatically mean that a child will have a history of child abuse. However, in the vast majority of families I have seen in counseling who have been (or are vulnerable to being) enlisted into the ADD discourse, some form of domestic violence and/or child abuse has occurred or is occurring. This can be obscured and looked over when the problem is presented as a child's neurological illness. ADD can even be used as a justification by an abusive parent for physical abuse of the child. A male child's "problem behavior" is often the boy's reproduction of an abusive father's behavior; as such, it is based in the dominant cultural practices of masculinity rather than biology. It is important, then, for the therapist not to accept the dominant construction uncritically as ADD, but to explore what experience of violence and abuse the family may have had or is currently having. It is, of course, then appropriate that this experience be addressed in counseling in its own right.

The violence and abuse that Paul and his mother had experienced were named and addressed with Paul in our meetings, as were many other issues. However, the mother's understanding of her experience of Paul was mediated by pathology rather than by the effects of abuse. She made it clear that she was not available to attending therapy with Paul; in her view, it was his problem, and she herself was already regularly meeting with a psychiatrist. As such, I was not able to attend to the place of mother blame in her experience, and I was only able to meet with Paul on his own and with the direct invitation to enter into the prevailing pathologizing construction of meaning. It was also clear that Paul's life was one in which he did not experience an understanding of what happened to him or around him, let alone any sense of effectiveness or control over it. He also experienced and expressed little knowledge of either himself or his life, which was evidenced by his frequently responding to questions by saying only, "I don't know." He was not hostile to our meetings and seemed quite happy to go along with events, which was his traditional approach to life. It just appeared to be that he really didn't know.

Clearly, no one piece of transcript can illustrate or demonstrate the full range of thinking and practice I have discussed here. So, in choosing a piece of transcript, I decided to privilege parts of a conversation that demonstrated the way in which the ADD construct, including the prescription of medication, was not experienced by Paul as either relevant or helpful to him—regardless of whether or not ADD can be regarded as a valid category. This transcript further illustrates the practice of creating a context in counseling that makes it possible for people to take charge of their lives, discover what they know about themselves, and reconnect with an experience of ability, competence, and strength. For Paul, this involved calling the "truth" status of the pathologizing of behavior into question; creating space for a description of Paul that was different from "disabled" or "less than"; and discovering and uncovering the ways in which he had experienced his ability to exercise a degree of control over the direction of his life. This then led to a further exploration of areas of his life that were rich in competence, ability, and successful action. The transcript consists of excerpts from a meeting that Paul and I agreed would be a review of the events and understandings we had talked about in the first 6 months we had been meeting. Other interviews and conversations could have been chosen that would have illustrated different aspects of this work.

IAN: Is it right that you have had a lot of involvement with doctors and pediatricians?

PAUL: What's a pediatrician?

IAN: A pediatrician is a doctor that specializes in seeing young people and children.

PAUL: Oh! Like a psychiatrist or something?

IAN: Well, it's a doctor for children.

PAUL: Like Dr. B?

IAN: Is Dr. B a pediatrician?

PAUL: I don't know. He's the one that described me as ADD and all that.

IAN: Right.

PAUL: I'm off medication now, and you know how Mum said that I'm not allowed to have Coke and all that because I'm hyperactive?

IAN: Yes.

PAUL: I've been having Coke and all, and I'm not hyperactive.

IAN: So can I talk to you about all that?

PAUL: About what?

IAN: About being ADD and hyperactive. When did you first hear about these things?

PAUL: About 18 months ago my mum took me to see Dr. B, and within a few minutes he said I've probably got ADD, and I ended up going on medication.

IAN: So around about a year and a half ago you went to see this doctor, and he said you had ADD. Had you ever heard of it before?

PAUL: Yeah, I knew a little bit before.

IAN: And what did you understand about it?

PAUL: Nothing.

IAN: Do you know what it stands for?

PAUL: Attention deficit disorder. But I didn't know it then.

IAN: So what do you understand about it now?

PAUL: Well, it's a chemical imbalance in the brain—it's the liquid in your brain that's not equal.

IAN: And what does that chemical imbalance mean? What happens?

PAUL: They find it hard to learn, getting on with other kids, self-esteem, all that sort of stuff. That's what I think it is.

IAN: So did you know all that at the time, or is that what you have learnt since then?

PAUL: Well, Mum told me all what it was, and I was quite worried about taking the medication. I was told it was a drug like speed or whatever, and, umm . . .

IAN: And what's speed?

PAUL: It's a drug.

IAN: And what effect does that have on you?

PAUL: I don't know, how am I supposed to know? I've never taken it. (*Laughs*)

IAN: So you've never taken speed?

PAUL: No way.

IAN: But this drug that you needed to take for ADD is like speed?

PAUL: Yeah. It's Ritalin, and he said it's like speed, but I wasn't too keen on it at first.

IAN: Why were you not keen on it at first?

PAUL: I don't know. You kind of hear "speed" and think of the illegal drug, and back then I was 12, 13 . . .

IAN: So you thought you were being asked to take an illegal drug. Did you think you'd be on to heroin next?

PAUL: (*Laughs*) Yeah. I kept asking Mum questions about it.

IAN: What questions did you ask her?

PAUL: I don't know. That was ages ago.

IAN: Why do you think you wanted to know more about it?

PAUL: I don't know—just to see if it was safe, I suppose.

IAN: So you were kind of worried about what kind of effect this would have on you?

PAUL: Yes.

IAN: What kind of effect did this drug have on you?

PAUL: When I started to take it, it took away my appetite a lot when I was getting used to it. But it worked; it helped calm me down a bit. But then, because I got used to it, it didn't work.

IAN: What else happened?

PAUL: Nothing really. It just helped me concentrate.

IAN: How did you notice that?

PAUL: I didn't. My teachers and that told my mum about it, and my mum told me. I don't know anything about what happens to me. I have to be told because, like, it's a bit hard to know what's happening if you don't even know if it's working or not.

IAN: Yes. That's why I was asking, because I was wondering if you had noticed any difference. You're saying . . .

PAUL: No, I never noticed a thing.

Taking a critical position in relation to the dominant medical and psychological discursive construction of ADD and tackling it head on can seem a bit like stepping out in front of a big truck with arms raised, carrying a little red sign with the word "stop" written on it. You are liable to get run over. So when a therapist is working with families that have already been enlisted into the ADD discourse and have a belief in the diagnosis and the efficacy of medication, arguing against that belief or attempting to deconstruct the notion without the preparation of an acceptable alternative understanding is likely to increase any sense of guilt, frustration, or hopelessness that made them so vulnerable to accepting the "biological basis of behavior" construct in the first place. For parents subjugated by mother blaming, denying the "rightness" of the interpretation of their problem as the results of ADD, without first deconstructing mother blaming as a cultural practice, will almost certainly serve to subjugate them further—because in the mother-blaming dichotomy, if a problem does not have a biological basis, then a mother must be to blame. For children who experience their motives and intentions through the "mad–bad" dichotomy, challenging the notion that they are ill may only leave them with the idea that they are "naughty" or fundamentally bad children, unless another understanding is available to them.

Consequently, challenging the ADD construct is not about arguing or debating with parents and children, or attempting to persuade them to see the error of their judgment (Nylund & Corsiglia, 1996). As I am not a psychologist or psychiatrist and therefore do not diagnose, test, or medicate, the chances are that if these approaches resolved the problems, the families I see would not be seeking my involvement as a therapist. If this is the case, then those areas that are not accounted for by existing or past intervention can become a focus of inquiry. It is also often the case that parents and children are in fact struggling against the toxic ideas of the pathologizing of behavior, the infantilization/growing down of children, and mother blaming, and are resisting the pressure to diagnose and medicate the children. Or, if this has already occurred but they are having serious doubts about its helpfulness or "rightness," then I find that joining with them in their doubts or critiques can provide a turning point in helping them to deconstruct the ADD discourse themselves. In fact, when I am able to invite them on a satirical exposé, it can be downright fun. Many parents have discovered the benefits of disattending to ADD. So, instead of attempting to convince them of the negative effects of pathologizing and ending up in a debate in which we are likely to discover our oppositional defiance with each other, I have found that I can join in helping parents and children support each other in an "oppositionally defiant" stand against the effects of pathologizing, labeling, and blame.

With regard to Paul's experience, as can be seen from the transcript, the question of whether ADD "exists" or not was an irrelevance, as it completely failed to engage him. It was more an experience that had been applied to him. Regardless of whether a meaning is "right," it must at least be experienced as helpful if a problem is to be successfully addressed. For Paul, the diagnosis was something that happened *to* him. It did not in any way engage his ability to know whether it was effective or not, or even how he would know if he knew if it was effective or not. As such, this practice facilitated two things: It externalized responsibility, and it grew Paul down. It externalized responsibility because he was no longer an effective player in his life. That role had been assigned to the medication. He did not have any system of knowing about himself; that knowledge came secondhand from teachers and his mother. It grew Paul down because he was not being engaged in discovering ways to take responsibility in his life or in learning to exercise good judgment—the stuff of maturity. He was being invited into a view of himself as not being able to take full responsibility for himself because of a neurological disorder, and as not being able to function adequately in his life without psychostimulants. Through the asking of certain questions, then, the construct of ADD was quickly established as an irrelevance if we were to address the issue of Paul's getting in charge of his life and establishing a connection to his self-knowledge.

IAN: So you were told that you had hyperactivity and you were told that you had ADD, and what that meant was that you had to start taking Ritalin, and you were not allowed to have much sugar, or red cordial [a sugary drink], or dessert. And what you're telling me now is that in the last month you have stopped taking Ritalin and you're eating a lot more sugar, and you say that things are no different from before a month ago.

IAN: Yeah.

IAN: So do you think that hyperactivity and ADD are two descriptions that fit you or don't fit you?

PAUL: Don't fit me.

IAN: So neither of them fit you?

PAUL: No.

Bateson (1972) has identified how "beliefs of restraint" can act to hold people from taking action to resolve the problems that beset them. Poststructuralist thought has demonstrated how belief systems survive and operate within a political context and can be subjected to the practice of deconstruction. The work of family therapists Michael White and David Epston (1989) has provided us with a process of therapy for deconstructing discursively based beliefs that are subjugating and impoverishing of persons, such as racist, sexist, classist, and heterosexually dominant belief systems. As previously discussed, the toxic ideas of pathologizing, infantilizing, and mother blaming are three such subjugating and impoverishing beliefs; thus, they need to be deconstructed in their own right. Again, there is little chance of challenging the construction of the problem as ADD unless these ideas are deconstructed first, as the strength of this construction is dependent upon the existence of the beliefs that underpin it. In the conversation with Paul, instead of struggling with the restraining and subjugating beliefs that surround a person identified as "being ADD," he shed the description that no longer described him. This allowed us to explore other areas of Paul's experience that fit with competence and personal agency, without contradicting his views or beliefs about himself.

IAN: So did it seem to you like you were in charge of your life, or did it seem more like what happened to you was up to chance or other people?

PAUL: I didn't know much about what was going on, and with behavior stuff and medication . . . I didn't recognize anything.

IAN: So did that mean you felt able to do anything about it, or did that make you feel, "Well, if I don't know anything about it, I can't do anything about it"?

PAUL: I don't know. I just tried to do my work and stuff, and whatever happened happened.

IAN: So did you feel active or passive in that?

PAUL: What do you mean, "passive"?

IAN: Okay. Well, "passive" is when you don't really do anything. You just go with the flow. You know, if you're in a river—you know rivers have currents . . .

PAUL: Yeah, I was in one.

IAN: Yeah? You've been in one, you've been in a current?

PAUL: Yeah, saving someone.

IAN: Yeah? What happened?

PAUL: It was a rip [riptide], actually.

IAN: Really, a rip?

PAUL: Yeah. He was getting dragged out to sea and stuff. We were boogie-boarding, and he got caught out, and I swam out and got him in. He was a long way out. I just swam with the current, you know, and went out with the board. I was just paddling and stuff and trying to get faster. I eventually caught him, you know, he was half choking and all, umm . . . So I put him on the board, hung on and kicked, and swam back in.

IAN: Wow! So you swam with the current out to where he was . . .

PAUL: And then I swam against it . . .

IAN: And then you managed to swim against it to save . . .

PAUL: . . . it wasn't that strong. He was quite small. About 10 or something, and he wouldn't have been able to swim back in.

IAN: So what would have happened to him if you hadn't been able to swim out to him?

PAUL: I don't know. He'd probably be floating out at sea right now, dead or picked up, or . . .

IAN: So you saved this boy's life?

PAUL: Yeah, probably.

IAN: That's pretty special.

PAUL: Yeah. It wasn't that far out, so it wasn't that big a deal, but it was a fair way out. Miles over my depth.

IAN: So he would have died, you saved his life, and it was way out of your depth, but it was no big deal.

PAUL: Yeah. It wasn't that far out, but it was deep enough for a really, really big humpback whale to go down, pick up speed, and show all its body out of the water (*using his hands and arms to illustrate the point*). It was that deep. But I don't know . . .

IAN: And there was a humpback whale there?

PAUL: No (*laughs*). If there was, I'd be swimming for my life.

IAN: So what would have happened if you had just sat there in the current and not done anything? That's what I mean by "passive."

PAUL: I went into it to get him. I didn't know there was one.

IAN: So, what would have happened if once you got out to him, you'd done nothing? Like being passive is when you don't do anything.

PAUL: We both would have been dragged out to sea.

IAN: So if you had been passive, you both would have been dragged out to sea.

PAUL: Yeah.

IAN: But you were active and you swam against it.

PAUL: (*Nods*)

IAN: Well, that's interesting because I was wondering whether, in your life, you feel you are active or passive. Whether you feel you are passive and you do nothing and you get carried along with the rip, or whether you are active and you swim against it to go in the direction you want to go in.

PAUL: I don't know. I was really trying when I was first on the Ritalin and all that, but then I ended up giving up and just going with the flow.

IAN: So at the beginning of the year you were active. You were kind of swimming against the flow. You were moving your life in the direction you wanted it to go in, and then later on you were passive.

PAUL: I suppose I went with the flow.

IAN: You went with the flow. The rip kind of carried you out in your life.

PAUL: Yep.

IAN: So what do you want for this year?

PAUL: I don't know. I want to try and not get into trouble and try to get on with all the kids and staff, because I've only got 2 years before I have to find a job, get a car and license, and . . .

IAN: So you have some plans for your life.

PAUL: Yep.

IAN: So these plans you have for your life—do they mean that you'd need to be active or passive in this?

PAUL: Active.

IAN: You'd have to be active in this?

PAUL: I want to be able to get a car, find some money and rent out a caravan, find a job, and live there. . . . I don't know when.

IAN: So, Paul, if you were being active in life rather than passive, how would you know you were being successful in being active in your life?

PAUL: I'd probably be able to find a job better, because my resumé would be of a couple of years of working in the school canteen. I've worked there for about half a year now. I'd probably be able to get a job in a canteen or a deli or something like that.

IAN: So has working in the canteen for that half a year . . . does that fit more with you being passive in your life and being carried out in the rip, or . . .

PAUL: No.

IAN: . . . or does that fit more with you swimming to the shore?

PAUL: Active! It more fits with being active.

IAN: So how have you been able to do that?

In combining the practice of deconstruction with the application in therapy of a narrative metaphor, Michael White (1991) has created a context in which both therapists and clients can engage in the challenging and deconstructing of those limiting and oppressive cultural and self-narratives whose "truth" status has dominated the clients' understanding of their lives. Through the practices of externalizing—which is, in effect, the opposite of internalizing pathology (White, 1989)—and the discovery of unique outcomes in a person's life that contradict the dominance of the problem narrative, then another narrative, a competence-based narrative preferred by the person, can be allowed room to develop into the narrative that becomes the dominant understanding of the person's experience of his/her life.

When ADD is the dominant narrative, it acts to internalize the problem by pathologizing the behavior, and to externalize responsibility and personal agency by investing the Ritalin with the ability to solve the problem. When a narrative and deconstructive approach is applied to this context, the ADD label itself can be externalized. Unique outcomes that accent the child's taking effective action against the effects of ADD can be located. For example, the child may be on a constant dosage of Ritalin, but the problem has begun to resolve without a corresponding rise in medication; or the problem may only occur at home and not in school, or vice versa; or the problem may not have worsened during a "holiday" from the drug. Curiosity about these inconsistencies can lead to the discovery of competence and personal agency in the child. This approach to the role of medication has been described in relation to therapeutic work with the label of schizophrenia (White, 1987).

With regard to my conversation with Paul, we did not have to directly deconstruct ADD's version (dominant story) of Paul's life, or to search within that context for evidence of protest, resistance, and contradiction. That was achieved in Paul's situation through rendering ADD irrelevant to him and effectively starving it of attention, by moving on to areas and experiences of his life that were more relevant to his achieving what he wanted in his life. As a result, he was able to realize that he had plans and the ability to achieve them. Although as counselors with children and young people we may often experience a strong imperative (from whatever source, including ourselves) to accept ADD's conceptualization of the problem and the language that is available in creating meaning around that problem, this conversation with Paul illustrates the potential worth of refusing to let the ADD construct set the agenda.

Finally, let me pose some questions for ourselves as therapists.

WHAT DID WE DO BEFORE ADD WAS INVENTED?

How, as family therapists, did we respond to children before ADD was invented? Did we not attempt to put the presentation of any given problem into a context? Were we not aware that some children, especially boys, were vulnerable to reproducing male violence and aggression when they had been subjected to abuse and violence in their lives, particularly by men? Did we not think that this was the reproduction of some of men's ways of being rather than genetic inheritance? Were we not aware of the ways in which children expressed emotional distress (often but not always as a result of abuse), and of how these expressions were experienced and described by parents and professionals as "behavioral problems"? If children had learning difficulties, did we not have ways of assessing and naming those and providing additional learning supports without pathologizing and infantilizing the children? What does the invention of a new pathology give us that we did not have access to before? If psychostimulants have an effect on us all, regardless of diagnosis, why does the use of medication need to be predicated on children's being defined as neurologically and psychologically "less than"? If ADD no longer existed as a construct, would we as therapists be any less effective in our attempts to help children and families overcome problems? Would ADD have a life if dominant Westernized culture no longer perpetuated mother blame, pathologizing of behavior, and the infantilization of children? If time and money were not cultural imperatives, would medical interventions based on drug treatment be a first choice?

EDITORIAL QUESTIONS

Q: *(CS) I feel you have presented a humorous, well-considered, and compelling case for us to re-examine some of our routine assumptions about ADD. Your workshop example (asking how many of the group members have problems attending, fidgeting, etc.) reminds me of your point about the importance of context in terms of how personally engaging or boring a child's environment is. I've never quite been satisfied with biological/medical explanations for why the same child who can't stay still in a classroom can be riveted and almost motionless in front of a computer game for hours!*

I understand that Paul's mother didn't want to see you in therapy and had her own therapist. It seemed from your helpful vignettes that your re-authoring questions helped Paul entertain a new story that he could actively influence his life without medications and without thinking of himself in ADD terms. If this process continued, and yet his mother (perhaps with the psychiatrist's support) wanted him to stay on his medication and spoke to Paul about his "still being ADD," how might you have responded? Would you have invited Paul to explore ways to respond to his mother's concerns? Could you elaborate on this.

Q: *(CS) I really resonate with your concerns that the ADD diagnosis can potentially distract us from considering contextual factors such as abuse, mother blame, and so forth. As you aptly discuss, I also am quite concerned that medication can be seen as the "locus of control" and that children may view themselves as "disabled." In addition to these concerns, I am trying to take into account other experiences I've had where teachers and parents have reported that medication such as Ritalin has been highly effective in helping children calm down and attend. One of the things that Dave Nylund and Victor Corsiglia (1996) talk about with parents who sincerely want to pursue medication is exploring the family members' ideas about medication before referring them for a medication evaluation. They ask questions such as these: "Would it concern you if Johnny received the message that he is damaged? What could be a useful way of telling Johnny why medication may be helpful?"*

Suppose a parent came to you because her son's teacher strongly urged her to get medication and therapy for her son. Let's further assume that you've done the sorts of things you mentioned about deconstructing the ADD discourse, but the parent remained convinced that the teacher was right and medication was needed. Would you ever consider the sorts of explorations described above for parents who really were convinced that medication was needed? What other reactions do you have on this? Are you concerned that medication should never be used for "ADD," or are you more concerned about the possible implications of using medications in this situation?

A: Thank you for your comments and the two questions that you have asked. They have been helpful to me in more directly considering some of the elements of this work. In beginning a response to your questions, I would like to address the second one first. The literature is fairly clear with regard to the use of psychostimulants, in that they "are not specific in their effects on individuals with ADHD," and furthermore that "finding[s] proscribe any diagnostic conclusion on the basis of response to drugs" (Jureidini, 1996). This means that your experience of seeing Ritalin have a "calming effect" on some children in school would be duplicated for the entire class, regardless of the children's fit with any particular diagnostic category, and cannot therefore be taken as evidence that any particular child has "something" called ADD (Rapoport et al., 1980). That said, it is not my role to advise on whether or not any person take psychoactive drugs. As I am neither a psychologist nor a medical practitioner, I believe that it would be unethical for me to engage in psychometric testing, psychological assessment, medical diagnosis, and prescribing medication. If these are the services that are required, then it would be unlikely that the parent and teacher you are supposing would in fact be consulting with me. However, if the parent in question was interested in counseling, then I would proceed in the way that I have described in this chapter.

This then relates in part to your first question, in that the practices of discovering and privileging people's ability to engage actively in their lives does not need to be predicated upon the prior deconstruction of an existing construct. It was my intention that this point be demonstrated by the transcripted conversation with Paul. Similarly, a parent, a teacher, or anyone else for that matter does not need to forswear her/his beliefs before being able to witness the emergence of another person's competence in life. Within narrative-influenced practice, the very act of creating space for the development of a person's alternative story is in itself a direct challenge to the dominant story's right to speak for that person.

REFERENCES

Advertiser [South Australia]. (1996, November 29).

American Psychiatric Association. (1994). *Diagnostic and statistical manual of mental disorders* (4th ed.). Washington, DC: Author.

Australian Doctor. (1996, October 1). Debate: Attention deficit disorder—controversies in medicine.

Bateson, G. (1972). *Steps to an ecology of mind.* New York: Ballantine.

Foucault, M. (1965). *Madness and civilization.* New York: Random House.

Foucault, M. (1979). *Discipline and punish: The birth of the prison.* New York: Peregrine Books.

Freer, M. (1997). Taking a defiant stand against sexual abuse and the mother blaming discourse. *Gecko, 1,* 5–28.

Jureidini, J. (1996). Some reasons for concern about attention deficit disorder. *Journal of Pediatrics and Child Health, 32,* 201–203.

Messenger [Adelaide, South Australia]. (1994).

Nash, H. (1994). *Kids, families and chaos: Living with attention deficit disorder.* Adelaide, South Australia: Ed-Med.

Nylund, D., & Corsiglia, V. (1996). From deficits to special abilities: Working narratively with children labeled "ADHD." In M. Hoyt (Ed.), *Constructive therapies* (Vol. 2, pp. 163–183). New York: Guilford Press.

Rapaport, J. L., Buchsbaum, M. S., Zahn, T. P., Weingartner, H., Ludlow, C., & Mikkelsen, E. J. (1980). Dextroamphetamine: Its cognitive and behavioral effects in normal and hyperactive boys and men. *Archives of General Psychiatry, 37,* 933–943.

Reid, R., Maag, J. W., & Vasa, S. F. (1994). Attention deficit hyperactivity disorder as disability category: A critique. *Exceptional Children, 60*(3), 198–214.

Wallis, C. (1994, July 18). Life in overdrive: An epidemic of attention deficit disorder. *Time,* pp. 42–50.

White, M. (1987). Family therapy and schizophrenia: Addressing the "in the corner" lifestyle. *Dulwich Centre Newsletter,* No. 1, 14–21.

White, M. (1988–1989). The externalizing of the problem and the re-authoring of lives and relationships. *Dulwich Centre Newsletter,* No. 2, 3–20.

White, M. (1991). Deconstruction and therapy. *Dulwich Centre Newsletter,* No. 3, 1–22.

White, M., & Epston, D. (1989). *Literate means to therapeutic ends.* Adelaide, South Australia: Dulwich Centre Publications.

Zametkin, A. J., Nordahl, T. E., Gross, M., King, A. C., Semple, W., Rumsley, E., Hamburger, S., & Cohen, R. (1990). Cerebral glucose metabolism in adults with hyperactivity of childhood onset. *New England Journal of Medicine, 323,* 1361–1366.

12

From "Cold Care" to "Warm Care"

CHALLENGING THE DISCOURSES OF MOTHERS AND ADOLESCENTS

KATHY WEINGARTEN

In a culture that promotes the values of autonomy and independence as relentlessly as European-American culture does, it is a political act for a therapist to see parents and adolescents together. Or, as I prefer to call it, it is an act of "cultural resistance" (Weingarten, 1995, 1997). The dominant cultural messages bombarding adolescents and their parents at every turn trivialize their relationship, valorize the adolescents' relationship with peers, and encourage silence instead of voice in relation to each other. In the work that I do, which I describe in this chapter, I am trying to counter these dominant messages in favor of others that make room for, accept the value of, and support parent–adolescent interaction through the developmental transitions that both adolescents and parents make. I heartily believe that as clinicians, we have the opportunity in every encounter either to promote the parent–adolescent relationship as a resource or to denigrate its value. We do the latter to the peril of us all.

In this chapter, I describe a consultation interview with two mothers and their daughters, which demonstrates the way I work with adolescents and the theoretical principles that underlie my approach. I tend to see adolescents with their parents. A discourse-analytic framework, which I describe below, provides the conceptual rationale for this practice. I also listen carefully to both what is said and what is not said; I am impressed by how much adolescents communicate both in words and in silence. During moments of silence, I try to understand whether their words have vanished or whether the perception that there is receptivity for their words has. Finally, I try to make room for the voice of the adolescent in preference to my own voice. As I discuss below, a postmodern narrative practice is ideally suited for this purpose.

In this chapter, I use my annotations of the transcript not only to show the ways certain interactions served the model I use with adolescents, but also to indicate places in the interview where I swerved from the model I wanted to be using. By proceeding in this fashion, I hope to recreate the interview as a work in progress, engaging the reader—with his/her own theoretical and clinical issues currently holding sway—as a participant in the creation of an emerging text (Penn & Frankfurt, 1994).

THEORETICAL ORIENTATION

Postmodern Practice

In the fall of 1993, at the time this interview was conducted, I based my work on postmodern principles, using discourse analysis as a primary theoretical tool and the narrative metaphor as my primary clinical orientation. The difference between a modernist and a postmodern paradigm for clinical practice has been described by several authors (Freedman & Combs, 1996; Gergen & Kaye, 1992; Hare-Mustin, 1994; Lax, 1992; Madigan, 1996).

In my work, I notice the difference in the following ways: I no longer believe that my task is to observe persons; to compare their thoughts, feelings, and behaviors against pre-existing normative criteria; and then to explain, advise, or intervene as a means to bring their responses in line with these criteria. These three related actions are consistent with a modernist paradigm. Instead, I believe that normative criteria participate in the creation of the very dilemmas from which persons suffer and seek to escape. I see my task as the creation of a conversational context in which persons can notice aspects of their experience that contradict the restrictive views of themselves, others, and the problems that beset them. When this occurs, choices for the development of new stories about their lives become possible and preferable. Since the stories we tell about ourselves are constitutive of our experience rather than represent it (White, 1995), persons who are telling new stories about themselves are creating paths for new thinking, feeling, and action. Thus, noticing, searching for, generating possibilities for, questioning about, and developing alternative story lines replace explaining, advising, and intervening as the modes of therapeutic action within the postmodern paradigm.

Postmodern practices, with their emphasis on the development of the clients' voice rather than the assertion of the therapist's voice, seem particularly useful for work with children and adolescents. Their stories are particularly vulnerable to colonization; their voices are particularly vulnerable to silencing. A postmodern practice can guard against the imposition of meaning on persons who, like children and adolescents, are less powerful than adults and whose stories may be less precisely formed (Stacey & Loptson, 1995).

Although the distinctions between modernist and postmodern practices are quite clear to me, and although I have a definite preference for postmodern practices, I am aware that in any one interview I may slip from postmodern to modernist practices. This happened on several occasions in the interview I present and discuss here. By annotating these occasions, I hope to illustrate how small shifts can make clinical work more consistently postmodern when this is a goal.

Discourse Analysis

Many conceptual systems are consistent with a postmodern paradigm. I have been strongly influenced both professionally and personally by ideas about discourse and discourse analysis (Hare-Mustin, 1994; Scott, 1990; Weingarten, 1995, 1997). These ideas form the conceptual background of the consultation interview that I present.

It has been important to me to try to understand how certain kinds of negotiated meanings operate either to subjugate, marginalize, or trivialize people's experience, *or* to allow it to be fully represented. The idea of discourse helps me understand the mechanisms by which some people's experience becomes dominant and other people's experiences—often those of women, children, people of color, homosexuals, and people who are differently abled—are pushed to the edge.

I use the concept of "discourse" the way social historian Joan W. Scott (1990) defines it—that is, as a "historically, socially, and institutionally specific structure of statements, terms, categories, and beliefs" (pp. 135–136) that are embedded in institutions, social relationships, and texts. Some discourses are made dominant and others are marginalized through the operation of these mechanisms. This meaning of discourse allows me to make sense of what Jerome Bruner (1990) calls the ways "culture forms mind" (p. 24).

At the time of this consultation, I was trying to understand the related discourses of mothers and adolescents (Weingarten, 1997). By reading popular and professional texts about adolescents, by observing mothers and adolescents in clinical settings, by listening to professional and lay conversations about mothers and adolescents, by watching media representations of the mother–adolescent relationship, and by noticing the ways schools both involved and sidelined parents of adolescents, I was trying to answer this question: What meanings about mothers and adolescents are given "truth" status and why?

I identified several "truths." Separation is seen as the primary developmental task for adolescents (and their parents); mothers are seen as the people from whom it is most essential that adolescents separate; and the "normal" separation process is believed to be inevitably conflictual (Bly, 1990; Dickerson & Zimmerman, 1992, 1993; Lazarre, 1991; Steinberg & Levine, 1990; Weingarten, 1997). Adolescents are encouraged to "find" an identity, as if there is one "right" self, and mothers who are still "searching" for theirs are considered to be negative influences. These "truths" are predicated on psychological theories of growth and change that value autonomy and individualism above interdependence and connection (Jordan, Kaplan, Miller, Stiver, & Surrey, 1991; Gilligan, Rogers, & Tolman, 1991); confuse closeness with intimacy (Weingarten, 1991, 1992, 1997); and promote a belief in a single, unified, "container" self (Gergen, 1991; Sampson, 1993).

All of these "truths"—and the host of others cascading from them—exert powerful influences. Persons experience their influence both in direct, explicit ways (e.g., it is common to hear two adults talk about a youngster in her/his presence, saying, "Can you imagine if she [or he] is this way now, what her [or his] adolescence is going to be like?") and in subtle, indirect ways (e.g., there is little or no advertising that shows mothers and adolescents together).

In my clinical work, at that time and still now, I set myself the task of challenging the limiting and constraining influence of these "truths" and of making these challenges serve as a springboard for alternative knowledges to surface and perhaps to become the bases of new stories. As a clinician, it is clear to me that every interview with a mother and adolescent provides multiple opportunities to do just that. In the interview that follows, I annotate those practices that I believe challenged or undermined the hold of these "truths" on the lives of the mothers and daughters who talked with me.

By seeing adolescents with their parents, I am also challenging the dominant ideology of separation that pervades standard mental health practice. Within the mental health context, this ideology is often expressed as "Adolescents need privacy to work in therapy." By meeting with adolescents and their parents together (in this interview, mothers and daughters), I am counterposing this idea with others: that a parent and adolescent can benefit from hearing each other's stories, and that each may be a resource for change for the other.

Narrative Metaphor

Always I am guided by the narrative metaphor, emphasizing multiple points of view rather than normative or expert ones (Dickerson & Zimmerman, 1996; Tomm, 1992; Zimmerman & Dickerson, 1994). During any interview, I am mindful that a re-authoring process can evolve from the opening of a new story or the narrowing of an existing one, and that many kinds of interactions create opportunities for the emergence of what Roth and Epston (1996) call "narratives of contrary experience." In this interview, listening intently, asking questions, making distinctions, introducing and emphasizing novel affect, and sharing personally can all provide potential paths to the development of new stories about the self, others and the problem.

CONSULTATION INTERVIEW

Background to the Interview

Timothy Nichols and Cheryl Jacques—the director and social worker, respectively, at a residential facility for adolescents—asked me to interview a group of four mothers and their daughters about whom they were particularly perplexed.[1] All four daughters had been "running" from the residence, engaging in high-risk behaviors while they were away. On the day of the interview itself, two of the daughters had "run," and so the interview took place with only two of the mothers and daughters present.

Tim and Cheryl spoke to me initially while Bonnie and Roberta, the two mothers (both European-American women in their early 30s), and Maryann and Tara, the two daughters (ages 16 and 12, respectively, and also European-American), listened in the same room.[2] Tim spoke first:

"We've had a lot of teenaged girls getting into trouble in ways that are very dangerous and self-destructive. One of the common de-

[1]For a description of the narrative work that they do at the residence, see Nichols and Jacques (1995).

[2]Both the mothers and the daughters have given permission for this material to be used. Their names have been changed to protect confidentiality.

nominators in these situations is that for one reason or another, the daughters and mothers have had disruptions in their relationships. Then, in recent years, as the mothers and daughters have tried to get their relationships to work in a healthier way, all hell has broken loose. More specifically related to Maryann and Bonnie and Tara and Roberta, Maryann has been with us for 6 months and is about to go home. But there still seems to be tension between Maryann and Bonnie. We think that a key to insuring success for Maryann is going to be improving her relationship with Bonnie. [We think this is true] for Tara and Roberta as well. There seems to be a lot of strong—angry—feelings between them."

I summarized what I had heard Tim say. Next, Cheryl spoke:

"I think it would be helpful to figure out what's the helpful part and what isn't in working with these families, so that if these families come in with the goal of wanting to strengthen their relationships, which most of the time they do, I can be helpful to them in reaching that goal. I've seen a lot of despair in a lot of the moms, like "I just don't want my daughter to go through the same thing I did, or the same thing that my mother did," and it's a heavy despair."

I nodded to Cheryl, indicating that I understood her concern. Asking whether they wanted me to know anything else before I met with Bonnie, Maryann, Roberta, and Tara, I moved to change everybody's places when they said, "Not for now." Tim and Cheryl went behind the one-way mirror, and I repositioned the chairs so that now just five of us were in the room—five persons and a large pad of paper, propped on an easel. This pad of paper turned out to play a significant part in the unfolding effects of the conversation that followed.

The Interview

I began the interview by asking whether each woman knew the other two women in the room (besides her own mother or daughter). As I suspected, not only did they not know me, they didn't know each other. I asked everyone present to take care to speak only what she was comfortable speaking in that unusual context. By doing so, I introduced the idea that they could take care of themselves. This assumption now floated in the room alongside Tim's observation that the daughters were behaving self-destructively. I explained that I would ask each of them questions, probably weaving my questions among them as the conversation evolved.

Because she was sitting at the far left of the group, I started by asking Maryann who else beside Bonnie was in her family? She replied that she had a sister (actually a half-sister), Annie. I asked Maryann, "What kind of kid is she? What's she like?"

MARYANN: I think she's . . . she's kind of violent.

KATHY: She's kind of violent?

MARYANN: Uh-huh . . . in my opinion.

KATHY: Okay. Give me some examples.

MARYANN: She punched me in the face the other day.

KATHY: Is that right?

MARYANN: Yeah. She's done it, like, a few times now.

KATHY: Okay. Now, when she punches you in the face, what do you do about it?

MARYANN: I hit her back.

KATHY: And does that help? Does that make her stop? Or what happens?

MARYANN: No. I get in trouble for it.

KATHY: Who gets you into trouble? (*She points to her mother.*) Okay. Do you think that Bonnie sees Annie as violent the way you see Annie?

MARYANN: No.

KATHY: So that might be one of the places that we would start from. Would you say that Annie is starting to show signs of getting into trouble? [I am introducing the language that Tim has used in his opening comments and that Maryann has just used herself.]

MARYANN: Uh-huh.

KATHY: You would. Okay. And what about your mom? Do you think she sees that? (*Maryann shakes her head "no."*) So from your point of view, Annie's already showing signs of getting into trouble. [By inserting the phrase "So from your point of view," I am aligning myself with the idea that there can be multiple views of reality. By not asking the two women to discuss their two views of Annie, I'm countering a conventional notion that differences must be resolved rather than coexist.]

KATHY: How old were *you* . . . well, first of all, do you agree . . . with the people at the residence that you have gotten into trouble?

MARYANN: Yes, I was umm . . . 11.

KATHY: That was the first time that if somebody had been really paying really good attention, they would have known that you were starting to get into trouble? Eleven or . . .

MARYANN: Eleven.

KATHY: Eleven. Okay. So that was starting. And what did you first notice about yourself?

MARYANN: I was drinking.

KATHY: You were drinking? That's what you first noticed. Did you notice anything before you started drinking? Like any feelings you were having that made you want to drink—that if somebody had been paying really good attention, they would have noticed that you were feeling something, that you were then going to start drinking? [Unfortunately, this hypothetical question sets up the possibility for blame. As the interview unfolds, I become aware of this, and I work to mitigate the possible effect of blame—in this case, mother blaming, which is a particularly pervasive and insidious element of the discourse of mothers in Western cultures (Caplan, 1989).]

MARYANN: I was extremely depressed and suicidal.

KATHY: So you started drinking after you were feeling really depressed and suicidal. And who was around at the time who might have noticed that? Or did notice? I don't know whether anybody noticed that. Did anybody notice it?

MARYANN: My mom [could have].

KATHY: Okay. Were you living with your mom and your stepfather at that time? And they . . . they didn't notice that you were depressed and suicidal. Did they notice when you started drinking?

MARYANN: Uh-huh.

KATHY: And that started at age 11. So tell me when you think somebody first noticed that you were getting into trouble. Because we've got 5 years to account for here. When did somebody first notice you were getting into trouble?

MARYANN: Um . . . 14 or 15.

KATHY: And who noticed? Who do you think noticed first?

MARYANN: My mom . . . I think my mom.

KATHY: Okay. Can I ask her what she noticed?

MARYANN: Uh-huh.

KATHY: (*To Bonnie*) Now you may not agree that you first noticed at 14 or 15, and I'll ask you when you think you did notice. But from Maryann's point of view, it was around 14 or 15 that you first noticed. What—at 14 or 15, what did you notice about Maryann that made you think she was in trouble?

BONNIE: She was very withdrawn, real quiet, slept a lot . . . she'd have real emotional outbursts; she was doing very poorly in school.

KATHY: So those were all signs to you.

I then used this pattern of questioning with the other three women—first Tara, then Roberta, then Bonnie. I asked the questions in the same order: whether the person believed she was in trouble now, at what age she thought she started being in trouble, what she noticed then, when others first noticed, and what they noticed at that time. By including the mothers in the same line of questioning during the interview, I was challenging several beliefs and making room for others. First, I was challenging the notion that mothers should be selfless and storyless—empty vessels for their children to fill with the stories of their lives (Weingarten, 1997). I was acting as if I believed that girls can listen to their mothers' stories and may be interested in doing so.

Second, I was challenging the idea that when mothers self-disclose, they are undermining generational boundaries that are already problematic in families in which teens are "acting out." I was acting as if I believed that telling one's story to another has the potential for an experience of shared meaning making, which itself can promote a feeling of intimacy (Weingarten, 1991). I was acting as if I believed that intimacy of this kind is possible between mothers and their daughters, and that there is little or no risk that this kind of sharing will interfere with important parenting tasks, such as specifying rules and setting limits.

Finally, I was taking the idea of trouble and contextualizing it by asking the women to provide a history and description of its manifestations when trouble was known only to them, to a few people, and to many others. In this way, an externalizing conversation formed without an explicit externalization of trouble (White, 1988–1989). I was able to get each woman to think about her long-term relationship with trouble. It was possible, however, that the phrases "starting to get into trouble" or "signs of trouble" might work against my purposes because they might promote an internalizing perspective. If so, questions such as "How old were you when trouble made its first appearance in your life? Who else do you think noticed trouble? How did trouble keep itself so well hidden from others? What changed to make trouble visible to others? How did trouble first appear to them?" and the like might have been more consistent with my intention of developing an externalizing conversation.

Tara told me that she was 4 when she first got into trouble; looking back, she knew this because she was "at my friend's house, hanging out with people who were, like, smoking joints and shooting heroin and stuff like that." Unlike Maryann, Tara felt that someone did notice right from the start—a sister of her mother's, Auntie Karen—but that her mother didn't believe Karen.

Roberta chimed in: "What was I doing?" Tara, however, was reluctant to answer her mother's question, and so Roberta did herself: "I was using drugs throughout the whole thing. Tara was real out of control, I was real out of control, and, like Tara said, there wasn't a lot of supervision that was going on."

Throughout the interview, I was putting the information I was getting on the large pad of paper. Each name was on the pad, and there were columns of numbers representing the ages when the women first knew they were in trouble, someone had noticed, and many people had noticed. Now, talking to Roberta, writing her ages on the pad, I asked her to help me: "So help me with this. What kind of mark could I make that would signal that you were out of it? Or that . . . I have an idea. What about a mark that would show that you were in trouble, too?" Roberta chose an exclamation mark. I then went back to the numbers already written on the page and entered exclamation points. The paper itself was now telling a story.

Roberta told me that she was 9 or 10 when she first knew that she was in trouble, but 13 or 14 when others began to notice. The "big-time" trouble began for her when she was 25 to 28 years old. Roberta also told me that all of her sisters either were in trouble now or had been in trouble also, most with problems of alcohol or drug abuse.

Now it was Bonnie's turn to talk. She told me that she was 14 when she started to be in trouble, and that soon after she realized it, others did too. She told me that she began to get out of trouble with alcohol and drugs "2 years after Maryann was born . . . it actually started when I got pregnant with Maryann."

MARYANN: It didn't stop then.

BONNIE: Well, it started to, though. I think it was a few years after that that I completely stopped.

KATHY: All right. And was there something about having . . . about becoming a mother, or taking care of Maryann, that helped you to stop?

BONNIE: Yeah.

KATHY: Is that something that you've ever told her [Maryann]?

BONNIE: We've ... I think it's come up. I mean I continued to smoke pot occasionally, and I suppose there were ... there were different instances where I would go ... um ... on kind of like ... partying, you know, where I would go out every weekend type of thing? But the drugs ... um ... I'm trying to think, when was the time you said you were going to call the police (*laughs*)? Around 9?

MARYANN: No, I was older than that. I was around 12.

BONNIE: But that was just occasional joints here and there. It wasn't anything as heavy-duty as it was when ...

MARYANN: You had a plant in the house ... in my room, so Peter's parents wouldn't know it was yours.

BONNIE: But that was just a plant.

MARYANN: Oh, it was just a plant. Ma, the plant was bigger than me. ... I said, "What's that?" "It's a fern." "No, it isn't, it's pot."

BONNIE: See, I'm comparing it to when I was in really bad shape ... where I was doing a lot of different drugs.

KATHY: And that was that time around 15 when you were doing a lot of drugs ...

BONNIE: Right. Until I got pregnant with Maryann.

KATHY: So that sounds like you were trying to get your act together and be responsible. ... But, Maryann, it sounds like and it also looks like ... you don't buy your mom's story. [I am commenting on the nonverbal communication, trying to determine whether Maryann can feel safe to say what she is thinking.] So do you want to ... it's not so much whether you can convince me, but maybe you could tell your mom something about what your point of view is about that. [Again, I am behaving in a way that promotes the idea that a goal of conversation can be mutual understanding not necessarily agreement.]

MARYANN: I've told you about 50 times: You don't live with you. You don't know what you're like. I do. I have to grow up with you. And I think I know when things were wrong.

KATHY: (*To Bonnie*) Are you interested in hearing from her point of view?

BONNIE: Sure.

KATHY: When ... so why don't you tell her straight out? You don't have to go like that (*Maryann has her head buried in her hands*), because she's ready to hear.

MARYANN: What am I supposed to tell her?

KATHY: You know—from your point of view, it didn't start getting better, your mom wasn't really not being in trouble, and it wasn't . . . it didn't stop being trouble for you until when?

MARYANN: I don't know. I don't think you stopped until a couple years ago, until yet met George [Bonnie's current boyfriend].

KATHY: Okay. So that's your reality, Maryann. That's your point of view.

BONNIE: Are we talking drugs?

MARYANN: Yeah. And alcohol. And all that stuff.

KATHY: (*To Bonnie*) Now, from your point of view, things were so much less . . .

BONNIE: Uh-huh . . .

KATHY: . . . starting when you got pregnant with Maryann that it's like . . .

BONNIE: She doesn't even know . . .

KATHY: She doesn't know what trouble was.

BONNIE: What trouble was (*laughs*).

KATHY: But that's . . . so that's a different comparison.

BONNIE: Right.

KATHY: Right? Okay. The comparison you can make that . . . what things used to be like and what they are now is like, that, this is—we're not even, we haven't even seen trouble. But from Maryann's point of view, she's saying, "Really, for me, it started to feel different 2 years ago. And up until then, things . . . I . . . things were hard for me because of the way you were using." (*To Maryann*) Am I saying . . . am I . . . putting your point of view out there in the right way?

MARYANN: Uh-huh.

KATHY: So you think that things started to look up with your mom at age 32. Have they started to look up for you? Are you still in trouble, or are you getting out of trouble now?

Maryann told me that she was trying to get out of trouble, but that it was hard. "I've . . . pretty much been sober for about a year. Well, I've had to be. It's not my choice, but I have to be." Tara said that she was trying to get out of her trouble, which was anger, but that this was hard as well. As Roberta told me that she was about 30 when she began breaking free of trouble, Tara interrupted.

TARA: No . . .

KATHY: What do you think?

TARA: You started at 28 . . .

ROBERTA: Well, 27 was when I got clean.

KATHY: Okay. I'm gonna try to . . . I'll go like this (*making a mark on the pad*). Twenty-seven to 30, kind of, was the start. Okay. Now that was 5 years ago. And this is when people started noticing that . . . that's the same thing. Did your mom start noticing, when she started getting clean, that you were in trouble? Is that sort of how it happened? [My marks on the paper lead me to notice a convergence of dates and ages.]

KATHY: (*Both Roberta and Tara nod their heads*). So you started noticing, but now we have these 5 years you've been noticing, Roberta. And Tara, you're still in trouble even though your mom's been on your case—been on it for 5 years. So that's something we're going to need to try and get . . .

TARA: Well, she hasn't really . . . she didn't really, like, still care or anything.

KATHY: So she noticed, but she didn't really care.

TARA: Yeah.

KATHY: Does she care now?

TARA: No.

KATHY: Okay. So here . . . that's a big thing I'm gonna . . . put here. (*I write the word "CARE" on the pad in big block letters.*) I'm gonna ask some pretty hard questions about this caring, although I want to find a little bit more about sisters and Mom here. But I'm just going to say something. I'm gonna . . . and I'm not going to check it out with anybody, yet, but . . . noticing when somebody is getting into trouble may not make a difference in helping them get out of trouble until the person who's in trouble feels like the . . . the grownup or the parent or somebody really, really cares, and really understands their experience. And that may be very different for the grownup, who may feel like they really care, and the child may feel like the grownup doesn't really care. And that may be one of the problems we have about people getting out of trouble, is that if you don't feel that somebody's really caring, you may not want to get yourself out of trouble. So we need to know a little bit about that for Bonnie and Roberta, with your sibs and with your moms, because I want to know who in your lives was noticing. So, Bonnie, do you have any siblings?

I was excited by what Tara said, and I dropped my usual way of conducting myself in an interview. I anticipated my own concern about what I was about to do when I said, "I'm not going to check it out with anybody, yet, but..." I believe now that I was observing myself slide from postmodern into modernist practice. To be consistent with postmodern practices, to create space for Tara's voice and not mine, I could have developed questions to amplify the significance of Tara's observation, rather than make a statement of my own. For instance, I could have asked, "What difference do you think feeling that someone cares would make? How can you tell when someone cares? Would caring be on trouble's team or another team? What would the name of the other team be?" Had I asked these questions, or others like them, I would have engaged the four women in the performance of their own thoughts about the effect of caring on their lives.

Not surprisingly, Tara's comment, and perhaps mine as well, created a sea change in the interview. The tone was quieter and more reflective. I asked Bonnie about her siblings, and they too had been visited by trouble. I then asked about her mother and learned that her mother died at age 38. I was taken aback.

KATHY: She was 38? [I'm putting this age on the board and drawing a diagonal line through the circle that represents her mother. This gesture fills me with sadness.] What did she die of?

BONNIE: Cancer.

KATHY: Wow. I'm really sorry about that. How old were you?

BONNIE: I was 14.

KATHY: Oh. Your trouble. [Writing the numbers on the board, I again notice the convergence of ages.] Hmm ... Had you thought your mom cared?

BONNIE: Uh-huh.

KATHY: And when she died, did it feel like no one cared any more? Was your dad looking?

BONNIE: My father was too drunk.

KATHY: Okay. So . . . there was a lot of trouble there.

BONNIE: Um . . .

KATHY: And he wasn't able to show he cared.

BONNIE: No.

KATHY: And you stopped feeling as if anybody cared, and you started using and got into trouble big time? Would it have been different if your mom had lived?

BONNIE: Yup. Very.

KATHY: I'm really sorry about that. Really sorry. [I pause and look directly at Bonnie. We are both near tears. Without being conscious of it, we are both showing care, the very subject we are discussing. Turning to Maryann, I pose a long hypothetical question to her.] So supposing that she did have you, Maryann, but she had never used. And her mother was alive and was still caring about Bonnie. And if Bonnie had been cared about and had been a young mother who'd been supported by her mother and wasn't using . . . wasn't doing drugs, would she have noticed? Would you have gotten to age 11 feeling depressed and suicidal?

MARYANN: Uh-huh.

KATHY: How come?

MARYANN: Because she married an asshole.

KATHY: Your dad is an asshole?

MARYANN: No, Peter is . . .

KATHY: Is Peter your bio-dad?

BONNIE: Annie's father.

KATHY: Annie's father. Okay. And so you've had trouble come from Peter. Does Peter live in the house?

MARYANN: No, not now.

KATHY: And is that something that the two of you have talked about . . . the kinds of . . . the kinds of ways that Peter was an asshole?

MARYANN: Uh-huh.

KATHY: And is that part of the work that happens in the residence, do you talk about that? Or you've talked to counselors about that? (*She nods.*) Okay. So that's another really important piece of it, which is that sometimes . . . stepfathers, and even fathers, can create terrible problems for girls. Really terrible problems. Now, we don't know anything about your dad, Tara. Has he created . . . is he part of the trouble for you?

I made the decision not to ask Maryann to give us details about what happened between her and Peter. From her nonverbal communication, I had the impression (later confirmed by others who knew) that she had been sexually abused by him. I didn't think that it was appropriate to ask Maryann to describe this in front of Tara and Roberta, who she didn't really know.

Tara told me that her father had been part of the trouble in her life, although she hadn't seen him for many years. He too abused alcohol and drugs.

KATHY: Have there been other men in your mom's life since your dad left that have caused trouble?

TARA: Uh . . . yes.

KATHY: What would we call them? Friends? Boyfriends?

TARA: Boyfriends.

KATHY: Okay. [I am writing the words "stepfathers/boyfriends" on the pad, and as I am writing I turn to Bonnie and say, "Well, we know you had problems with your father," at which point I add the word "father" to the list. Then I turn to Roberta.] What about you?

ROBERTA: Yeah. My, uh . . .

TARA: She didn't know her father.

ROBERTA: So I don't know who my father is, or . . . why he is, or . . . my stepfather, who, uh . . . I think died believing that I was his daughter, sexually abused me from age about 9 till about 17, so yeah, there was . . . and he was an alcoholic.

Again I was writing on the paper. I think we all saw simultaneously that Roberta's sexual abuse had begun the year she told us she first knew she was in trouble. I knew I was feeling a combination of outrage and compassion. I was also aware of the time remaining in the interview. I was softly tapping the pad of paper and telling people, "We need to get some ideas about what to do about all of this," gesturing with my hand across the entire pad.

KATHY: . . . I mean, I mean, I get—I sort of feel outraged about it. I don't want any of you to go on living with this. You know? It sucks. [This is not a planned show of feelings to model caring, but rather a spontaneous outburst that reveals my distress and concern. As it happens, I do think that it expresses caring in a way that Bonnie later describes in the interview. Tara indicates a wish to speak.] Yes?

TARA: We have, like . . . like when there are birthday parties . . . like, we, um, some of us, like, just sit down and talk about it and stuff, like what happened.

KATHY: Some of you in the family?

TARA: We've asked, like . . . sometimes we call my grandmother, but she don't want to talk about it.

KATHY: So that's one thing—getting sort of strong together by talking together about the hard times—*and*, I think you're saying something else, which is facing it. Not being in denial, but really looking at it, facing it. Okay. What other ideas? Anybody?

ROBERTA: Um . . . recovery.

KATHY: Recovery. Yeah. Right. It's awfully hard to get out of trouble if you're in trouble. And drugs and alcohol are trouble. What else besides recovery? Staying with it . . . (*I turn to Maryann, whose head is in her hands again.*) Maryann? Do you have any ideas?

MARYANN: Unh-unh.

KATHY: Are you out of it here? How come?

MARYANN: Because . . . I don't know . . .

KATHY: Does this whole thing leave you cold?

MARYANN: Uh-huh.

KATHY: So we're not . . . we're not talking in a way that's . . . um . . . does it make sense to you but it doesn't matter? (*Maryann nods.*) Okay. So we've got something that makes sense, but it doesn't matter. Do you think that your heart has stopped allowing you to let things matter?

MARYANN: Uh-huh.

KATHY: Is your heart cold?

MARYANN: What do you mean by that?

KATHY: Well, I mean as an image. You know, hearts that can feel are warm, as an image. And hearts that can't feel any more are cold. So I'm really asking you, is your heart cold?

MARYANN: No.

KATHY: Okay. (*I flip over the paper on which I have been drawing and draw a heart shape that fills the page.*) I'm going to draw a heart here. Can you just show me . . . would you do this? Show me how much of your heart can feel, and how much of your heart you have . . . you're keeping cold because it hurts too much. (*Maryann slowly leaves her seat, goes over to the pad of paper, and draws a line diagonally across the heart shape that I have drawn.*) Is that half? Or is it . . .

MARYANN: Not even half.

KATHY: Not even half. Which is the smaller half? Then . . . yeah. (*Points to the smaller segment*) But is it the feeling or not feeling?

MARYANN: (*Mumbling and in a very low voice*) Smaller.

KATHY: The smaller half is the feeling?

MARYANN: Uh-huh.

KATHY: So . . . we've been talking about trouble, but one of the other parts of the trouble has to do with recovering feeling. Because you're not going to be able to stay out of trouble—we'll do it this way (*using my arm, I make a sweeping gesture across the entire heart shape*)—until this is all feeling. Tara, that's true for you, too. I'm going to ask you to do the same thing, okay? I'm going to give you a heart, and you tell me . . . you draw, like Maryann did, how much of your heart is feeling, and how much of your heart is not feeling. And which side's which. (*Tara draws a diagonal across her heart and labels the larger segment "feeling."*) The smaller half is not feeling. Okay. Well, you're younger, and we really, really want the direction—you look up here, Tara—we want the direction to be moving . . . so that this is feeling.

This section evolved from my introducing the image of a heart to Maryann. I can't think of a single other time I have looked at a person and thought of his/her heart. Maryann was looking forlorn, and she was not participating, as Tara, Bonnie, and Roberta were, in talking about steps that could be taken to overcome the effects of trouble on their lives. I suspect that I was aware of my *own* "heart"—aware, perhaps, that my heartstrings were being pulled—and so I asked Maryann about *her* heart.

I didn't let Maryann's quiet demurrals rebuff my efforts to engage her. By continuing to ask her questions, I thought that I was communicating that I believed she wished to be in dialogue and that she did want things to matter. However, my embedded assertion that she was keeping her heart cold because it hurt too much was an assertion of "truth" in a situation in which I didn't know that to be so. By making this assertion—by dropping the stance of curiosity (Cecchin, 1987) and "not knowing" (Anderson & Goolishian, 1992)—I foreclosed (at least in that moment) learning why *Maryann* thought part of her heart was cold.

This first embedded assertion signaled a shift in paradigm. I had moved out of a postmodern paradigm into a modernist one. Watching the tape of the interview and remembering what I felt at the moment, I am now able to reconstruct why the shift took place. First, let me identify other signs. As I was looking at Maryann's delineation of the part of her heart that could not feel, I made a link that had not been made by anyone else: I imposed meaning, ironically engaging in an activity that I myself have written about as an example of a way that nonintimate interaction is produced (Weingarten, 1991, 1992). I asserted that until all of her heart could feel, she could not get out of trouble. Next, I informed Tara that the same was "true" for her. Finally, I made a "command" statement, the only one in the interview, requesting that Tara look in my direction.

All of these "moves" were modernist in this context, and they were based on two modernist tenets. First, I was using a psychological metaphor, locating the problem in Maryann (Dickerson & Zimmerman, 1995). Second, I was taking an expert position, implying that I had privileged access to expert knowledges about the nature of her problem.

I suspect that the reasons I moved from a postmodern to a modernist paradigm at this point in the interview are similar to the reasons it happens to me on other occasions. I knew I was nearing the end of our allotted time together, and I was silently reviewing whether or not I had "done enough." Critical self-evaluation told me that I had not—that I should have "done" more. Of course, there are many possible ways of interpreting "doing." I believe that in this moment I was influenced by the discourses of mothers and traditional psychotherapy (working in tandem) to conceptualize "doing" as doing *for* others. Thus, my attention was drawn to my ideas and to assessing whether or not they might have been useful. My attention was drawn away from what I could do to create a conversational context that would engage Maryann in a dialogue in which new meaning would develop as a "function of the relationship" and as a "byproduct of mutuality" (Anderson & Goolishian, 1992, p. 31).

My shift to a modernist paradigm, with its bias toward pathology and deficit-based models, also contributed to my not noticing an available resource for developing an alternative story line. Despite a portion of her heart's having no feeling, Maryann had managed to stay in recovery for 1 year. I could have asked her questions such as these: "How have you accomplished this? What does having accomplished this tell you about yourself? Are you aware of anything about yourself that might have predicted your ability to do this? What might others have noticed about you that would have led them to believe in this new development in your life?"

I then asked Tara and Maryann, "What may make the feeling part of your hearts grow bigger?" Neither girl answered, and there was a moment of silence. Bonnie spoke up.

BONNIE: I think it has to do with the care.

KATHY: You do?

BONNIE: Uh-huh.

KATHY: Tell me how.

BONNIE: I think if they feel that nobody cares, then that's where the not feeling comes in.

KATHY: But both of you moms, you're saying you do care . . .

BONNIE: Yeah, but they don't even feel . . .

KATHY: And they don't feel it?

BONNIE: Right.

KATHY: So that's really what we've got to work on, that they . . . that the residence is going to have to work on.

BONNIE: Right.

ROBERTA: I know for Tara, her attitude is "You don't care, why should I?"

TARA: Yeah.

ROBERTA: You know? And I do care, and part of my caring is having her in where she is, and she looks at that as I don't care. You know, quite the opposite of that . . .

TARA: You put me in one place and you don't go any place.

BONNIE: I think our way of caring . . . we, the mothers' way of caring is kind of almost a cold caring because of the way we were brought up.

ROBERTA: Right.

BONNIE: So even though we can sit here and say we care, but it may not be enough of a feeling for them because we don't even know how . . .

ROBERTA: Exactly.

BONNIE: . . . or what it feels like.

KATHY: All right. Okay. So, now, what would happen if you moms had a . . . either like a group of moms where you got to talk about how to have warm . . . how to be able to show warm caring when you didn't get enough warm caring yourselves . . . maybe that would be helpful as something to add into the treatment plan, here. So I'm going to put that up here as well. "Help moms to show warm caring." Okay. We're going to need to stop because I have until 12 and I need to talk with Tim and Cheryl, but this is something, you know, I do at the end of meetings, which is . . . Can you just sort of wrap your chairs around . . . ?

BONNIE: Okay.

KATHY: Um . . . the person who is holding this [a small Lucite cone]—it can be any object—what we do is we pass it around until nobody has anything more that they want to say. But the person who's holding it can say whatever she wants. And she can speak until she's finished and no one can interrupt her. Okay? [I am describing a variation on a reflecting method (Andersen, 1986, 1991) that I have used with Sallyann Roth in a number of teaching contexts, and also in a group of mothers and their daughters in which I was a participant. The object is used in a manner similar to the use of the "talking staff" (Roth, 1993). This change of format helps us shift to reflect on what has been said, what has not been said, what we are experiencing now, and what we can imagine for ourselves in the future.] So I'm going to start, and I'm going to say that I was really scared coming into this interview today, because I didn't know, you know, what you all were going to be like, and I know that I'm going to leave today feeling that this is one of the best experiences, clinically and meeting people, that I've ever had. And, um . . . (*My voice begins to waver; it sounds like—and it does—have tears in it; and then I am unable to speak for a few seconds.*) I feel like you've really taught me a lot, and I feel really . . . um . . . I feel really . . . both sad and touched, and I'm really glad you let me talk with you so honestly. Thanks.

ROBERTA: Um . . . I don't know. I . . . I'm willing to do anything to help me help Tara, help generations, whatever, and um . . . it's real hard to hear . . . to talk about it. It's real hard to, um . . . I try to stay real straight-faced, like it was no big deal and let it roll off my back, and it doesn't really feel that way. (*Roberta wipes a tear from her cheek.*) And sometimes I feel like I need to be that way for Tara. Um . . . I don't know. I just hope whatever she's got to go through turns out okay, you know? Because, like you're . . . like Cheryl said, my main concern is I don't want her life to be anywhere near mine.

Um . . . you know, not only with my pain and my using, but with my insecurity and my not liking myself, and you know, all that other stuff, too. But um . . . I don't know. It feels good to be here. I'm glad you guys shared with us, and, you know, I appreciate it. (*Roberta passes the object to Tara, who looks at it and slowly passes it to Bonnie.*)

BONNIE: Um . . . I think it was great to know that we're not alone. That there are other people out there that are going through a lot of similar things. That, um . . . and it's been an interesting year. It's been a year for us. And it's been an eye-opener to know what causes things to happen. And I agree with you, Roberta, that you don't want it to repeat. And whatever I can do so that that doesn't happen, um . . . and I think . . . I think this was great coming here, too. And doing this. And when you put it all down on a board and you can actually see it, um . . . you can see that I'm really not to blame. I mean, because all this time I have been blaming myself and saying, "Boy, I really screwed up." And now I know why I did. And, um . . . and that's been one of the hardest things for me to deal with, this past year, is that it's my fault. And, um . . . I may be able to make it a little easier for me to connect with Maryann. Knowing that our pasts aren't really that different. (*Bonnie passes the small Lucite cone to Maryann, who rubs it for a second or two and passes it to me. I pass it along to Roberta, and it travels among the five of us, in silence, until I place it on the floor.*)

KATHY: Thanks, guys. [We are clearly not "guys," but it is the word Roberta used, and the word that feels congruent to me at the moment.]

In the last 4 minutes of the interview, the reflecting format did promote a different kind of speaking and listening. Maryann and Tara did not speak, but it seemed to me then, as it does now, that their listening was keen. What is important to know, and what I cannot know for sure, is whether their not speaking represented a silencing of their voices or a preference for witnessing their mothers' voices and, perhaps, mine. The distinction is a critical one. The silencing of voice is usually an expression of marginalization, whereas witnessing—in silence or in words—is another form of participation (Ross, 1996). I would regret the former and celebrate the latter.

Bonnie, Roberta, and I reflected by speaking on the effect of the interview as a whole on us. I talked about and showed my feelings. By doing so, I was continuing to offer myself as a person who was making her concentrated presence available. I was showing that I placed value on "warm care"—a phrase that now, 4 years later, still circulates in my everyday awareness. From a postmodern narrative perspective, the intention behind—or the epistemological stance that informs—showing one's feelings is also an important distinction to draw (Griffith & Griffith, 1992). I hope that my self-disclosure served the purpose of what David Epston has named "transparency" (White, 1991). As Freeman and Lobovits (1993) write:

> Traditional concepts of self-disclosure, in the authors' view, involve revealing personal information in the hope of either increasing the client's identification with the therapist or providing some kind of model for the client on how to live his or her life. The purpose of transparency is to deconstruct that aspect of the therapeutic hierarchy that is based on unrevealed expert ideas about what is best for the client.

I was letting the four women know that their stories had affected me and that I was grateful to have taken part in the conversation in which these stories were told. Four years later, I can say that their words continue to have resonance for me and that I hear their voices in my work with other mothers and daughters.

Roberta and Bonnie both spoke about the effects of the interview on them. Roberta, uncharacteristically, cried. Perhaps the interview had deconstructed the meaning of "staying straight-faced" and allowed Roberta to question whether she needed to act as if everything rolled off her back to be helpful to Tara. By crying, she might have been showing that some aspects of their life story were a big enough deal to shed tears over—and a big enough deal for her to invest time and energy to stop another generation from feeling "insecure" and "not liking themselves."

Bonnie had learned that she was "not to blame." She told us that the hardest part of the year for her had been to feel that Maryann's problems were her fault. The board's graphic display of "reasons" released Bonnie both from the immobilizing clutches of blame and from the constraining belief that she and Maryann were different. She speculated that she might now be better able to connect with Maryann.

Follow-Up

At the time, these "outcomes" seemed impressive to me. Tim and Cheryl, the director and social worker at the residence, were very pleased with the information and felt that they would go back to work with clear next steps to take. Three months later I got a call from Tim, providing a follow-up. Using the information he provided in our conversation, I decided to write Roberta and Bonnie a letter. I am including the letter that I wrote, annotated with the changes that I would make now. The letter chronicles and reflects on some of the events that have taken place in the four women's lives.

My letter was warm and sincere. I also again, at times, authorized myself to tell rather than ask and to pronounce rather than to consult. Given my commitment to postmodern ideas, my extensive exposure to them, and the fact that I teach them, I must conclude that the pulls toward modernist practices are powerful; that there are pervasive incentives to hold an expert rather than a co-authoring stance; and that the reinforcements for operating with professional expert knowledges are omnipresent and compelling.

January 27, 1994

Dear Bonnie and Roberta:

I spoke with Tim a couple of nights ago, and he brought me up to date about some of the recent events of your lives and the work that you are both doing alone and in the group. I was really touched that you asked Tim to keep me posted. I know that I am carrying with me my connection to each of you, to your daughters, and to your relationships with each other. So I was pleased to learn that you also think about me and our conversation.

First, let me tell you how pleased I am that you have started a parents'/mothers' group. It takes time, commitment, and courage to do that. It is [Is it] part of the work of resisting what has been in favor of what can be.[?] It is [Is it also] about daring to hope.[?] [If so,] I would like to join my hopes with yours.

Next, Tim told me that Maryann had revealed, and been willing to follow through on, her experience of being sexually abused by her pediatrician this August. I feel a combination of grief and outrage on her behalf, and also admiration that she was able to talk about it and hold him accountable. In this way, she begins the process of healing not just for herself but for others. [Do you think that speaking out is part of Maryann's healing process? If Maryann speaks out, will this help others?]

Bonnie, I understand from Tim that this has been very hard for you. There is so much we have to learn about mothers' experiences when their children have been sexually abused. I'm sure [Do you think] that as you speak about your experience, you will help many others become clearer about the kinds of feelings that mothers of victims [young persons who have been abused] feel and the kinds of support that are helpful.[?]

Roberta, Tim said that Maryann's abuse has made you recall your own incest experience and that this may become an opportunity for you to work with your experiences in a different way, perhaps by supporting Bonnie. Incest—abuse— is so damaging, and yet there are moments when something we have experienced can be helpful to someone else. I hope that on balance, Roberta, you find that talking with Bonnie is more healing than hurtful to you. I think that you were brave to offer help. [Do you think that, on balance, talking to Bonnie will be more helpful or hurtful to you? What do you think that you were drawing on to offer help? What does this tell you about yourself?]

Tim also told me specific points that you wanted him to convey to me. Of course, I would be honored to meet with you again, whenever you decide the time is right, and in whatever grouping you think makes sense. Tim said that you felt less blamed; that your interactions with your daughters feel more open; and that they seem more genuine in their expressions of feeling. I wonder whether they were moved by how genuine you each were during the interview—whether your courage in sharing your own histories so authentically paved the way for their genuineness?

Tim told me that you had said that the interview helped you know "stuff we knew but didn't know we knew." Wow! That was so exciting for me to hear. That really says in a nutshell what I most value in a therapeutic process. I am really grateful to both of you that we worked together so that this could happen for us all. The interview made me feel more confident about the value of mothers' sharing themselves with their daughters. I practice this in my own life, but your feedback makes me feel stronger about taking that position publicly. I thank you for that.

Finally, I am really excited about the power that we as mothers can feel in our lives when we join with each other to know ourselves so that we can help our daughters to know themselves.

Yours in the power of shared/sharing experience,

Kathy

As noted in the letter, with the help of people at the residence, Bonnie and Roberta started a parents'/mothers' group. I know from Tim that the group continues to meet; thus, they created institutional change. Maryann, Bonnie, Tara, and Roberta continued to make significant gains in their relationships. In the summer of 1995, I visited the parents' group and spoke to five women, Bonnie and Roberta among them, about their experiences in talking to their teenagers about love and sex. Bonnie reported that she and Maryann were close, and that now that she was (at last) in a loving relationship, Maryann was talking with her about how she accomplished this because she wanted a loving, safe relationship for herself. Roberta also reported a close relationship with Tara; in fact, she told us she could only stay for part of our meeting, because she had promised Tara she would watch a videotape with her that evening. About an hour into our conversation, Roberta was beeped. She returned from the phone with a big smile on her face: "Tara called just to tell me she loves me."

CONCLUSION

In this chapter, I have annotated this edited transcript of a first consultation interview in three ways to demonstrate the three primary ways that I work with adolescents. The first type of annotation shows challenges to dominant discourses regarding mothers and adolescent daughters. The second type of annotation shows a close attention to words and silences. The third type of annotation shows my effort to make the work consistent with a postmodern narrative practice.

There is another way that I have tried to make this work consistent with a postmodern practice, and that is in the construction of the chapter itself. Typically authors present examples of cutting-edge work—often interviews that elegantly illustrate their approach to clinical work. This tactic, I believe, functions like a dominant discourse about how to do professional writing and presenting. In this chapter, I have attempted to resist this dominant discourse, seeing it as yet another location in which modernist rather than postmodern practices can take hold. I have preferred instead to position myself in relation to the reader with evolving rather than expert knowledges. In doing so, I hope that I contribute to the "flattening" of the hierarchies among those who teach, write about, practice, read about, and engage in therapy (Freedman & Combs, 1996; Madigan, 1993).

Reflecting back on work that I did 4 years ago, I am gratified that I no longer find the work congruent. This tells me that I am continuing to evolve as a therapist. My professional life is filled with daily struggles to bring my work into line with my beliefs, commitments, and intentions. It is this struggle that makes me feel empathically connected to the adolescents and their parents whom I see. It is also the struggle that I wish to share and from which I hope readers will find something to learn.

EDITORIAL QUESTIONS

Q: *(CS) I was taken by your courage as a seasoned therapist—as I was in your book* The Mother's Voice *(Weingarten, 1997)—to be so open with the reader about your own struggles with what you said or didn't say with these families. I think we all have these doubts, but your contribution invites us to let down our professional guard and take a reflective view toward our own work.*

As I read your chapter, I found myself oriented toward your productive, task-oriented discussion of how the teens and parents stayed out of "trouble." I was also thinking of the two residential staff members sitting behind the mirror watching you work, and thinking of the pressure I might feel in a similar context to "stand and deliver"—to make sure, as you say, that I have "done enough," particularly in regard to the presenting concerns. I think that this pressure is even more likely in a one-time consultation with an outside agency.

I was struck as well by your mention that your goal was to "create a conversational context" for dialogue to occur. Your transcript also demonstrates to me that you accomplished this. But what I struggle with are those moments where this conversational context and dialogue may not show a direct or apparent connection to the presenting concern. You speak at one point of shared meaning making promoting intimacy. Are there times when you orient yourself more exclusively toward this intimacy, toward whatever the clients wish to dialogue with each other about, and other times where you become more focused on particular themes/problems (e.g., "trouble") and particular solutions to these problems? If we become focused on particular themes rather than on creating dialogue wherever this goes, how do we know when this is "doing for others," and how do we know when this is justified? How do you sort out when you wish to help clients critique particular themes or stories, and when you are oriented to increase understanding, dialogue, and intimacy between participants?

A: In both my personal and my professional life, I have been enormously helped by the idea of discourse. As I have written previously, understanding the ways in which prevailing discourses of mothers, adolescents, and mother–adolescent relationships affected my family allowed me to make radical changes in our family life that I believe have stood us all in good stead (Weingarten, 1997). These changes have promoted greater intimacy and more dialogue among us.

In your question, there are several embedded dichotomies that I wish to comment on: theme versus dialogue; a focus on problems versus a focus on promoting intimacy; and critiquing discourse versus increasing understanding, dialogue, and intimacy. In my personal and clinical experience, I don't find that I have to choose between doing the one or the other; there is a flow or criss-crossing between all of these conversational possibilities.

For instance, I try to conduct an interview in such a way that the process of critiquing discourse does not happen in an academic or abstract way. I believe that in this interview, Bonnie deconstructed negative premises that are associated with a discourse of mothers. At the end of the interview, she said that she knew now "that I'm really not to blame. I mean, because all this time I have been blaming myself and saying, 'Boy, I really screwed up.' And now I know why I did. And, um . . . and that's been one of the hardest things for me to deal with, this past year, is that it's my fault. And, um . . . I may be able to make it a little easier for me to connect with Maryann."

I believe that Bonnie was now able to "see through" the discourse of mothers that would label her a bad mother. She had come to understand that the perspective from which she could be judged "bad" is one that would strip away the contexts of her life and fail to include her own subjective experience. In addition, the discourse of mothers that would produce Bonnie as the person who could be blamed for the troubles experienced by her daughter is one that also holds mothers ultimately responsible for the actions of their children. This discourse arose at the same time that mothers were "given" exclusive responsibility for child care—a feature of North American family life that developed in the late 19th century, in response to changing economic and social conditions (Weingarten, 1997, in press). The residential staff's interest in working collaboratively with these two families undermined the proposition that mothers should be solely responsible for their children.

As I was participating in the interview, I was challenging several assumptions that are embedded in multiple discourses. For instance, the discourse of adolescents promotes the idea that mothers should back off when their children are teens. By encouraging the mothers as well as the daughters to share their life experiences, I was challenging this assumption. Another assumption that I was challenging is that adolescents do not care if their parents understand them or not. By acting according to the idea that most people want to feel understood, I behaved in a way that "naturalized" this possibility.

I believe that in interviews such as this one, by acting from assumptions that challenge dominant discourses of mothers and adolescents, I am creating opportunities for understanding, problem solving, and dialogue to take place. Likewise, I believe that with more dialogue, more moments of intimate interaction are likely to occur (Weingarten, 1992). From this point of view, no dichotomies exist; each conversational practice enhances every other. The work thus feels all of a piece.

Q: *(CS) Were the two residential staff members included in the reflections, or were they to remain in the observing position for the remainder of the session? What was your thinking about including or not including them in the final reflections?*
A: The two residential staff members returned to the interview room, and there was a brief conversation with them. They commented particularly on the ways they could help the mothers and their daughters follow through on initiatives that were mentioned in the interview. The director, Tim Nichols, indicated that he would get in touch with me in a few weeks, and he did do that. Little did he or I guess that we would stay involved in relation to these mothers and their daughters for many years.

Q: *(CS) At various points, you refer to the marks you made on the pad as the mothers and daughters were responding. At one point you state, "The paper itself was now telling a story." Could you elaborate on this? What were you hoping for in using this pad? Was this more for you, them, or both? Does the use of this pad relate at all to the thematic versus dialogic focus in my first question?*
A: I mean that "The paper itself was now telling a story" in a literal sense: Just as a genogram tells a story, so too did the markings on this paper. I was not drawing a formal genogram, but rather diagramming, or rendering in a mutually agreed-upon code, the information about their families and events in their lives that the four women provided. As I made notations, patterns were revealed. We all noted coincidences (e.g., the relationship of Bonnie's trouble to her mother's death; the relationship between the trouble in Roberta's life and her stepfather's sexual abuse of her).

The paper became a "player" in the conversation. The mothers and Tara were gesticulating toward the paper throughout the interview. I had the experience of hearing what the women were saying, registering it on the paper, and then seeing what "connection" jumped out at me or them. Writing on the pad was part of the gestalt of this particular conversation, and as such it contributed to the creation of new awareness and to possibilities for new understanding and interaction.

REFERENCES

Andersen, T. (1986). The reflecting team: Dialogue and metadialogue in clinical work. *Family Process, 26,* 415–428.
Andersen, T. (1991). Guidelines for practice. In T. Andersen (Ed.), *The reflecting team: Dialogues and dialogues about dialogues.* New York: Norton.

Anderson, H., & Goolishian, H. (1992). The client is the expert: A not-knowing approach to therapy. In S. McNamee & K. J. Gergen (Eds.), *Therapy as social construction*. Newbury Park, CA: Sage.

Bly, R. (1990). *Iron John: A book about men*. Reading, MA: Addison-Wesley.

Bruner, J. (1990). *Acts of meaning*. Cambridge, MA: Harvard University Press.

Caplan, P. (1989). *Don't blame mother: Mending the mother–daughter relationship*. New York: HarperCollins.

Cecchin, G. (1987). Hypothesizing, circularity, and neutrality revisited: An invitation to curiosity. *Family Process, 26,* 405–413.

Dickerson, V. C., & Zimmerman, J. L. (1992). Families with adolescents: Escaping problem lifestyles. *Family Process, 31,* 341–353.

Dickerson, V. C., & Zimmerman, J. L. (1993). A narrative approach to families with adolescents. In S. Friedman (Ed.), *The new language of change: Constructive collaboration in psychotherapy*. New York: Guilford Press.

Dickerson, V. C., & Zimmerman, J. L. (1995). A constructionist exercise in anti-pathologizing. *Journal of Systemic Therapies, 14,* 33–45.

Dickerson, V. C., & Zimmerman, J. L. (1996). Myth, misconceptions, and a word or two about politics. *Journal of Systemic Therapies, 15,* 79–88.

Freedman, J., & Combs, G. (1996). *Narrative therapy: The social construction of preferred realities*. New York: Norton.

Freeman, J. C., & Lobovits, D. (1993). The turtle with wings. In S. Friedman (Ed.), *The new language of change: Constructive collaboration in psychotherapy*. New York: Guilford Press.

Gergen, K. J. (1991). *The saturated self: Dilemmas of identity in contemporary life*. New York: Basic Books.

Gergen, K. J., & Kaye, J. (1992). Beyond narrative in the negotiation of therapeutic meaning. In S. McNamee & K. J. Gergen (Eds.), *Therapy as social construction*. Newbury Park, CA: Sage.

Gilligan, C., Rogers, A. G., & Tolman, D. L. (Eds.). (1991). *Women, girls, and psychotherapy: Reframing resistance*. New York: Haworth Press.

Griffith, J., & Griffith, M. (1992). Owning one's epistemological stance in therapy. *Dulwich Centre Newsletter,* No. 1, 5–11.

Hare-Mustin, R. (1994). Discourses in the mirrored room: A postmodern analysis of therapy. *Family Process, 33,* 19–35.

Jordan, J. V., Kaplan, A. G., Miller, J. B., Stiver, I. P., & Surrey, J. L. (1991). *Women's growth in connection*. New York: Guilford Press.

Lax, W. D. (1992). Postmodern thinking in clinical practice. In S. McNamee & K. J. Gergen (Eds.), *Therapy as social construction*. Newbury Park, CA: Sage.

Lazarre, J. (1991). *Worlds beyond my control*. New York: Dutton.

Madigan, S. P. (1993). Questions about questions: Situating the therapist's curiosity in front of the family. In S. Gilligan & R. Price (Eds.), *Therapeutic conversations*. New York: Norton.

Madigan, S. P. (1996). The politics of identity: Considering community discourse in the externalizing of internalized problem conversations. *Journal of Systemic Therapies, 15,* 47–62.

Nichols, T., & Jacques, C. (1995). Family reunions: Communities celebrate new possibilities. In S. Friedman (Ed.), *The reflecting team in action: Collaborative practice in family therapy*. New York: Guilford Press.

Penn, P., & Frankfurt, M. (1994). Creating a participant text: Writing, multiple voices, narrative multiplicity. *Family Process, 33*, 217–231.

Ross, V. (1996, March 16). Witnessing.mftc-L@MAELSTROM.STJOHNS. EDU

Roth, S. (1993). Speaking the unspoken: A work-group consultation to re-open dialogue. In E. Imber-Black (Ed.), *Secrets in families and family therapy*. New York: Norton.

Roth, S., & Epston, D. (1996). Consulting the problem about the problematic relationship: An exercise for experiencing a relationship with an externalized problem. In M. F. Hoyt (Ed.), *Constructive therapies* (Vol. 2). New York: Guilford Press.

Sampson, E. E. (1993). *Celebrating the other: A dialogic account of human nature*. Boulder, CO: Westview Press.

Scott, J. W. (1990). Deconstructing equality-versus-difference: Or, the uses of poststructuralist theory for feminism. In M. Hirsch & E. F. Keller (Eds.), *Conflicts in feminism*. New York: Routledge.

Stacey, K., & Loptson, C. (1995). Children should be seen and not heard: Questioning the unquestioned. *Journal of Systemic Therapies, 14*(4), 16–32.

Steinberg, L., & Levine, A. (1990). *You and your adolescent: A parent's guide for ages 10–20*. New York: HarperCollins.

Tomm, K. (1992). Therapeutic distinctions in an on-going therapy. In S. McNamee & K. J. Gergen (Eds.), *Therapy as social construction*. Newbury Park, CA: Sage.

Weingarten, K. (1991). The discourses of intimacy: Adding a social constructionist and feminist view. *Family Process, 31*, 285–305.

Weingarten, K. (1992). A consideration of intimate and non-intimate interactions in therapy. *Family Process, 31*, 45–59.

Weingarten, K. (Ed.). (1995). *Cultural resistance: Challenging beliefs about men, women, and therapy*. New York: Haworth Press.

Weingarten, K. (1997). *The mother's voice: Strengthening intimacy in families*. New York: Guilford Press.

Weingarten, K. (in press). Sidelined no more: Promoting mothers of adolescents as a resource for their growth and development. In C. Garcia Coll, J. Surrey, & K. Weingarten (Eds.), *Mothering at the margins: Voices of resistance*. New York: Guilford Press.

White, M. (1988–1989). The externalizing of the problem and the re-authoring of lives and relationships. *Dulwich Centre Newsletter*, No. 2, 3–30.

White, M. (1991). Deconstruction and therapy. *Dulwich Centre Newsletter*, No. 3, 21–40.

White, M. (1995). *Re-authoring lives: Interviews and essays*. Adelaide, South Australia: Dulwich Centre Publications.

Zimmerman, J. L., & Dickerson, V. C. (1994). Using a narrative metaphor: Implications for theory and clinical practice. *Family Process, 33*, 233–245.

13

Re-Considering Memory
RE-REMEMBERING LOST
IDENTITIES BACK TOWARD
RE-MEMBERED SELVES

STEPHEN MADIGAN
WITH COMMENTARY BY LORRAINE GRIEVES

The self is an act of grace, a gift of the other.
—BAKHTIN (1986, p. 4)

On a recent family trip to Ireland, my 5-year-old nephew, Frankie, asked me to help him find his lost soccer ball. Taking his request on as a serious matter, I proceeded with the following questions: "Did you leave the ball on the beach? Is the ball at the back of the house? Did you leave the ball in Grandad's room?" At this last query he jumped up with excitement, and together we made trails toward my father's room. To our great relief, we found the soccer ball resting on the night table.

The soccer ball's rediscovery was of great comfort to Frankie, and it left me to question who it was that could claim responsibility for this act of memory. Was it Frankie's remembering? Was it a memory that came from inside of me? Did it somehow involve a joint action of re-membering between the two of us? I wondered where to locate this act of remembering.

REMEMBERING MEMORY

Throughout my familial, religious, and academic training, I was consistently taught that *my* memories were *my* own. If I forgot a thought, it was merely a matter of thinking "hard" enough, and I could remember anything; it was all a matter of willpower. My experience with Frankie has moved me toward a reconsideration of how memory is constructed.

To cerebrate the act of the soccer ball's rescue from a social constructionist, poststructural, or postmodern framework invites a re-evaluation of Western psychology's central tenet that memory is a personal act (Hoagwood, 1993). The infrastructure this psychological tenet rests upon is of the Enlightenment project, and situated within ideas of absolute truths, linear progress, and the expert planning of ideal social orders.

Within psychology's conceptual domain, memory is contained within the individual and is his/her responsibility. From this vantage point, memory is treasured, tortured, mystified, and privately owned by the individual citizen. Supporting this particular knowledged view of memory are specific sets of relationship practices, be they therapeutic, political, or religious. The practice sets are what have acted to hold, support, honor, and obey this modernist belief of memory over time.

Psychological practices stationed within a privatized idea of memory are being challenged on many postmodern fronts. For example, social psychologist Edward Sampson (1993) suggests that memory is not the sole right and creative property of an individual, as psychological science would have us believe. He claims that memory can be viewed as socially constructed and jointly shared within the embedding discourse.

Sampson (1993) believes it necessary for mental health practitioners to "disabuse" the idea that remembering is simply and entirely a matter of calling forth a "stored trace located somewhere in the mind of the individual" (pp. 128–129). Congruent with Shotter's (1990) and Billig's (1990) earlier work in the area of the social construction of memory, Sampson writes that when we remember something, "we are not calling up a trace laid down somewhere in our inner computer banks; rather, we are engaged in a process of constructing an event in a current situation" (p. 131). It is within the specifics of a consensual (and not necessarily agreeable) social conversational process that memories are "jointly constructed" (Billig, 1990) and recalled.

Bakhtin writes that "neither individuals nor any other social entities are locked within their boundaries . . . a person has no sovereign internal territory" (p. 83). From this perspective, memory is situated within a dialogic context and *not* placed under individual sovereignty. Billig (1990) endorses the notion that the social process in which memories are recollected is frequently in the form of a dialogue, where participants collectively construct "the positions for and against the topics of which they are talking" (p. 69). Middleton and Edwards (1990) suggest that memory is a "collective remembering," since remembering and forgetting are inherently social activities.

These alternative positions have led me to speculate that the found soccer ball was not a matter of Frankie's bringing forth a "shy thought" from a long and forgotten part of his "memory bank." The memory of the soccer ball's lost location can be considered within a domain of collaborative, participatory remembering, co-constructed by Frankie and myself. The soccer ball's recovery can be viewed as a joint remembrance *through* Frankie, myself, and the embedding relational discursive context.

My experience with Frankie and the rediscovered ball has led me to ponder other questions and other contexts of influence regarding memory. For example, I have been considering the many different memories of who I might be as a person, which seem to shift and change depending on the given situational context. If, for example, I were to compare lying down on an analyst's couch with lying down on a friend's couch, I would predict that memories would be constructed differently according to the context. All that influences the discursive particulars of these contexts; all of everything the analyst, the friend, and myself bring to the contexts of our past, present, and ideas of the future; and all that influences our locations in culture, class, gender, race, sexual preference, age, and so on—all these elements would have some bearing on our co-construction of, and meaning given to, memory.

How I perceive the contexts of either analysis and friendship, and how the contexts perform the culture in these contexts, would be shaping of what I may or may not remember and/or forget about my self(s). Memory may not be as simple and as straightforward as the structural humanists have led us to believe. Remembering may not be just a matter of memory coming back *up* from the depths of a skin-bound self. "The" memory we speak of may not be a singular noun or a particular isolated thing at all, but rather a part of a relationship action embedded in and negotiated through cultural discourse.[1] The subject site of psychology's interest would maneuver toward discussing how and through what means memories are internalized, and discerning how and through which cultural discourses specific and preferred memories are brought forth and maintained.

When memory and the act of remembering are situated within cultural discourse, the domain of possible remembering is vast and is di-

[1]Discourse can be viewed as what can be said, who can say it, and with what authority.

rectly influenced and restrained by the discursive "perspective." Who, what, where, how, and why memories are remembered are directly figured through the influence of the other. What and how we remember through a cultural discourse begins to call into question many essentialist memory notions, such as denial, transcendence, and transference.

From one conversational context to the next, the particular self one may or may not remember or forget is greatly affected by the dialogic situation. In the next section, I explore the discursive relationship between the memories of who our identities are and the context both memories and identities are negotiated and maintained within.

RENEGOTIATING PROBLEMS AND IDENTITIES

Foucault (1982, 1989) maintains that the conversational domain through which we come to know our many selves is dictated by fields of power and discourse that command what is allowed to be said, who gets to say it, and with what authority (Law & Madigan, 1994). What we do remember about our selves is negotiated and distributed through a complex web of the community's most dominant (and agreed-upon) discourse (Madigan, 1996).

"Identity," says feminist Jill Johnson (1973, p. 18), "is what you can say you are, according to what they say you can be." Identities, like memories, are not freely created products of introspection or the unproblematic reflections of a private inner self. They are conceived within certain ideological frameworks constructed by the dominant social order to maintain its interests. Identities are negotiated and distributed.

Identities and memories, and our remembrances of our identities, are profoundly political, both in their origins and in their implications. For example, a remembrance of a night "on the drink" might evoke memories of shame, of cultural tradition, or of "reverie," depending on the context. Our distributed selves and the selves we normally remember is influenced by and reproductive of cultural and institutional norms. As contributing members of this community of discourse, we experience ourselves within the relational politics of these dominant norms.

NARRATIVE IDEAS AND THERAPEUTIC PRACTICE

Through a translation of Foucault's (1982) ideas on the insurrection of alternative versions of who we might be as persons (Madigan, 1992)— versions that live outside the dominant discursive norm that dictates who should be—therapists David Epston and Michael White have translated the idea of multiple other remembrances of self into a therapy practice guided by a narrative metaphor (White & Epston, 1990). Of central importance to Epston, White, and others who practice narrative therapy is the bringing forth of re-remembered alternative selves that are experienced outside the realm of a specified problem identity. The so-called problem identity is not considered a fixed "state," nor is it located within the person. The problem identity is viewed within a context of intricate negotiations that take place inside complex fields of power and discourse.

The consequences of a culturally biased commerce of problems regularly finds a person's constructed identity very misrepresented and underknown by dominant-knowledged sets of "thin conclusions" (M. White, personal communication, October 1995). Both the process of pathologizing and the technologies imported to implement the discourse of pathology speak volumes about the dominant signifying mental health culture, but little of the person being pathologized (Caplan, 1995).

A narrative therapeutic interview is concerned with (1) how the "known" and remembered problem identity of a person has been manufactured over time; (2) what aspects of the social order have assisted in the ongoing maintenance of this remembered problem self; (3) which cultural apparatuses keep this remembered self restrained from remembering alternative accounts and experiences of lived experience; (4) how the person can begin to re-remember alternative identities of self that live outside the problem's version; (5) how dialogical space can be created to "stand up for" the performance of this re-remembered and preferred self; and (6) who else in the person's life might be engaged to offer accounts of re-remembrance and provide the person safety in membership.

Problems, identities, and what information a person remembers are constitutive (White, 1995) and are constructed through an intricate dialogic interchange of power and community discourse (Madigan, 1996). For practitioners introducing narrative ideas into therapy, change occurs through recognizing and locating persons, memories, and problems within the dominant norms of the social domain. This, of course, runs contrary to the last 100 years of psychological thought.

Persons entering into these re-remembering conversations are offered opportunities for alternative and reclaimed remembrances of who they are, who they have been, who they would prefer to be, and who they might be in a possible future. The person who has been wrongly totalized, personified, and misrepresented within a problem's type, diagnosis, or pathology enters into a substitute dialogic context. Entering into the performance of an alternative re-remembering conversation is constitutive of lives and relationships (White, 1995).

RE-REMEMBERING

A personal act of re-remembering that has inspired me to ponder the power, context, and constitutive performance of remembering was on the occasion of my mother's death in November 1992. It was a time of immense grief. In the 6 months leading up to her death, I felt completely filled up with fear, sadness, anger, and confusion. It became more and more difficult for me to re-remember my mother as she was prior to the onset of the cancer that eventually killed her. I had lost my ability to locate our relationship historically. My healthy view of her was temporarily and temporally forgotten.

Along with the copious amounts of food and drink that arrived at our home during the time of my mother's wake, numerous letters and "Mass cards" began to show up. Cards and letters were sent to my family from my mother and father's neighborhood friends and work associates. Notes of remembrance poured in from my own and my sister's friends. Each person wrote to recall a specific story of their relationship to my mom. They outlined the wonderful ways in which she had affected their lives, and they constructed and accounted for a variety of particular pasts, presents, and futures. My mom's letter writers shared our grief and recalled volumes of great stories.

These letters of re-collection summoned a series of collective "other" remembrances. The letters assisted me in the reconstruction of other memories of who my mother was through time (past, present, *and* possible futures). Within this dialogic context, it remained possible to reclaim the multiple versions of who my mother was as a person, beyond the story of loss and death I was immersed in.

It was through the re-remembering experience of my mother in my own life that the idea of therapeutic letter-writing campaigns first emerged in my therapy work (Madigan & Epston, 1995). Since her death, I have instigated numerous letter campaigns designed to recall the alternative other in persons struggling with a problem's restrained and oppressive description of them, and the institutionalized discourse that supports these negative descriptions.

RE-MEMBERING THROUGH LETTER-WRITING CAMPAIGNS

Over the last few years, I have worked at patching together the ideas of memory as a social phenomenon (co-constructed during the search for young Frankie's soccer ball), the powerful effect of re-remembering alternative accounts of persons through letter writing (through the funeral Mass cards sent to my mom), viewing discourse within an analysis of power and knowledge (Foucault, 1980) and separating problem identities from person identities (White & Epston, 1990).

What allows the above practices a sense of cohesion is situated in my experience of working and learning alongside my colleague David Epston (1989), who does beautifully novel and well-documented work with therapeutic practices of the written word. Together, all of these ideas and experiences form the ideological base for what have become known as "therapeutic letter-writing campaigns" (Madigan & Epston, 1995).

Therapeutic letter-writing campaigns assist people to *re-remember* lost aspects of themselves. The campaigns assist persons to be *re-membered* back toward membership systems of love and support from which the problem has *dis-membered* them.[2] Letter-writing campaigns have been designed for persons as young as 6 and as old as 76. They have assisted persons struggling with an assortment of difficulties, including anxiety, bulimia, depression, perfection, and fear. The campaigns create a context where it becomes possible for people struggling with problems to bring themselves back from the depths of total isolation, and from acts of self-harm and suicide attempts (Madigan & Epston, 1995). Persons receiving letters[3] rediscover a discourse of the self that assists them to re-member back into situations from which the problem has most often dis-membered them. These include claiming former membership associations with intimate relationships, school, sports, careers, and family members, and reacquainting themselves with aspects of themselves once restrained by the problem identity.

Over the years, I have encouraged massive international writing campaigns that net literally hundreds of responses, and have had equally successful three-person problem blockades. Over this time, letters of support have arrived from some very curious authors. For example, family dogs, teddy bears, cars, dead grandparents, unborn siblings, and movie stars are among the variety of encouraging campaign contributors. (See "Campaign Contributors," below.)

Letter-writing efforts can take on a variety of shapes and forms, but the most standard campaigns involve the following:

1. The campaign emerges from a narrative interview when alternative accounts of who the person might be are questioned, revived, and

[2]See Barbara Myheroff (1982). I would like to acknowledge personal communications with Michael White, Imelda McCarthy, and Nollaig Byrne on the subjects of re-membering and dis-memberment.

[3]Campaign contributors also include pictures, collages, audiotapes, videotapes, and poems.

re-membered. The person is also asked to consider whether there are other people in her/his life who may regard the person differently from how the problem describes her/him. These different accounts are then spoken of. I might ask the following questions: "If I were to interview _____ about you, what do you think they might tell me about yourself that the problem would not dare to tell me?" Or "do you think your friend's telling of you to me about you would be an accurate telling, even if it contradicted the problem's tellings of you?" Or "Whose description of you do you prefer, and why?"

2. Together, the client and myself (along with the client's family/partner, friend, therapist, etc., if any of these are in attendance) begin a conversation regarding all the possible other descriptions of the client as a person that she/he might be but has forgotten to remember because of the problem's hold over her/him (as I have outlined above in "Narrative Ideas and Therapeutic Practice"). We dialogue on who the client might be, who the client would like to be, and who the client used to be well before the problem took over her/his life. We recall the alternative lived experiences of herself/himself that the client has forgotten through the problem's restraining context.

3. We then begin to make a list of all the persons in the client's life who would be in support of those alternate descriptions. Once the list is complete, we construct a letter of support and invitation (see Madigan & Epston, 1995).

4. If finances are a problem, I supply the envelopes and stamps for the ensuing campaign.

5. If privacy is an issue, we use Yaletown Family Therapy as the return address.

6. The client is asked to bring the letters into the therapy session and to read them aloud. (Sometimes a letter writer is invited into the session to recite a letter in person and to act as a witness to his/her own letter and the letters written by others.)

7. I will offer to read the letters back to the client and/or the letter writer, so that either or both may experience a textual re-telling of these written accounts (other support persons might be asked to come to the session as witnesses to this re-telling re-remembrance).

8. The client is asked to go through the collection of letters as a way of conducting qualitative re-search on herself/himself. A re-search model based in grounded theory is used: The client is asked to scour through each letter and begin to establish familiar themes and categories commonly found within the letters. These categories are then to be produced and written into a return letter to all the people who took part in the campaign. One young person who was taking her life back from bulimia stated during the re-search portion of the cam-

paign, "I get it—the categories are beginning to tell me who I really am!"

CAMPAIGN CONTRIBUTORS

The repercussions of many problems will often push persons to dis-member themselves from the support systems that surround them, and will coerce them toward isolation, detachment, and withdrawal. Similarly, problems may compel support persons to move away from the persons struggling, by encouraging hopelessness, anger, and despair.

Our experience has shown that once support persons have received a letter inviting them to contribute to a campaign, they will often feel compelled to write more than once (three and four letters is not uncommon). Customarily, contributors have had the experience of feeling "left out" of the helping process. Being left out will often leave them with the opinion that they are "impotent" and "useless." Frequently they report feeling "blamed" and "guilty" for the role they believe they have played in the problem's dominance over the person's life. They describe that these "impotent" and "useless" feelings are often helped along by various professional discourses and self-help literature.

Letter campaign authors explain that their contributions have helped them feel "useful" and "part of a team." In addition, the writing of a re-remembering text offers family members and other support persons with an opportunity to break free of the problem's negative dominance in their own lives, and allows for an alternative and active means for renewal and hope. As one older man who committed himself to an anti-depression campaign for his newly retired friend explained, "The letter campaign helped me to come off the bench and score big points against the problem so my friend could pull off a win . . . in helping him I helped myself."

Therapeutic letter-writing campaigns act to re-remember alternative accounts of a person's lived experience that a problem will often separate them from. The campaign encourages the person to become reacquainted with the membership group or groups that the problem has separated him/her from (e.g., family, friends, school, sports teams, etc.).

Therapeutic letter-writingcampaigns are designed as counterpractices to the dis-membering effects of problem lifestyles, and form a dialogic context of preferred remembering and meaning. The following is an account of one such campaign.

RE-MEMBERING A LIFE BACK
FROM DIS-MEMBERMENT

Mickey[4] was a 16-year-old girl who found herself on the brink of an anorexically inspired death and could not re-remember herself as anything but a "less than worthy" person. The problem had formed a wedge between Mickey and all of the persons who wished to love, help, and support her. Mickey's mother and father experienced feelings of being "cut off," "paralyzed," and "anguished" at being forced to watch her "slow and painful death." They experienced "frustration," "bitterness," "anger," and "hopelessness." All persons in Mickey's support system—parents, siblings, cousins, extended family, friends, teachers, family doctors, and helping professionals—were affected by anorexia's grip on her.

Mickey had found herself in anorexia's grip since the age of 12, and had had numerous hospital admissions. Her identity, as she had come to know it over the last few years, was ascribed according to the manner of the embedding community of discourse—in her own and in the discourse of the professional system (and more recently at home and with her friends), she was referred to as "manipulative," "bitchy," "depressed," "controlling," and "chronic." I asked her which label concerned her the most, and she stated, "The chronic one is the worst thing to be called, because this means I am a hopeless case."

In my first interview with Mickey, I questioned her about the many ways in which anorexia had acted to "dis-member" her from her life, community, and other memories of who she might be. I engage her in an externalizing conversation that sought to understand the internalized problem discourse (Madigan, 1996).

MICKEY: I just stay by myself now a lot.

STEPHEN: Are there ways in which you think that anorexia has separated you from the things you enjoy the most?

MICKEY: Yes.

STEPHEN: Can you name some of them.

MICKEY: I am not in school any more. I don't do my art, or read, and I haven't played piano in about a year. . . . I used to play volleyball and field hockey, but not any more.

STEPHEN: Did you have any idea that anorexia would take all this away from you?

[4]All names have been changed and permission has been given to use this interview.

MICKEY: No, I actually thought I would get more friends . . . it's weird.

STEPHEN: Has anorexia allowed you to keep up with your friends?

MICKEY: No, they have all left me behind—they hate me . . . they can't deal with my anorexia.

STEPHEN: Has anorexia in some ways formed a wedge between you and your friends?

MICKEY: Yeah, I guess—it doesn't make any room for anyone else . . . there is no time for anyone else.

STEPHEN: Would a good friend do this to you?

MICKEY: No, not really.

STEPHEN: In what ways has anorexia formed a wedge between you and your friends?

MICKEY: It tells me that they hate me, that I am no good . . . that I am less than them, that they only like me because I have this disease . . . you know? That they will not be there for me when I get better—that I am a loser and they pity me and don't like me.

Anorexia's problematic assault on a person's life will often act to bring forth isolation, negative comparison, perfection ideals, and feelings of being less than worthy and not measuring up (Vancouver Anti-Anorexia League, 1995). It is important to situate the problem's rhetoric, tactics, and cultural support systems within a community context as a way of emphasizing the problem's location and person's identity within the larger discursive domain.

MICKEY: I just don't ever seem to be good enough or measure up to other people's expectations of me.

STEPHEN: Who do you think believes that you don't measure up?

MICKEY: Well, sometimes my parents and my friends never call any more . . . I don't know, sometimes I just think I would be better off dead, you know? Just get it over with and stop all the pressure that I feel to be somebody, to measure up to this and that.

STEPHEN: Do you think that anorexia has in some way tricked your mind into a belief that somehow you haven't quite measured up?

MICKEY: I just don't seem to ever do anything right—my body is fat; I'm not as smart as I should be.

STEPHEN: Who do you think it is that holds the yardstick of who you should and shouldn't be?

MICKEY: *Cosmopolitan* [the magazine] (*laughs*). I don't know ... it's just that wherever you look, you see people all advertised and better than I am ... and don't eat this and how to lose 5 pounds and who I should be. ... It is really frustrating to have all this thrown at you all the time. ... I just feel like I want to run away and hide ... it's easier this way.

STEPHEN: Do you think that many young women your age are anorexically trained to feel that they never quite measure up, even if they are measuring up and feeling okay?

MICKEY: Yes! It really bugs me, because all of us ... all of my friends feel like shit and can't see themselves and get all bent out of shape over the slightest things.

STEPHEN: How does anorexia blind all of you young women ... all of your friends away from seeing the good aspects of who you are, and direct you only towards what you are not and perfection ideals?

MICKEY: Exactly. We get caught up in comparing ourselves. Anorexia always talks down to me and tells me who I am not, and I get to the point of getting so confused that really I just feel like I am losing myself.

STEPHEN: Would you be at all interested in regaining back parts of yourself?

MICKEY: Yes.

During the latter part of the second session, I outlined the letter-writing campaign to Mickey and her family. She said that she would try anything once, but first outlined her conditions of participation: (1) that she alone would pick the respondents in the campaign; (2) that she would decide which letters would be read out loud in the session; (3) that each member of her family had to write "a really honest letter" to her (4) that she would agree to respond to each person who sent a letter, even if "the letter was bad"; and (5) that she would hold onto and "be the keeper of the letters."

Mickey's letter-writing campaign was designed to assist in the re-re-membering of unique aspects of her life, now restrained by the anorexia. I likened her campaign to a eulogy or obituary put together on her behalf while she was still living. Mickey thought this was "a bit morbid but true." Members of her family, her friends, two teachers, and a few professionals were asked to assist Mickey in a re- remembering process through written accounts that outlined their memories of their relationship with her, separate from the problem's relationship to her. By docu-

menting alternative versions, the letters were to be designed to counter-
act the infirming effects of the problem story. We all agreed that these
textual accounts could hold a tremendous potential for the re-storying
of Mickey's life and could loosen anorexia's grip on her.

Mickey and I constructed the following letter for campaign distribution. The words in quotation marks are verbatim remarks that Mickey
made during our sessions. Written on my office letterhead, it read:

> Dear Friends of Mickey:
>
> Hello, my name is Stephen Madigan, and I am a family
> therapist who is working alongside Mickey in her battle to go
> free of anorexia. As you may already know, anorexia has
> been pushing Mickey around for close to 4 years of her
> young life. What you may not know is that anorexia tells
> Mickey that she "would be better off dead,"[5] that she "has
> no friends and nobody likes her," that she "doesn't measure
> up," and that "you only like her because you feel pity."
>
> Did you also know that anorexia pushes Mickey into
> "isolation" and "despair," and sometimes has her convinced
> that she is "better off dead"? Anorexia has waged its best
> efforts to kill Mickey, but somehow she remains alive and
> wants to "find a way to be free."
>
> Mickey believes that the time has come for her to "reach
> out" and ask her family and friends to write her a letter of
> support that may counteract anorexia's claims against her. Is
> it possible for you to write Mickey a note that outlines a story
> of (a) what you remember most about her, (b) who you think
> she really is as a person that lives outside of anorexia's
> description of her, (c) what you think is in store for her future
> once she goes anorexia-free, and (d) what you think your
> relationships will be like with her once she gives anorexia the
> slip. Mickey insists that you "tell her the truth with no BS,"
> and she will *really* understand if you don't want to write."
>
> We want to thank you in advance and let you know that
> Mickey intends to return all correspondence with her return
> letter of acknowledgment. THANKS!
>
> Yours in Anti-Anorexia,
>
> Mickey and Stephen

Mickey had compiled a list of 18 names for the initial mailout. As
the weeks went on and campaign letters began arriving, she thought of
12 new persons for letters to be sent out to. At last count, 44 letters, all

---

[5]Words in quotation marks are Mickey's actual phrases taken from the session and insert-
ed into the letter.

of them recalling counter versions of who Mickey was as a person, arrived to play their role in the anti-anorexic letter campaign.

We met for 8 more therapy sessions, (5 times alone, twice with her parents, and once with her two closest friends). Our sessions were based on recalling and retelling the news of her newly revived and re-remembered self. Mickey and I would take turns reading aloud. She would seize opportunities to reread her "favorite letters," and take time to expand upon the narratives being told by her "community of concern" (Madigan & Epston, 1995).

My last "official" contact with Mickey came 5 months after the first letter arrived. At this time I realized that Mickey was well on her way to stealing her life back from anorexia. Working alongside her community of concerned letter writers, Mickey slowly began performing qualities of her re-remembered self into anti-anorexic action. Anorexia's description of her was beginning to fade into an unsupported memory.

Recently, I spotted Mickey walking down the main shopping street of Vancouver in the company of three girlfriends, two of whom I recognized from the campaign. I tried to get her attention; however, she seemed too involved in the laughter and dialogue at hand.

COLLECTIVE RE-MEMBERING

The idea that memory is socially constructed poses many questions to the taken-for-granted bias of modern psychology's theory and practice. Memory's location within the social domain is in concert with narrative therapy's practice of locating so-called "psychological" problems and persons' identities within the cultural domain and relational politics of community discourse (Freedman & Combs, 1996; Madigan, 1996; Tamasese & Waldegrave, 1990; Waldegrave, 1996; White, 1995; Zimmerman & Dickerson, 1996). The negotiation and distribution of what constitute problems and personal identities include the effects of gender, class, and race on the shaping of problems, and identity (see Madigan, 1996). I would like to add to a narrative therapeutic ideology the idea that problems, identity, *and* memory are co-created, jointly "owned," forever liminal, and always "betwixt and between" the dialogic context.

Sampson (1993) writes that "human freedom involves the rights of individuals collectively to determine their mutual fates" (p. 168). Mickey was able to find a revived sense of her life through the collective re-membering of her community of others. The dialogic context of the campaign intimately wove together countless stories of a young person whom anorexia had helped her forget. Her community's recollected re-remembrances assisted her re-entry into a vast catalogue of other remembered lived experiences formally restrained by anorexia. This sense of renewal and hope seems to have rendered the discourse of anorexia helpless.

The many voices contained within the letters points us to remember that we share a collective responsibility for one another. This responsibility creates problems as easily as it affords freedom; it can promote a re-membering toward community or support the dis-membered isolation that problems often bring. Mickey and other persons I have worked on campaigns with have taught me that it takes a community of collaboration to imagine a memory.

When I was growing up, my mother would always dialogue with a particular saint when anything went missing in our household. To our great surprise, this means of re-remembering appeared to be failproof. Although I left the faith and its practices behind me some time ago, "in a pinch" I still find myself in consultation with the saint when things go missing. The mystic counsel brings forth a feeling of calm; however, I am presently stymied, as I have lost my keys and can't seem to remember the saint's name. Perhaps young Frankie will help to construct a re-remembrance.

COMMENTARY BY LORRAINE GRIEVES

In commenting on this chapter, I will draw from my experience of viewing memory and re-membering practices in similar ways to those which were clearly mapped out by Stephen in this Chapter. I will draw from my personal experience and from my work within the community as an advocate for people struggling with anorexia, bulimia, perfection, and depression to provide some reflections, thoughts, and queries.

Because problems tend to thrive in isolative environments, the idea of initiating a collective re-membering campaign can perforate a very dark environment with the light of multiple possibilities for everyone involved. As Stephen mentioned, those who are being affected by the problem can be recruited into ideas of hopelessness, helplessness, and "impotence." When allied as a community in support of the person struggling to move away from the problem, new hope for "strength in numbers" can and most often does emerge. For many people, finding a community that is in support of their moving away from the problem and into preferred activities and interests has been an important step in their journey—especially when the problem has been a strong influence for a number of years.

Through my experience with letter-writing campaigns, I have witnessed new stories about individuals who burst forth to provide visions that the problem-saturated story never would have allowed. A community of voices that supports the multiple possibilities that can be afforded a person as he/she moves away from the problem, can act as a great agent to form a bond of hope. I have seen this work very successfully in the context of the Anti-Anorexia/Anti-Bulimia League where people often share their experience and call upon a community of support. The glimmers of hope that appear when various people have read and remembered forgotten passions, talents, interests, and hopes will provoke tears of grief for all that the problem has taken from them and will often provide a renewed sense of vigilance to resist the problem's influence. Remembering to not forget each of our unique attributes, talents, and interests can be strongly reinforced by letters, videos, pictures, etc. Looking back at these archives of support and resistance can render the problem more transparent as it displays tactics that are repetitive and often predictable.

I am encouraged to see these ideas documented in a solid written account because this provides the opportunity for myself and for others to reconsider taken-for-granted notions of memory, re-remembering, and re-membering. As I viewed these ideas I found myself reflecting on ways that I may have supported problem-induced amnesia with people I have met with over the years. I think that this "amnesia" becomes increasingly prominent when people are labeled "chronic" and "resistant to treatment," as stories of hope are usually long forgotten at such points in a person's struggle. I am hopeful that these ideas invite helpers to support the emergence of alternative stories that are saturated with aspirations rather than hopelessness. Ideas of "collective remembering" have left me inspired and very intrigued and I wonder what yet unimagined ways these ideas can and will be utilized? It seems that the possibilities may be endless.

EDITORIAL QUESTIONS

Q: *(DN) Stephen, reading your chapter was very moving for me. I particularly admired how you situated your therapy ideas and practices in your own personal experiences (your mother's death and Frankie's lost soccer ball). I also appreciated reading the transcript of your work with Mickey. Making the internalizing problem discourse visible and explicit appeared to assist Mickey in separating and opposing oppressive cultural discourses. I view externalizing the internalized problem discourse as an act of cultural or political resistance. In what ways does a letter-writing campaign represent another practice of cultural resistance?*
A: If we were to view "resistance" as an experience of deconstructing

and taking action against dominant and taken-for-granted discursive practices, letter-writing campaigns could be considered an act of cultural resistance. They represent possibilities for change and offer one particular form of collaborative uprising to dominant discursive practices. It is also important to realize that if there were no resistance, there would be no power relations, because life would simply be a matter of obedience. Power relations are obliged to change when there is resistance.

One of the most important ways to situate the discourse of problems in persons' lives and relationships is looking at how to "resist." And we must be clear that *to resist is not only a negation to power.* To say "no" is the minimum form of resistance, and of course at times this is very important. However, there are many other practices of resistance that can break us out of misrepresented and oppressive discursive practices. I am happy to report that acts of therapeutic and cultural resistance are very creative and very generative in their experience!

ACKNOWLEDGMENTS

I would especially like to thank the Vancouver Anti-Anorexia League for the ideas they continue to imagine. As always, I am inspired by David Epston and my comrades at Yaletown Family Therapy: Heather Elliott, Ian Law, Colin Sanders, Jennifer Sigman, and Vanessa Swan. I would especially like to thank my very favorite 6-year-old cheeky monkey—the one and only *Frankie*!

REFERENCES

Bakhtin, M. M. (1986). *Speech genres and other late essays.* (V. McGee, Trans.). Austin: University of Texas Press.

Billig, M. (1990). Collective memory, ideology and the British Royal Family. In D. Middleton & D. Edwards (Eds.), *Collective remembering.* London: Sage.

Bordo, S. (1994). *Unbearable weight: Feminism, Western culture and the body.* Berkeley: University of California Press.

Caplan, P. (1995). *They say you're crazy: How the world's most powerful psychiatrists decide who's normal.* New York: Addison-Wesley.

Epston, D. (1989). *Collected papers.* Adelaide, South Australia: Dulwich Centre Publications.

Epston, D. (1994). The problem with originality. *Dulwich Centre Newsletter,* No. 4.

Foucault, M. (1982). The subject and power. In H. Dreyfus & P. Rabinow (Eds.), *Michel Foucault: Beyond.* Chicago Press.

Foucault, M. (1989). *Foucault live: Collected interviews, 1961–1984* (S. Lotringer, Ed.). New York: Semiotext(e).

Freedman, J., & Combs, G. (1996). *Narrative therapy: The social construction of preferred realities.* New York: Norton.

Hoagwood, K. (1993). Poststructuralist historism and the psychological construction of anxiety disorders. *Journal of Psychology, 127*(1), 105–122.

Johnston, J. (1973). *Foucault live: Collected interviews, 1961–1984.* New York: Semiotext(e).

Law, I., & Madigan, S. (Eds.). (1994). Power and politics in practice [Special issue]. *Dulwich Newsletter,* No. 1.

Madigan, S. (1992). The application of Michel Foucault's philosophy in the problem externalizing discourse of Michael White. *Journal of Family Therapy, 14*(3), 13–35.

Madigan, S. (1996). The politics of identity: Considering community discourse in the externalizing of internalized discourse. *Journal of Systemic Therapy, Spring,* 47–63.

Madigan, S., & Epston, D. (1995). From spy-chiatric gaze to communities of concern: From professional monologue to dialogue. In S. Friedman (Ed.), *The reflecting team in action.* New York: Guilford Press.

Middleton, D., & Edwards, D. (Eds.). (1990). *Collective remembering.* London: Sage.

Myeroff, B. (1982). Life history among the elder: Performance, visibility and remembering. In J. Ruby (Ed.), *A crack in the mirror: Reflexive perspectives in anthropology.* Philadelphia: University of Pennsylvania Press.

Sampson, E. (1993). *Celebrating the other: A dialogic account of human nature.* Boulder, CO: Westview Press.

Shotter, J. (1990). The social construction of remembering and forgetting. In D. Middleton & D. Edwards (Eds.), *Collective remembering.* London: Sage.

Special Double Issue on Eating Disorders. (1993). Eating disorders and sexual abuse [Special issue]. *Eating Disorders: Journal of Treatment and Prevention, 1*(3–4).

Tamasese, K., & Waldegrave, C. (1990). Social justice. *Dulwich Centre Newsletter,* No. 1.

Vancouver Anti-Anorexia, Anti-Bulimia League Newsletter. (1996). Newsletter, *2*(2).

Waldegrave, C. (1996). Keynote address presented at Narrative Ideas and Therapeutic Practice: The 4th Annual International Conference, Vancouver, B.C., Canada.

White, M. (1995). *Re-authoring lives: Interviews and essays.* Adelaide, South Australia: Dulwich Centre Publications.

White, M., & Epston, D. (1990). *Narrative means to therapeutic ends.* New York: Norton.

Zimmerman, J., & Dickerson, V. (1996). *If problems talked: Narrative therapy in action.* New York: Guilford Press.

14

Voices of
Political Resistance
YOUNG WOMEN'S CO-RESEARCH
ON ANTI-DEPRESSION

DAVID NYLUND
KATHERINE CESKE

My heart yearns for love that no longer exists. I'm unable to receive
feelings that remain. Yet they don't remain in any world of mine.
Why am I all alone? How can this be? So misunderstood and still
never gotten the benefit of the doubt. No one accepts me for me
except me. Some say: I have no respect, no courtesy, no love, no
common sense. How would they know? Do they feel what I feel? See
what I see? Hear what I hear? Why does my voice have to be
silenced? I just want to scream: Look at me, hear me, be me. Am I
the only one who perceives life as unfair? A double standard?
Hypocritical? I'm tired of meeting up to everyone else's
expectations. What about my own? Why can't I live the way I want?
Does everyone really know what's best for me? Don't underestimate
me. Take my word just this once . . . *I am capable.*

—MEL, a 16-year-old woman battling depression

DEPRESSION AMONG YOUNG WOMEN:
A POSTMODERN VIEW

Increasing numbers of adolescent women are being diagnosed with depression (Pipher, 1996). From a traditional psychiatric and psychologi-

cal viewpoint, depression is located within the adolescent. This perspective is grounded within modernist language traditions of functionalism and structuralism (Madigan, 1996). Modernist therapy privileges the clinician's voice over the client's voice. These traditional practices typically focus on a client's deficits. We are concerned about the effects of modernist practice, particularly in work with adolescent women. When modernist ideas dominate, the focus is shifted away from the cultural conditions that place teenage girls at risk for depression. This shift in attention privatizes the problem to the adolescent, while ignoring the inequities of race, class, and gender that may promote depression (Madigan, 1996). In addition, since young women's voices are particularly vulnerable to being marginalized (Gilligan, 1982; Gilligan, Rogers, & Tolman, 1991; Weingarten, 1995), a modernist practice of the therapist-as-expert imposing meaning on the adolescent can lead to colonization and further silencing (Stacey & Loptson, 1995).

Our practice is situated within a postmodern and narrative framework, specifically the work of Michael White and his colleagues (Freedman & Combs, 1996; White & Epston, 1990; Zimmerman & Dickerson, 1996). Informed by postmodern ideology, our aim is to render transparent the societal discourses that may support the life of problems in persons (Hare-Mustin, 1994; Madigan, 1996; Weingarten, 1991). We think that various discourses encourage depression among adolescent girls. These discourses are situated within a patriarchal society that influences young women to conform to the dominant conventional image of the perfect girl—one who is thin, controls her sexual desire, silences her voice, and is "nice," "feminine," and accommodating. In addition, the discourse of separation/individuation, which privileges individualism over connection (Dickerson, Zimmerman, & Berndt, 1994; Gilligan et al., 1991; Weingarten, 1994), may support depression. The separation discourse can recruit adolescent females into feeling that they have to carve out a "true" identity on their own and be cut off from important relationships with adults, especially their parents. In addition, parents can fall victim to parent blaming (particularly mother blaming) if they do not push their children to become independent. These discourses place young women in a double bind. If they subscribe to the dominant ideas of what it means to be a young woman, they may silence themselves to maintain relationships; the effects of this censoring can be depression or eating disorders (anorexia nervosa, bulimia nervosa). However, when adolescent girls try to stand up for themselves, they can be excluded and labeled as "troublemakers."

In our therapeutic conversations with young women, we seek to unmask, identify, and externalize the discourses that leave them vulnerable to depression. These dialogues help counter the privatization of problems by locating depression in a cultural and sociopolitical context (Madigan, 1996). We then invite young women to challenge discourses that may be subjugating and limiting. Kathy Weingarten (1995) refers to the act of subverting constraining discourses as "cultural resistance." Another author who has had a major influence on our work, Carol Gilligan, similarly names the practice of challenging dominant discourses as acts of "political resistance" (Taylor, Gilligan, & Sullivan, 1995). Taylor et al. explain: "A healthy resistance and courage lead girls to take action against social or cultural conventions that encourage them to disconnect from themselves and others. This political resistance challenges the idealization of relationships and images of bodies that require girls not to experience their feelings and desires, or not to know what they know" (1995, p. 26).

CREATING COMMUNITIES OF CONCERN THROUGH CO-RESEARCH

Michael White (1995) talks about how problems have a way of dismembering people from their own knowledges. Problems can also use the culture to get the upper hand (Zimmerman & Dickerson, 1996). For instance, anorexia nervosa uses Western society's emphasis on thinness (via advertising billboards, magazines, and the rest of the mass media) to gain influence over young women's lives. A narrative practice seeks to de-privatize the effects of problems such as depression (Madigan, 1996). When young clients' voices are privileged and the problem is located within a sociocultural context, the young persons can separate from dominant cultural ideas that support depression and begin to re-member their own special abilities and knowledges. Madigan and Epston (1995) refer to "communities of concern," which are created or expanded through such practices as letter-writing campaigns, anti-problem leagues, "consulting your consultant" interviews, and co-research. These practices lead to clients' circulating their solution knowledges to other clients who have experienced similar problems.

Consistent with our idea of honoring young women's voices and moving away from expert knowledge, we have included the transcripts of our work with Claudia and Linda[1] both of whom have resisted depression. The interviews were conducted as co-research projects. Lobovits and Seidel (1994) identify four characteristics of a therapist who engages in co-research: fostering a collaborative attitude, valuing

[1]Confidentiality has been preserved. KC (Katherine) was the therapist working alongside Claudia. DN (David) was the therapist working with Linda.

emotional experiences and reflections, engaging in empowering relationships, and diminishing the effects of existing hierarchies. From a co-research posture, we invited Claudia and Linda into an inquiry about the effects of depression, cultural and gender prescriptions that promote depression, and countertactics they have used to subdue depression.[2]

Claudia's Co-Research

Claudia, 16, had a long-standing relationship with "depression" when she was transferred to me (KC) by a colleague. She remembered depression's entering her life around the time of her parents' divorce. Since that time, it had encouraged her to become involved with drugs. Eventually the depression attempted to convince her to take her own life. Claudia exhibited a great degree of compassion and emotion. Society tried to persuade her that these attributes were flaws rather than virtues. In addition, she possessed a rather large amount of artistic genius, which depression did not want her to value or acknowledge. Therapy focused on honoring her own unique skills and talents versus valuing those qualities society labeled as desirable.

KATHERINE: I'm wondering about the effects of depression on your self-identity—how it made you think of yourself as a person.

CLAUDIA: It made me feel like I was less of a person—like everyone else was better and I didn't measure up. Like, you know, they were these wonderful people with all these friends and this good life, and there's me all depressed. It's kind of like you realize you're depressed, you know that you're not happy, but you don't realize how bad it is.

KATHERINE: It fools you.

CLAUDIA: Yeah, you don't realize that it's there, but you kind of know it's there. It's like you're not happy, but you don't realize how bad it is.

KATHERINE: So it kind of keeps that hidden.

CLAUDIA: Yeah.

KATHERINE: Has that been dangerous?

---

[2]The co-research interviews with Claudia and Linda were the culmination of many prior conversations that externalized depression. As Linda and Claudia experienced further separation from depression, they were each able to locate the problem in the larger, sociocultural context. This needs to be stated so as to not imply that these co-research interviews occurred early in therapy.

CLAUDIA: Yeah.

KATHERINE: What direction did depression want to take your life in?

CLAUDIA: Down.

KATHERINE: Down. If it had its way, where would you be now?

CLAUDIA: Dead.

KATHERINE: Dead. It does not mess around. What strategies did it use to try to kill you?

CLAUDIA: Just takes over your thoughts, your actions, your body.

KATHERINE: What kind of thoughts did it place in your head?

CLAUDIA: That you're not a good person. That others are better. That you shouldn't be there. That you're just a mistake or something. That nobody cares, and if you were gone, nobody would even notice or care. Or, if they did notice, they would be happy.

KATHERINE: Wow. Could it be pretty convincing?

CLAUDIA: Very.

[Later in the interview:]

KATHERINE: What particular pressures do you think young women face that makes them particularly vulnerable to depression?

CLAUDIA: Looks.

KATHERINE: Looks. How so?

CLAUDIA: A lot of it has to do with looks, I think, because you just want to look like everyone else, fit in, and there is so much pressure from society that you have to be beautiful and have to look this way and act this way.

KATHERINE: Yeah. So there's a lot of pressure in society to look this way and act this way. Who promotes that?

CLAUDIA: TV and magazines.

KATHERINE: How does that affect young women?

CLAUDIA: They see the magazines saying that this is what you got to look like to be beautiful. It gets a lot of girls to be anorexic and stuff. I never had the problem, though.

KATHERINE: You've never had that problem, but depression had you?

CLAUDIA: Yeah.

KATHERINE: How did it do that?

CLAUDIA: It kind of made me feel bad about how I looked.

KATHERINE: So that was one more lie that depression could tell you?

CLAUDIA: Yeah.

KATHERINE: What other things do you think particularly young women face that make them vulnerable to depression?

CLAUDIA: There's a lot of sexual pressure.

KATHERINE: Sexual pressure. Can you tell me more about that?

CLAUDIA: Like thinking that a guy would only stay with you if you have sex with him and stuff.

KATHERINE: So a lot of pressure that the young women get, not the young men necessarily.

CLAUDIA: Yeah. And then if they do have sex, they're considered sluts, but if they don't, they think the guys will leave them.

KATHERINE: So how does that contribute to depression? What does that do?

CLAUDIA: Makes you feel bad. Makes you feel like you have to do it, but you shouldn't do it. Like you have to do it, but you're not supposed to.

KATHERINE: So really a double bind there. And so depression wins no matter what.

CLAUDIA: Yeah. If you don't do it, you lose; if you do it, you lose.

KATHERINE: Do you think that depression is rooted in our culture? In some respects, people feel that depression is within themselves and it's somehow a problem that they have created. Sometimes people see that there [are] a number of cultural influences that really push depression along.

CLAUDIA: I think it has to do with each person. [For] some people, it's something that happened; [for] some people, it's society.

KATHERINE: So it really depends on the person and how depression enters their lives?

CLAUDIA: Because it can enter in all different ways. [It could] just be there, or something could happen—an accident or something terrible could happen. Or society could do it.

KATHERINE: How could society do it? I'm curious about that.

CLAUDIA: I think it's mainly the looks stuff that society contributes to.

KATHERINE: That's a biggie. So you're saying depression can team up with anorexia?

CLAUDIA: Yeah.

KATHERINE: It can feed that. Does that pressure get teenage girls to start doubting themselves or questioning themselves or evaluating themselves?

CLAUDIA: Yeah.

KATHERINE: Yeah. How so? Like, how did it get you to do that?

CLAUDIA: Maybe just like they see all these beautiful girls on TV, all these super-skinny girls that are, like, sizes you can never fit into no matter how hard you try. All these super-skinny girls and they have all this perfect skin because [of] all the makeup they have on. But you can't see it and just think, "Wow, that's what I'm supposed to look like." So you just see it on TV and they start out in the commercials. It's mostly commercials, I think, saying, "Look like this, buy this, be like this."

KATHERINE: So what effect does that have on you?

CLAUDIA: It brings you down.

KATHERINE: How does it do that?

CLAUDIA: It makes you feel you are not up to standard.

KATHERINE: So it gets you to not appreciate the gifts you have? Appreciating the shape you have?

CLAUDIA: Yeah. It makes you think you could always be better.

KATHERINE: That sounds like it's not a helpful message.

CLAUDIA: And some girls, they try to look up the message and then, like me, said, "I'm never going to be like that. Why even try?"

KATHERINE: How did that affect you?

CLAUDIA: It made me give up, not caring about anything, not care about myself.

KATHERINE: So it really had far-reaching effects.

CLAUDIA: Like, I would just throw any clothes on, would not brush my hair or anything. I wouldn't put makeup on or anything. I would just look like a total slob.

KATHERINE: Was that your choice, or [was] depression choosing that for you?

CLAUDIA: At the time I felt it was my choice, but I think I was influenced by depression.

KATHERINE: I guess I ask that because sometimes people have learned to protest some cultural ideas on how you should look. I don't know if you felt like wearing those clothes was a protest, or was more a sign that depression was getting at you.

CLAUDIA: At first, a protest.

KATHERINE: So do you appreciate your ability to protest cultural ideas of how a woman should look?

CLAUDIA: Yeah.

KATHERINE: What do you think depression thought of your protest?

CLAUDIA: I don't think depression liked it too much!

KATHERINE: So how did you protest depression? What strategies did you discover that really worked for you?

CLAUDIA: First of all, I stopped hanging around with my friends who did drugs, and then I stopped doing drugs on my own and started getting involved in stuff.

KATHERINE: Like what stuff?

CLAUDIA: Like getting a job or joining a club or something.

KATHERINE: How did that affect depression?

CLAUDIA: It kind of made you forget about it, kind of pushed it out of the way, like, "Okay, I've got something to do now."

KATHERINE: Yeah. And were these clubs coed, or were they with young women, or . . . ?

CLAUDIA: Well, I started a job and it was with a whole bunch of people, and just being around people, talking to people, meeting new people.

KATHERINE: So doing that was really helpful? (*Claudia nods "yes."*) So it kind of got you to forget about it. Did it do anything else for you?

CLAUDIA: It made me focus more on my life, like I was taking a new step into my future—that I was actually doing something instead of just sitting by and watching my life go by.

KATHERINE: So, really? I like that. "Taking a step into my future." Does depression like that? Does depression like you or others to think about their future?

CLAUDIA: Not really. It wants you think about it's going to [be] . . . horrible, terrible.

KATHERINE: So this was a real step away from depression?

CLAUDIA: Yeah.

KATHERINE: Wow!

CLAUDIA: It wants you to watch life go by instead of live it.

KATHERINE: So taking the first step to actually live your life according to your own design was an anti-depressive strategy?

CLAUDIA: Yeah.

KATHERINE: Did it lose its . . . when do you think was the point where depression lost its grip on you?

CLAUDIA: I think it still has a grip somewhat, and it will always have a little grip that will always be there lingering, ready to take you if you're willing to go.

KATHERINE: So how do you keep depression at bay?

CLAUDIA: Learn to accept who you are and to love yourself, and to not really listen to stereotypes, and don't think about stuff that's all around you. Just think about yourself and think, "Hey, if that person does not like what I'm doing, well, that's too bad." Just think I'm doing what I feel is right.

KATHERINE: How do you keep those ideas alive?

CLAUDIA: You have to work at it. You've got to be selfish.

KATHERINE: How do you mean that? That's a doozy. Is that something that a lot of young women, especially, are told not to be?

CLAUDIA: Yeah, I think so. You've got to be selfish and just make yourself a priority. Just think of yourself before others. Society and everyone says, "Think of others before you," but when it comes to your emotions and stuff, you should [think] of yourself and what's best for you. Like, if you do something, is it going to make you feel good, or is it going to make you feel bad? If it makes you feel bad, don't do it.

KATHERINE: Even if it means that it's going to upset somebody else?

CLAUDIA: Yeah. Even if it will get people made at you. You've just got to do what you think is right.

KATHERINE: How did you come to this?

CLAUDIA: Just work and time—a lot of time.

KATHERINE: Any coaches that helped you?

CLAUDIA: My mom helped me a lot—helps me, and was always there for me, supporting me.[3] There were a couple of good friends that

[3]An act of cultural resistance, as Claudia defied the separation/individuation discourse and remained connected to her mother. Her mother also acted as a political resister in encour-

always stood by me and are willing to listen, and just if I have a problem they would be, like, "Too bad." [They'd talk] about it with you and how to figure it out.

KATHERINE: So they would be there for you—girlfriends?

CLAUDIA: Yeah.

KATHERINE: Is there something to having other young women around to help you?

CLAUDIA: Yeah, you've [got] to be out doing something. Because if you're just getting bored, then it just gets your mind to wander and get depressed and start meddling on to stupid little things.

KATHERINE: Is that how depression enters—by picking at stupid little things?

CLAUDIA: Yeah, and then it goes from there.

KATHERINE: You were saying something that I was really struck with: "You've got to be selfish." You've got to think of yourself first and think about "Is it going to help me or hurt me?" I was wondering: Do you think that's a hard thing for young women, especially, to really realize?

CLAUDIA: Yeah.

KATHERINE: How so?

CLAUDIA: Just society again.

KATHERINE: What kinds of pressures do young women have along those lines?

CLAUDIA: Like, girls are supposed to be nice and stay home and cook and clean and be all neat.

KATHERINE: Yeah, and do for others?

CLAUDIA: Yeah. Do stuff for other people and be, like, a mother figure and stuff.

KATHERINE: So being mothers from age 2 and up.

CLAUDIA: Yeah.

KATHERINE: So does it really kind of go against tradition to really think of yourself?

CLAUDIA: Yeah. It was always, like, little girls are supposed to be sweet and nice. It starts when you're little. You're supposed to be sweet

aging Claudia to make her own needs a priority and maintain her voice as a young woman.

and nice, but boys are mean and rude to you, but that's okay because they are boys. Girls are supposed to be nice.

KATHERINE: How does that make teenage women vulnerable to depression?

CLAUDIA: Because they're really not that nice. They really don't want to just make other people happy.

KATHERINE: It kind of goes against what you want to be, what anyone would want.

CLAUDIA: You've got to realize the realization of what you want from life, and then you have to work at it and not let anyone try to stop you from getting what you want. Really, the only way to get to that is something you've to do on your own—something you've just got to reflect on who you are and what you're going to be 10 years from now. If you like how you are, or if you've just got to change what you're doing. Like, if you stop doing drugs, how your life will be in the future.

KATHERINE: So you have to take a cold, hard look at things and really set goals for what you want in life?

CLAUDIA: Yeah.

KATHERINE: Not what other people want you to do, but what you want to do?

CLAUDIA: It's what you want, what will make you happy, because only you know what's best for you.

KATHERINE: Is that a hard thing again for young women to realize? (*Claudia nods her head "yes."*) You're nodding your head.

CLAUDIA: Yeah. It's tough because some people, maybe boys, won't like you.

KATHERINE: Yeah. It's tough. Do you think depression likes it when you think of yourself?

CLAUDIA: It hates it.

KATHERINE: The depression didn't like it when you were in control of your life?

CLAUDIA: Yeah, it wanted to control you and tell you what to do and feel.

KATHERINE: Is it like a dictator?

CLAUDIA: Yeah. It likes other people controlling your life.

KATHERINE: So that can be parents planning your life out for you, or society telling you what to do or look like?

CLAUDIA: Yeah. Depression didn't like it when I took control of my life and started being selfish. It started looking for another victim!

KATHERINE: So it's always looking for someone vulnerable, and you're not vulnerable when you are in control?

CLAUDIA: Yeah.

KATHERINE: You said you are always going to have to have your eye out for depression. You think it's small, you think it's even almost gone, but you said you have to keep your eye out.

CLAUDIA: It's always to be there lingering in your past, and it could sneak up again. And so you have to look out for it and keep your control of your life, and just each morning know that you're going to have a good day.

KATHERINE: Yeah, you were saying that, each morning you would wake up. Can you say more about that?

CLAUDIA: That each morning you could wake up and decide if it's going to be a good day or a bad day.

KATHERINE: So, decide your own destiny?

CLAUDIA: That choice is yours—what kind of day you're going to have—and depression does not like it because your life is yours to live. But depression tries to live it for you.

KATHERINE: So what anti-depressive ideas would you like to pass on to other young women?

CLAUDIA: Well, the medication is a good start, but being active—not sitting around doing nothing—helps.[4] Even if its just like walking the dog or doing yardwork or going to a party.

KATHERINE: Anything else?

CLAUDIA: Don't take society too seriously!

Linda's Co-Research

Linda, 13, came to see me (DN) because of her struggle with depression. She was a very outspoken person who at times was pushed around by her anger. When she was younger, her forthrightness was considered an

---

[4]See Griffith and Griffith (1994) and Nylund and Corsiglia (1996) for discussions of interweaving medication into a narrative practice.

asset. As she entered her adolescence, however, her frankness began to be viewed by her parents and teachers as "defiance."[5] Linda began to feel that she either had to silence her voice and become depressed, or speak out angrily and be seen as rebellious. The therapy focused on ways that she could stand up for herself when doing so ran counter to societal discourse (Zimmerman & Dickerson, 1996). My work with Linda's parents included addressing their concerns that their daughter was not fitting with society's idea about who she should be.

[The interview begins with a discussion of "perfectionism."]

DAVID: How has perfectionism tried to influence you?

LINDA: I used to spend a lot of time in the bathroom. I think a lot of girls . . . now I'm not in it, but I was in it earlier, like the last year or so . . . makeup . . . it really makes your self-esteem go down, because you feel really ugly without it. You're like, "Oh, I can't leave the house without makeup," and stuff.

DAVID: How do you think perfectionism—the idea of having [to] look a certain way . . . that if you don't wear makeup, you're ugly—how do you think it affects young women in relationship to depression?

LINDA: I think a lot of it has to do with our appearance and, like, the pressure to be that way. It's like a conspiracy thing. They're trying to make it seem like "real people" are anorexic models on TV. You don't see real-looking people on TV, except for people they're making fun of, like old people that are grumpy. But not people that you would think, "That's somebody I want to be like," or whatever.

DAVID: So would you say that perfectionism and depression are like a conspiracy?

LINDA: Yeah.

DAVID: Did the conspiracy get you to compare yourself to the models on TV? (*Linda nods her head "yes."*) So, those images on TV that women become susceptible to, who's promoting the conspiracy? What sources are behind the conspiracy?

LINDA: I think it's been there for a long, long time, because I have a Sears, Roebuck and Company catalog from 1902 and there are all these white velvety things that are supposed to make your skin beautiful, and it's been there for like, forever. It would just be beau-

[5]We view adolescence as a social construction as opposed to a developmental "truth." Through our postmodern lens, we see teenage identity and the stage of adolescence as culturally manufactured (Madigan, 1996).

tiful. It's something that everybody wants to be, and, like—even people like Rosie O'Donnell, [who] says, "I'm happy and fat." Maybe she isn't depressed about it or whatever, but I'm sure [she] would much rather be skinny, in her mind.

DAVID: How do you think the pressure to look a certain way affects teenage girls?

LINDA: It makes us, like, really want to be like that, and I think it's a lot of—the big reason why people are depressed and stuff. We all can't look that way. We have these people around that make you feel ugly. I could get, like, a million compliments saying, "Oh, you're so beautiful," and stuff like that. But if one person says I'm ugly, or "You're breaking out," or something, it can just make it go all away. It's like it's a lot more powerful than the compliments.

DAVID: So it invites depression?

LINDA: Yeah, people ask me, like they come up to me and go, "Oh, what's wrong?" and stuff. They really don't want to hear everything, so I keep it inside. Then it all builds up and makes me sad.

DAVID: Lately you have been resisting perfectionism and these ideas, right? How have you done that?

LINDA: Well, my parents took away my makeup for a week once when I got in trouble. I was like, "Oh, my God, I'm going to die. I'm never going to go outside." During that time, I think my self-esteem got a little higher. I mean, at first I looked a lot worse, but now I put makeup on to enhance what I have or whatever, not make me look like a totally different person.

DAVID: How has that helped with your view of yourself?

LINDA: It makes me realize that, you know, like, I can be beautiful without it and stuff.

DAVID: Was this realization a strike against perfectionism? Was it an anti-depressive step?

LINDA: Yeah.

DAVID: What other pressures have you felt as a teenage woman that may have contributed to depression trying to take over your life?

LINDA: The pressure to have a boyfriend. Like, my friend . . . if she doesn't have a boyfriend, she gets depressed and says, "If I don't have a boyfriend, I get fat."

DAVID: Where do you think she gets that idea that you have to have a boyfriend or you're going to get fat?

LINDA: I think a lot has to do with not getting enough love at home or whatever. Also, movies always show women—almost every movie, even, like, action movies—having a boyfriend or husband.

DAVID: What are the effects of this pressure to have a boyfriend?

LINDA: You start looking for love so hard that you settle for anything.

DAVID: How might that idea of settling for anything promote depression?

LINDA: I think it's one of the big reasons why girls get depressed, and that's why I'm staying away from it, because it's bothered me before. It's made me sulk around the house and made me depressed [i.e., having no boyfriend]. Now I like being single. It makes me feel better. I mean, it makes me able to work on myself and not have to worry about other guys. I just, like, want to go out with myself, I guess, in a way!

DAVID: So you're developing an anti-depressive relationship with yourself?

LINDA: Yes, I'm trying to find out about myself, and I'd rather concentrate on that than anybody else right now.

DAVID: What other pressures do you think you and other teenage girls are up against that bring on depression?

LINDA: Well, there is pressure to have sex if you want a boyfriend. I think guys take advantage of that. I'm not saying that all men are dogs or anything, but there are the "mold boys." That's what we call them, the "mold boys."

DAVID: What's a "mold boy"?

LINDA: All the boys that are made into that little mold, and they have to be all the same—I guess from pressure from society. These mold boys don't care about you. They just want something from you. That's how they are. They go around, "Oh, yeah, I'm a player," like that's something good to be. Like, that's what I hate. Another thing I have is that [a guy] can have lots of girlfriends and he'd be all studly, or whatever, you know. But if a girl had more than one boyfriend, she's a slut or a "ho" [i.e., whore] or something.

DAVID: What do you think of that double standard? Is it a double standard that depression uses to its advantage?

LINDA: Yeah, I think so. I think it's wrong . . . how little things can make a girl have a reputation. You're slutty or whatever. So if you don't have sex, you might not have a boyfriend or be popular, but if you have sex, the guys talk about it and it gets around. She's a "ho."

DAVID: What effect do you think this double standard, this double-bind message has had on you and other young women?

LINDA: It's kind of hard. They learn one thing about you and form an opinion and never look at them twice.

[Later in the conversation:]

DAVID: Linda, I was wondering about some of the struggles you have had in maintaining your opinions, your voice. We have talked in the therapy about how you think there's a double standard there, right?

LINDA: Yeah. When I speak up in class or state my opinion or whatever, some of the teachers think I'm being difficult and stuff. You know what I mean? But if I was a boy, I would be seen as strong and standing up for myself.

DAVID: Is this fair? Is this another way depression uses the society to gain control of you?

LINDA: Yeah.

DAVID: Have you felt pressure to give up your voice, sort of?

LINDA: Yeah. Because when I speak up, I get in trouble.

DAVID: Why do you think you get in more trouble than a boy, for instance?

LINDA: Because girls are supposed to be "nice." It's not right, though.

DAVID: Do you appreciate that you stand up for yourself, even though society, teachers, even your parents tell you not to?

LINDA: Yeah. It's been hard, though.

DAVID: What about with your parents? Have you felt that they unintentionally pressured you to act "nice," more "feminine" . . . give up your beliefs?

LINDA: Sometimes. Not my mother. I can talk to her. She's pretty supportive and stuff.

DAVID: Do you value that about her? I'm thinking that some teenagers feel it's not cool to talk to their parents, that they have to go on their own. Do you value your connection with her?

LINDA: Yeah. My dad is hard sometimes. Like, he wants me to go to

Catholic Church and stuff, but I don't want to. It's not like I'm lazy or anything. I just have my own spiritual meetings with myself. My own religion that's different from my dad's.

DAVID: Is that something that you value about yourself? That you are carving out your own spirituality, even if it means upsetting others?

LINDA: Yeah. I think all girls should do something like talk to themselves. I live next to this levee, and I go out there and talk out loud. I don't know if I'm talking to God or whomever, but I'm talking to something, and depression goes away. I just feel a lot, like, totally cleansed, and my mind feels fresher and freer.

DAVID: So going out to nature is a spiritual experience. It sounds as if it's an anti-depressive tactic? You'd like to pass that on to other young women? (*Linda nods "yes."*) Any other thoughts or any advice you have for young women who are facing these pressures we've talked about?

LINDA: Just try to concentrate on yourself, and just maybe . . . there's going to be boys around forever. I mean, just take time off and just really concentrate and think about what's going on with you. Just think about some things you want to change about yourself and like to change. Just totally concentrate on yourself.

DAVID: So commit to yourself, as opposed to the ideas that women should put others first?

LINDA: Yeah. Just work on yourself, and I think it will build your self-esteem up. Just try to develop a love for yourself. Don't care so much what others, guys, think of you.

DAVID: What has focusing on yourself done to depression?

LINDA: It's shrunk it!

DAVID: Any other thoughts?

LINDA: Yeah, that perfection thing. I mean, you can do your hair and makeup, but do it for yourself. That's what I'm doing. Just concentrate on yourself. I'm not talking about building a wall around me. I mean, I still have boys for friends. But I think of me more now.

DAVID: Do these steps you're taking . . . are [they] like building a wall for yourself to keep depression from entering?

LINDA: Yeah! In a way, yeah. Let people in, but not depression.

DAVID: Okay, that's great. Thank you, Linda. I don't think depression and its allies liked this conversation!

LINDA: I don't think it did either!

CONCLUSION

In keeping with narrative philosophy, we refrain from concluding this chapter by quoting the "experts" in the field or by making declarations about the true nature of depression. Instead, we conclude it by highlighting some of the thoughts shared by the young women in this chapter that are most meaningful to us. We also discuss the societal forces that Claudia and Linda have identified as particularly evocative of depression.

Adolescent women struggle against certain patriarchal discourses that are embedded in our culture. This struggle, it is thought, makes adolescent girls particularly vulnerable to depression. Claudia and Linda cite several examples of such discourses. In particular, they point to the pressures to conform to a certain standard of beauty and feminine behavior. Claudia states, "A lot of it has to do with looks . . . there is so much pressure from society that you have to be beautiful and have to look this way and act this way."

Claudia identifies the mass media as important sources of this pressure to be beautiful. Furthermore, she states that the images of beauty presented to young girls are unrealistic and fabricated: "All these super-skinny girls that are, like, sizes you can never fit into no matter how hard you try . . . and they all have this perfect skin because [of] all the makeup they have on. But you can't see it and just think, 'Wow, that's what I'm supposed to look like.' . . . It makes you feel like you are not up to standard."

Linda adds that the media promote the misconception that one has to be beautiful to be admired: "They're [the media] trying to make it seem like 'real people' are anorexic models on TV. You don't see real-looking people on TV, except for people they're making fun of . . . not people that you would think, 'That's somebody I want to be like,' or whatever." Consequently, Linda states that girls use any means (makeup, cosmetic surgery, excessive dieting) to achieve the "look" that society guarantees will lead to love and admiration. Yet, Linda contends, the methods that girls use to achieve "beauty" serve instead to remind them that they are flawed, according to society's standards. "Makeup . . . It really makes your self-esteem go down, because you feel ugly without it," Linda poignantly articulates.

As a woman (KC), I found that re-reading the transcripts of Linda and Claudia's co-research had a strong impact on me. I was surprised by how constant the discourses affecting adolescent girls have remained over time. Despite rhetoric about Western society's emerging enlightenment in regard to women, many of the messages troubling teenagers today are similar to those that influenced me 20-some years ago. As Linda so eloquently states, "I think it's [the pressure for young women to be beautiful] been there for a long, long time, because I have a Sears, Roebuck and Company catalog from 1902 and there are all those white velvety things that are supposed to make your skin beautiful . . . I think it's a lot of—the big reason why people are depressed and stuff."

I especially remember the requirement for girls to define themselves by their ability to please others, principally men. Many teenage women spoke of being their own persons, yet a young woman's worthiness continued to be measured by her ability to attract the opposite gender. For example, one common impression among teens was that a girl had to be attractive to be popular. Girls were also expected to follow a certain behavioral protocol in order to be pleasing. As an adolescent, I felt pressure to be ebullient (anger was not tolerated), bright enough (but not smarter than my male counterpart), self-effacing, and self-sacrificing. At times I had to pretend that I didn't know what I knew (Gilligan et al., 1991). Moreover, I was expected to have opinions as long as they agreed with everyone else's. Finally, I recall pressure to be responsible for others' self-worth. This would often include comparing my talents unfavorably to theirs.

Through time, beauty and femininity have been clearly defined and yet unattainable standards to which all young women aspire. Furthermore, what is considered attractive continues to shift (e.g., dainty features and voluptuous curves gave way to a muscular body and full lips, and now there's the "waif" look). Girls are encouraged to attain one image of beauty, only to be required to reinvent themselves a few years later. In other words, teenage women are told by peers, parents, the media, teachers, and young men that they have "self-worth" only if they are able to attract boys. Girls are also advised that their ability to attract a boyfriend is dependent on their level of beauty. Yet the image of attractiveness is largely unachievable. Consequently, young women often receive the message that who they are, when defined by external measures, is never good enough. According to Claudia and Linda, depression exploits this belief.

Also according to Linda and Claudia, the mixed messages that girls receive about their sexuality are particularly deleterious. Linda explains that "there is pressure to have sex if you have a boyfriend. . . . if you don't have sex, you might not have a boyfriend or be popular, but if you have sex, the guy talks about it and it gets around. She's a 'ho.'" Claudia states that this double bind often invites depression by making a girl feel dirty or inadequate, regardless of her choice.

Linda and Claudia expose another discourse that depression employs to its advantage. This notion revolves around defining oneself by the impression of others. As Linda agrees in her interview, girls are often required to act "nice" or "feminine" and to give up their voice and beliefs. I recall how this specification influenced me into believing that the opinion of others was the most accurate measure of my self-identity. Hence I attempted to mold my actions, preferences, and opinions to what I believed would be pleasing to others. What I discovered, however, was that "people pleasing" was a trap. First, I could not ever win everyone's approval. This was an invitation to feel incapable. Therefore, I would try harder to please those who disapproved; however, I soon found that the more I tried to please others, the more distant from myself I became. This would lead to feelings of despair. I became dis-membered (White, 1995) from my own version of myself. Claudia contends that acting "nice" or "pleasing" subjects young women to depression because it is against their own preferences to be interminably sweet and agreeable: "They really don't want to just make other people happy."

In their interviews, Claudia and Linda allude to the consequences teenage women face if they shed the "nice girl" image and insist on keeping their own voices. The pressures to conform are often subtle, but are sometimes overt. For instance, Linda notes that she is often labeled "difficult" by teachers when she states her opinion. As a teen, I remember how girls who refused to relinquish their voices were ostracized. They were labeled "troublemakers" by adults and "bossy" or "weird" by peers.

Both co-researchers speak of the double standard society places on young women in regard to maintaining their own voices. Linda shares that the behavior others label as "difficult" is often viewed as a sign of strength and confidence in her male peers. She asserts that young women have two choices: conforming to society's mold of femininity and giving up one's sense of self, or insisting on one's own ideas and being chastised, insulted, or shunned by others.

Despite the sometimes painful consequences, both young women insist that fighting the pressure to conform and recognizing one's own uniqueness are powerful anti-depressive strategies. Each co-researcher has found her own way of resisting dominant culture and honoring herself. Claudia states that she found her way out of depression by learning to be "selfish." She defines this as "[making] yourself a priority. . . . Society and everyone says, 'Think of others before you,' but when it comes to your emotions and stuff, you should think of yourself and what's best for you." She also advises young women to choose friends who support their goals rather than society's. Linda adds that she fought depression in part by discovering her own spirituality. She proposes that other adolescent women should find ways to carve out their own unique, unconventional spirituality. Linda's and Claudia's stories enliven me as a therapist, particularly as a woman, to oppose dominant cultural and gender training. Their wisdom encourages me to pass it on to other young women who consult me. Both of us hope that Linda's and Claudia's knowledges will inspire others to engage in acts of political resistance.

EDITORIAL QUESTIONS

Q: *(CS) I appreciate your emphasis on having your clients both designated as "co-researchers"! I think this is such a positive new trend in psychotherapy research—treating clients as having valid perspectives on their own therapy that are worthy of recognition. I also like how you both use everyday, conversational ways of talking with Claudia and Linda.*

You explain that in your therapeutic conversations with Claudia, Linda, and other young women, you try to "unmask, identify, and externalize discourses that leave them vulnerable to depression." Could you talk about how you envision this making a difference in these girls' lives? When they leave the therapy office and go back out with their peers, for instance, what sorts of things do they say happen differently as a result of your conversations together? How do you understand this occurring? In other words, what do you see as a connection between identifying these social discourses and their ability to react in a different way?

A: By unmasking the discourses that may promote depression, we hope to counter young women's privatizing the problem to themselves—that is, seeing the problem as a reflection of their own identities. By externalizing and deconstructing, we invite young persons to consider that their depression is not the truth of their identity. Rather, depression is supported and maintained by patriarchal discourses. It is our experience that when young women view depression as a social construction and separate from themselves, they are better able to fight it effectively without self-blame. We then hope that the young women we work with will take the conversations they have with us and continue them with other adolescent women. This helps to break down the privatization of problems and to build support and community. Eventually, our hope is that locating the problem as social discourse will assist young women in more actively recognizing and resisting times when they feel their voices are silenced.

Q: *(CS) You speak briefly of additional ways to build "communities of concern" besides co-research, such as letter-writing and anti-problem leagues. You also point out how parents are sometimes inadvertently blamed or excluded from work with teens in a well-intended effort to help the teens individuate. How do you try to include parents in your work with teens? What sorts of reactions do they have to the sorts of conversations you had with Claudia and Linda? Are there ways you have discovered to help decrease the chances of polarization and increase opportunities for mutual connection regarding these controversial topics? Beyond family members, what sorts of support have the two of you invited (e.g., letters, etc.)?*

A: We like to include parents in the conversations. In fact, Linda's mother was present while I (DN) interviewed her. First, we like to ask the young women whom they would like to include in their meetings, and we try whenever possible to honor their choice. We may state that it may be important to include parents in at least some of the meetings, so as to bring them up to date with new developments. Most of the time, the young women think that it is a good idea to include the parents in at least some meetings.

We structure the meetings and the conversations in such a way that when one person (e.g., the young woman) is responding to our questions, the other person (e.g., a parent) is in a listening/reflective position and refrains from speaking at that time. This invites a parent or parents to hear their adolescent daughter in ways that they may not have heard before. In the past, they may have been too busy planning a response that would lead to unproductive, reciprocal patterns. This structuring of the conversations is intended to honor the young woman's voice.

We also encourage alternative conversations, through the practice of internalized-other questioning (Tomm, 1992; Nylund & Corsiglia, 1993). In this practice, each party takes on the identity of the other person while responding to a series of questions. This invites each participant to begin to understand the other's experience on an experiential level. Historically, family therapy has given more weight to the parent's voice. Narrative ideas help to balance the teenager's voice with that of the parents.

In addition to family members, we invite other audiences to respond to teens' struggles and triumphs over depression. The most common method involves the use of reflecting teams (Andersen, 1991). These teams are usually made up of our colleagues, and sometimes also of people who are significant to a teen (e.g., friends, doctors, or relatives). At times, "depression" is in attendance (sometimes a colleague will become/act as the voice of the "externalized" problem to add more voices to the dialogue/reflection).

We also help teens broaden their support network by inviting them to bring friends or adults who are particularly influential in their lives (e.g., coaches, teachers, pediatricians) to one or more of their therapy sessions. In addition, we work with teens to find their own creative ways of sharing their knowledge with others (e.g., advice letters or videotapes). In our experience, the act of advising others seems to solidify teens' stance against depression. We often collect and (with clients' consent) disseminate to other young clients the insights, observations, and anti-depression strategies of teens who work with us in therapy (clients' confidentiality is always honored and protected n these exchanges).

Lastly, we write letters to some clients (with their permission) in which we share our reflections about our recent conversation in therapy (White & Epston, 1990; Nylund & Thomas, 1994). This is yet another way that we can provide an audience for young women's triumphs against depression (especially when depression keeps them from acknowledging the more subtle gains).

Q: *(CS) I agree with you and your co-researchers that often women face powerful social invitations to accommodate to others at the expense of themselves. It also makes sense to me that this could be a recipe for depression, as you all demonstrate so effectively! You have persuasively documented some of the everyday pressures for teenage women to please others and ignore their own voices. Given that therapists' voices often carry special weight, what implications does this have for how you relate to these clients? Do you think that young women clients ever sense your own preferences for countering dominant social standards by the sorts of questions you ask? If so, how do you go about creating room for them to disagree with your own values, so that these don't inadvertently foster yet another standard for conformity? If a young woman stated her preference for prevailing gender stereotypes (e.g., using lots of makeup, dieting, etc.), how might you respond? How would you go about deciding whether to try to deconstruct and unmask this expression, or whether to honor and validate this as a genuine value preference?*

A: We are cognizant of the intentionality behind our questions about social discourses. We are also conscious of the fact that pushing a client to conform to a therapist's agenda is not respectful of the client, and therefore runs counter to our narrative philosophy. It is our opinion that therapists are not immune to communicating their philosophical biases to others. We feel that messages or therapeutic biases that remain invisible to the client have the most potential for harm. Therefore, we let our biases be known and invite the young women to evaluate and critique our ideas. Knowing that "people pleasing" is something young women are trained into, we invite them to disagree with us (another form of resistance!).

If a young person were to state her preference for practices in league with dominant discourses, we would be curious about how she has made that choice for herself and what meaning it has for her. We would remain open to the possibility that this is the young woman's own creative way of honoring herself (e.g., a young woman may be dressing up to please herself or wearing makeup as a means of personal expression and affirmation). We might state that sometimes it may be hard to know one's own choice, because dominant discourses are very powerful but sometimes invisible.

Our goal in questioning dominant cultural practices is not to censor young women's preferences, but to encourage them to broaden their repertoire of ideas and behaviors. Our intention is also to enhance teens' awareness of cultural messages that may have previously been invisible to them. Our hope is that this practice will give young women the freedom to choose which ideas they wish to embrace. Ultimately, we would honor a young woman's preference so as not to reproduce dominant cultural practices of power.

Q: *(CS) Before you heard of narrative therapies, how might you have worked with teenage girls dealing with depression? What were these ways like for you? For your clients? If you both were to imagine therapists from a more traditional background in working with teens reading your chapter, what sorts of reactions do you think they might have? If you were to reply to these imagined reactions from your heart, how might you respond?*
A: I (DN) worked from a strategic framework and would have primarily worked with the parents. I would have been interested in ways the parents were trying to respond to their daughter that became part of the problem. Then I would have been the expert who would advise the parents to "do something different" to break the problem pattern.

I (KC) would have been working from a cognitive-behavioral therapy perspective. My therapy would have focused on helping a young woman identify and then challenge "depressogenic beliefs." I would have educated her about the various "cognitive distortions" contributing to her depression, as well as possible strategies to combat them. I would then have given her homework assignments designed to reinforce the connection between cognitions and mood.

For both of us in our previous work, the discussion of depression would not have included an examination of cultural discourses. The work was decontextualized. In addition, we might have placed a great deal of importance on helping a teenager "get in touch with her feelings" (the catharsis discourse). Lastly, neither of us would have been transparent about our own knowledge, intention, or biases.

Our intention is not to attack traditional therapists' preferred ways of doing therapy, or to encourage them to stop doing what is working. Rather, we hope that our chapter will invite readers to incorporate a consideration of the larger sociopolitical factors supporting depression into their work; this is a neglected aspect of most therapy models. We also hope that our chapter invites readers to evaluate the possible effects, both positive and negative, of their theoretical orientations.

REFERENCES

Andersen, T. (Ed.). *The reflecting team: Dialogues and dialogues about the dialogues.* New York: Norton.

Dickerson, V. C., Zimmerman, J. L., & Berndt, L. (1994). Challenging developmental "truths": Separating from separation. *Dulwich Centre Newsletter,* No. 4, 2–12.

Freedman, J., & Combs, G. (1996). *Narrative therapy: The social construction of preferred realities.* New York: Norton.

Gilligan, C. (1982). *In a different voice: Psychological theory and women's development.* Cambridge, MA: Harvard University Press.

Gilligan, C., Rogers, A., & Tolman, D. (Eds.). (1991). *Women, girls, and psychotherapy: Reframing resistance.* New York: Haworth Press.

Griffith, J., & Griffith, M. (1994). *The body speaks.* New York: Basic Books.

Hare-Mustin, R. (1994). Discourses in the mirrored room: A postmodern analysis of therapy. *Family Process, 33,* 19–35.

Lobovits, D., & Seidel, E. C. (1994). *Relational co-research in narrative training and supervision.* Paper presented at Narrative Ideas and Therapeutic Practices: The 2nd Annual International Conference, Vancouver, B.C., Canada.

Madigan, S. (1996). The politics of identity: Considering community discourse in the externalizing of internalized problem conversations. *Journal of Systemic Therapies, 15*(1), 47–62.

Madigan, S., & Epston, D. (1995). From spy-chiatric gaze to communities of concern: From professional monologue to dialogue. In S. Friedman (Ed.), *The reflecting team in action* (pp. 257–276). New York: Guilford Press.

Nylund, D., & Corsiglia, V. (1993). Internalized other questioning with men who are abusive. *Dulwich Centre Newsletter,* No. 2, 29–26.

Nylund, D., & Corsiglia, V. (1996). From deficits to special abilities: Working narratively with children labeled "ADHD." In M. Hoyt (Ed.), *Constructive therapies* (Vol. 2, pp. 163–183). New York: Guilford Press.

Nylund, D., & Thomas, J. (1994). The economics of narrative. *Family Therapy Networker, 18*(6), 38–39.

Pipher, M. (1994). *Reviving Ophelia: Saving the selves of adolescent girls.* New York: Ballantine Books.

Stacey, K., & Loptson, C. (1995). Children should be seen and not heard?: Questioning the unquestioned. *Journal of Systemic Therapies, 14*(4), 16–32.

Taylor, J. M., Gilligan, C., & Sullivan, A. M. (1995). *Between voice and silence: Women, girls, race and relationship.* Cambridge, MA: Harvard University Press.

Tomm, K. (1992). *Interviewing the internalized other: Towards a systemic reconstruction of the self and other.* Workshop, California School of Professional Psychology, Alameda, CA.

Weingarten, K. (1991). The discourses of intimacy: Adding a social constructionist and feminist view. *Family Process, 31,* 285–305.

Weingarten, K. (1994). *The mother's voice: Strengthening intimacy in families.* New York: Harcourt, Brace.

Weingarten, K. (Ed.). (1995). *Cultural resistance: Challenging beliefs about men, women and therapy.* New York: Haworth Press.

White, M. (1995). *The life of the therapist: Inspiration in narrative therapy.* Workshop presented at Bay Area Family Therapy Training Associates, Cupertino, CA.

White, M., & Epston, D. (1990). *Narrative means to therapeutic ends.* New York: Norton.

Zimmerman, J. L., & Dickerson, V. C. (1996). *If problems talked: Narrative therapy in action.* New York: Guilford Press.

15

Sex, Drugs, and Postmodern Therapy
A TEEN FINDS HER VOICE

TOM HICKS

The intent of this chapter is to present some descriptions of a therapy that is consistent with the category "postmodern." In the postmodern spirit of diversity, I offer descriptions of a therapy loosely based upon some ideas of a postmodern, neopragmatist philosopher, Richard Rorty. Although I implicitly utilize many of the other ideas offered in this book, I hope that readers will find these additional assumptions useful.

Before describing any assumptive framework for therapy, however, I wish to emphasize that I seek to establish a collaborative context for therapy. This means deciding at each meeting, *along with the participants*, "Who will speak with whom about what?" (Andersen, 1991). This also includes consulting the clients about how they would want me to participate.

The chapter describes my conversations with Jody,[1] a 17-year-old female adopted teen with a history of rape, sexual molestation, drug

---

[1]This is a fictitious name to protect confidentiality, though she has consented to this telling of her story.

misuse, a very active sexual life, long-standing therapy, and resilience. She is also very intellectually gifted, having completed 2 years of college by age 16. Following an overview of my assumptive framework, the chapter is presented in two sections. In the first of these sections, I describe Jody's life up to the point before we began meeting together; I also present a theoretical discussion of our first eight meetings to demonstrate and explain my assumptive framework within various aspects of our therapy conversations. In the following section, to demonstrate my assumptions further, I provide a transcript of a portion of a recent meeting.

OVERVIEW OF ASSUMPTIVE FRAMEWORK

The claim that there is no neutral algorithm (any grid which can be referred to for deciding what knowledge can be considered to be objective reality) for deciding between beliefs in any given area is not equivalent to the claim that we cannot decide between beliefs. To deny the existence of such an algorithm is to argue merely that the reasons for or against a particular view cannot be determined in advance by reference to notions of truth, reality, or the moral law. They are rather determined in the course of conversation, with regard to the concrete advantages or disadvantages a given point of view has. Our reasons for taking up one scientific, political, or even aesthetic perspective as opposed to another are thus pragmatic rather than dogmatic; they are reasons debated in dialogue and open to revision or rejection depending upon what other options are advanced. . . . This means that issues are decided in discussion, in view of the importance of specific purposes and plans and hence in terms of what makes sense to the participants to the discussion themselves. The philosopher [read: therapist] as the ultimate arbiter of validity has no place. (Warnke, 1987, p. 152, describing the neopragmatist position of R. Rorty)

The therapeutic assumptions in this chapter draw heavily upon the quotation above. The chapter elaborates on and demonstrates three assumptions related to this quote, which can be very useful in helping therapists respond to their teen clients from a postmodern position. These assumptions are as follows: (1) Despite overwhelming obstacles, teens and those trying to help them are doing their best to make the teens' lives better; (2) teens should participate as fully as possible in therapeutic conversations, and should be consulted directly about the purposes and plans for their own lives and about which beliefs and ideas make sense to them; and (3) when teens are involved in such a dialogic speech context, the conversations evolve toward the teens' taking up more of a position of self-reflective agency in the discussions relating to their lives. Each of these assumptions is now examined separately below.

Assumption 1. Despite Overwhelming Obstacles, Teens and Those Trying to Help Them Are Doing Their Best to Make the Teens' Lives Better.

The first assumption has three separate parts to it. Each part delineates an important area of therapeutic conversation and is examined separately.

A. *"Despite overwhelming obstacles . . . "* What counts as an obstacle or problem for a particular teen should be determined by the teen in conversation with the therapist and others in the problem-organizing, problem-dissolving system (Anderson & Goolishian, 1988).[2] Some common obstacles that teens may cite may include rules, interference from adults in many areas of their lives, and having to attend school. A therapist does not educate or confront a youth about these, but instead tries to understand *how* this problem or obstacle is a problem for the teen. Despite giving an appearance of bravado, even teens who are told to go to therapy by others (e.g., parents, probation officers, school counselors) often feel like failures because they have not succeeded in contending with these challenging obstacles. While avoiding implicitly or explicitly blaming a teen, a therapist is empathetic in attempting to understand how the teen experiences these obstacles.

B. *". . . teens, and those trying to help them, are doing their best. . . ."* Despite the power of this feeling of failure on the part of teens and those around them, I assume that teens and those who care for them are doing their best to struggle against the obstacles or problems. Even when they appear to be completely defeated by these obstacles, teens are still trying their best not to allow these obstacles to defeat them further or to continue to "mess up" their lives. A therapist attempts to understand the magnitude of the obstacles that a particular teen is facing. After this, the therapist tries to appreciate and understand the teen's attempts to cope, or ways of coping, with the obstacles. I assume that teens are continually making these attempts. A therapist who is curious about these efforts will find many current attempts that the teen will say are having positive effects on his/her life and that can be further developed. Also, the thera-

---

[2]As stated by Anderson and Goolishian (1988), the therapeutic system is composed of those engaged in "relevant conversation" around a "problem or problems," rather than a social structure such as a "family system." Change is the evolution of new meanings through dialogue among those who make up the therapeutic system.

pist will identify along with the teen attempts the teen and others are making that are inadvertently producing effects the teen evaluates as making his/her life worse. The therapist can then invite the teen to consider whether these attempts are misguided and therefore obstacles to a better life.

    C. " . . . *to make the teens' lives better.*" A therapist and teen together can evaluate the "specific purposes and plans" the teen has for her/his life, and they can discuss whether the teen's attempts are producing positive effects that make her/his life better. When the teenager evaluates an attempt to struggle against the obstacle as itself making her/his life worse, then this attempt becomes viewed as an obstacle. For example, the youth may identify "not caring" as an attempt to deal with "parents who interfere," but may come to see after reflection that this "not caring" doesn't actually help the youth move toward what she/he wants in life. Once "not caring" is viewed as an obstacle blocking a better life, the therapist is curious about how the teen is trying, or would want to try, to struggle against this "not caring" in order to make her/his life better. Reflecting on what counts as a "better life" involves the teenager in becoming a self-reflective agent.

Assumption 2. Teens Should Participate as Fully as Possible in Therapeutic Conversations, and Should Be Consulted Directly about the Purposes and Plans for Their Own Lives and about Which Beliefs and Ideas Make Sense to Them.

The second assumption, in other words, is that teens become active participants in voicing their intentions, plans, and purposes for their own lives. They take an active part in the conversations that concern their future. In short, they are viewed as capable of participating in self-reflection, agency, and dialogue. This process can be very influential because teens can change the dialogue through their contributions to it and can be changed by it as well.

    Often teens' voices are not heard because they are not "rational." A modernist view of "rationality" suggests that assertions should be systematically justified with "objective" evidence. A postmodern view argues that the "rational" way is only one of the numerous ways in which humans can speak and by which they can become educated, informed, and enlightened. To disqualify another's or one's own speech because it is not "rational" means to limit one's own or another's prospects for "edification" (Rorty, 1979, p. 357). Our opportunities to be informed by others or to facilitate the self-informing of others or ourselves become restricted if we allow only "scientific" voices to be heard. To hear teens' voices, therapists must be willing to allow for parodic, poetic, or practical ways of speaking. They should listen for the sense rather than the non-sense in what has just been said, and should not close off potentially helpful ideas by not allowing "nonrational" voices into the dialogue. This attitude of acceptance from the therapist helps give birth to a nondogmatic speech context that invites dialogic creativity and thus facilitates the development of unexpected new meanings.[3]

Assumption 3. When Teens Are Involved in Such a Dialogic Speech Context, the Conversations Evolve toward the Teens' Taking Up More of a Position of Self-Reflective Agency in the Discussions Relating to Their Lives.

Dialogue is needed when an especially valuable kind of creativity is to take place. Dialogue constitutes the "field of answerability" in order to favor the open and free, the "unfinalizable"—the readiness for something new and original. So-called "objective," "scientific" discourses are constructed so as to restrict or ignore this dialogic possibility (Hitchcock, 1993).

To paraphrase Rorty (1979), for a teen to attempt to be different (i.e., not to comply with the norms of the day) without recognizing his/her own differentness (i.e., without understanding the prevailing norms) is madness in the most literal and terrible sense. So, as the dialogue proceeds, the teen moves toward increased self-reflection as the therapist invites the teen to understand, reply to, or answer the challenges of the "rational," "objective" voices in the conversation. These voices speak the current norms and expectations of our culture. Those who care for teens utilize these privileged cultural norms to evaluate how well adolescents are progressing in their lives.

Therefore, a therapist's aim is to assist a teen in understanding these norms—not in an attempt to encourage compliance to them or departure from them, but rather to assist the teen in *authoring a reply* to them.[4] Room is made in the conversation for preserving the legitimacy

---

[3]The work of M. M. Bahktin develops the notions of "dialogue" and "authorship," and is becoming a source of ideas for many postmodern therapists. Unfortunately, space does not permit the opportunity to explore in any detail Bahktin's ideas of how dialogue evokes new and unexpected meanings, and how monologue depends upon dogmatic authoritarianism to curtail dialogic possibilities (Hitchcock, 1993).

[4]This is very much an oversimplification of Bahktin's notion of "dialogism" and the relational nature of "selfhood." As Hitchcock (1993, p. xv) states, "The importance of the concept of **dialogism** is that it emphasizes the specific situations of dialogic exchange. The addressor, as Bahktin so ably showed, is strongly attentive to the perceived audience or addressee. . . . [dialogue] in its basic form denotes a relational capacity to selfhood (the addressor co-authors and is co-authored by the addressee)." [Italics added for emphasis].

of the teen's evolving preferences within a developing self-reflective position, which takes into account the norms and traditions currently voiced in the conversation.

In addition, teenagers initially experience obstacles as forces outside themselves (e.g., "They are making me unhappy," "School is making me unhappy"). But by reflecting on unsuccessful ways of coping with these obstacles, adolescents are able to shift their focus from outside forces to how they are coping with such forces. This can result in their resisting nonproductive reactions and further developing more helpful ones.

A BRIEF HISTORY OF JODY'S LIFE, AND A THEORETICAL DISCUSSION OF OUR FIRST EIGHT MEETINGS

History

Jody's mother described her from the age of 2 on as "manic," as having an extreme temper, and as constantly having outbursts. A videotape still exists that shows Jody at age 2 becoming frustrated and "pitching a fit." The notion that Jody was "manic" or somehow "mentally ill" followed her from this very young age, and at age 13 she saw her first psychiatrist. In fact, from the ages of 13 to 16 she visited several psychiatrists who described her in different ways, including "schizophrenic," "schizoaffective," and "manic–depressive." She told me that she heard voices at age 13 and that she was very scared by this. She was medicated with Thorazine and many other medications. The voices stopped shortly after they started and while Jody was taking Thorazine.

At age 10 Jody was molested by a neighbor for a period of months. At age 14 Jody was raped in a hotel room by three Marines. Shortly following this incident, she was raped again by an older male. After this she became very sexually active and began using drugs, mostly crystal methamphetamine. For the next 2 years (ages 14–16), Jody was engaging in promiscuous sex and using a variety of drugs. She also received various psychotropic medications in psychiatric treatment.

Jody dropped out of high school at age 14. However, because she is extremely intelligent, she got a general equivalency diploma, entered college, and was able to complete 2 years by age 16. Jody became pregnant at this age. Upon learning she was pregnant, she immediately discontinued all use of drugs and her sexual behaviors. She also immediately married the baby's biological father and quit college.

Approximately 6 months after Jody became pregnant, she came to see me for counseling. She came in because she "felt pretty good," despite never having "dealt with" being raped at age 14 or molested at age 10. Also, she said she had never "dealt with" the rest of her "past" (i.e., her history of drug use and promiscuous sex). Having spent considerable time in the psychotherapy culture, her primary thought at this time was that she might be "repressing" and "dissociating" her true feelings about her "past" and the traumas that occurred. Her mother strongly encouraged Jody to go to therapy because she understandably was very concerned that Jody was not "dealing with" the traumas and with her past problems.

The story that Jody was "mentally ill" was very powerful, and it suggested that "feeling pretty good," given everything that had been going on in her life, was probably a sign that something was deeply wrong with how she was coping with things. There was also an idea circulating that Jody's doing well now was the result of a hormonal change related to her pregnancy, which was masking a bipolar disorder; according to this idea, when she was no longer pregnant, she would again "go manic–depressive."

Theoretical Discussion of Our First Eight Meetings

This subsection integrates our first eight therapy conversations with the three assumptions discussed earlier.

Assumption 1

Part A. From the history above, it is obvious that Jody had many obstacles to contend with in her life. She coped with the trauma of molestation and two rapes through promiscuous sex and misuse of drugs. Upon reflection, Jody said that these ways of coping complicated rather than helped her situation. In addition, Jody's adoptive mother and father viewed her as "mentally ill," most probably "manic–depressive." From my perspective, her parents' story was a well-intentioned attempt to make sense of Jody's life and to try to make her life better by helping her get psychotherapy. Her "mental illness" was now being viewed by Jody and her parents as interfering with Jody's "working through" her traumas. But the only real evidence that she had not "worked through" these traumas was that she did not want to think about them or remember the details; she would rather put them out of her mind. Other than this, she felt she was doing well. When I asked her whether her mom and dad or her husband had other concerns right now, in addition to her not wanting to discuss or remember these details, she said they did not. But she did feel guilty because she had not "fulfilled her potential" in life, and because her family thought she was "mentally ill." From the perspective that she was mentally ill, if she did not "work through" her resistance to remembering and talking over the details of her traumas, she would become even more ill and would further fail to live up to her potential. Therefore, she was nervously seeking out help to talk about these traumas so she would not become "sicker," on the one hand; on the other hand, she was hoping to get her family "off her back" by at least coming to therapy. All of these factors contributed to her obstacles.

Part B. Jody felt that her overwhelming obstacles included (1) sexual molestation and rape, (2) a history of drugs and promiscuous sex, and (3) mental illness. I wondered what Jody and others were doing about these things. Jody said that she just "stopped drugs and sex" because she became pregnant and she wanted her baby to have a good life. She said that doing this was easy because she felt so strongly about her baby starting out life right.

As far as the sexual molestation and rape were concerned, she said she just did not think about them. But she said that part of what she did was to "get guys to like me and then just blow 'em off—hurt 'em real bad—it was like I had what they wanted and I had the power, and it felt good to make them suffer like I had to suffer." But she said that continuing this would be bad for her child, so she stopped it.

I wanted to know whether she had to fight hard against her "mental illness" for it not to mess up her life completely. She said, "No. It doesn't really bother me much. I'm thinking maybe it was more when I was younger, but now I feel fine. I really do." Then I thought out loud that maybe this notion that she was "mentally ill" was an outdated way to try to help or to make sense of things and didn't really make sense any more; maybe she was just a very resilient person who was able to handle what had happened to her sexually when she was younger. We then reviewed some obstacles in her life, with the idea in mind that maybe she was very resilient and a "forward-moving-type person." For example, Jody is part African-American and her adoptive parents are European-American. How had she handled this obstacle? "By not paying much attention to it," she said. We talked over how the videotape of her "pitching a fit" could be seen as her being very "strong" about knowing what she wanted and "persistent" about getting it. This strength and persistence showed up in how she tried to make herself feel better about the sexual traumas by getting revenge, even if now this did seem misguided. But could someone who was "mentally ill" just stop all this in order to give her child a good life?

The more we talked like this, the more it seemed to Jody that mental illness was not really one of her obstacles. However, she felt the story that she was "mentally ill" would be an obstacle that would limit her chances for a better life.

Jody liked these new ways of thinking about herself. They felt "true." She began to feel that she had lots of tools to try to make a good life for herself, and was feeling quite hopeful after a few meetings.

Part C. I invited Jody to evaluate the effects of her attempts (such as being forward-moving, strong, and persistent). Did these attempts produce effects that helped her have the kind of life she would want for herself? She was obviously a very determined and strong person; was she putting these qualities to use in a way that was getting her where she wanted to go? What was she doing that was making her life better, and what was she doing that was making it worse? Her basic reply was that she did not feel like reviewing everything (which fit with being forward-moving), but that she knew she was strong. She thought that maybe she was very emotionally upset in her life, but she was not mentally ill. She felt she knew that moving forward and trusting her strength was the thing to do, and that to go back and explore the traumas of her past right now would not be good for her.

Assumption 2

Jody wanted to work individually with me, because she felt that her parents were very invested in the idea that she was "mentally ill." Since Jody was married, I was able to do this without legal difficulty and to maintain the confidentiality that she felt was important. I did not speak with her parents until after the fourth session. After our fourth meeting, Jody wanted to have her parents in to see how her new ideas about herself would fit with their understandings. Jody wanted both of us to talk with her parents and get their perspectives, and then she would see what, if anything, she wanted to say to them about where her views might be different from theirs.

Both parents were very concerned about Jody, but encouraged at how well she had been doing. They gave a detailed history, highlighting those episodes that pointed to the idea that Jody was "ill," probably "manic–depressive." The mother explained that Jody might be doing better now because she had read that during pregnancy the biochemistry changes; after the baby was born, Jody could become "manic" again. We all discussed possibilities to try to make sense of Jody's "problems," including that perhaps she developed "dissociative identity disorder" at age 13 (because the voices she heard were experienced by Jody as coming from outside her head) as a result of her molestation at age 10. I suggested that perhaps she "integrated" these voices when entering adolescence, because she never heard the voices again after taking Thorazine. This idea seemed more promising, as her "sudden integration" put mental illness in the past, and both parents were open to it.

Jody sat back and listened; she did not challenge her parents' views at this time. She decided to wait and think about how to respond to this story her parents still held in their attempt to make sense of her. She felt it was understandable that her parents would hold this view of her, given her past, their values and beliefs, and the prominence of this framework in our culture for interpreting behavior. Jody also came to think that this story would continue unless she was able to have some "successes of my own."

Previously, her successes (including completing 2 years of college) had been interpreted as her parents' successes, because they helped so much that the credit for any success was given to their helping rather than Jody's efforts. In this way, their well-intended efforts to help made it more difficult to see her successes rather than her "mental illness." She became determined to identify some activities she could do on her own that would demonstrate both to herself and to her parents that she was not "sick." Jody's new sense of herself as "strong" and "forward-moving" was giving her the confidence she needed to attempt to overcome the obstacle of the *story* that she was "mentally ill."

Assumption 3

For conversations to move from monologues to true dialogue, the prevailing voice in the conversation must be answered by the voicing of a perspective that can account as well or better for the "brute facts" and yet is inconsistent with the prevailing voice. In many conversations in the West, the prevailing or dominant voice is the voice of "objective, scientific truth." This voice describes persons from the privileged perspective of expert knowledge, turning the persons and their lives into objects to be described. People's lives are authored by this "all-knowing" voice, and their utterances are subjected to its evaluation. But, instead, viewing a teen as a subject who is capable of generating valid self-descriptions that are inconsistent with the prevailing discourse, and then subjecting these self-generated descriptions to the teen's evaluations (rather than judging them against "objective" knowledge), bring the teen's voice into the conversation in an attempt to assist her/him in authoring a reply to the prevailing, disqualifying voice of so-called "objective" knowledge.

Jody planned to have her baby, doing as much as possible on her own, so that "I can know I did it and so my parents can see that too." In addition, she decided to do more problem solving on her own, although she would seek out her parents' input if she felt she needed it. She also began to assert to her parents that even if she had been mentally ill in the past, she wasn't now, and so they should just treat her as "normal." Her self-generated descriptions of being "forward-moving," "strong," and "determined" felt like a better account of her life, and she was able to "answer" the categorical descriptions generated by the prevailing story that she was "mentally ill." Finally, she was able to talk about the traumas as a way of demonstrating to herself and to her parents that she wasn't "repressing" them. Jody and I then took a long break from therapy after eight sessions.

TRANSCRIPT AND DISCUSSION
OF A RECENT MEETING

The portion of transcript presented here covers the last 15 minutes of our second session upon Jody's return to therapy after a 9-month break. She was now wondering how to deal with her concerns about her weight. I have selected this portion to demonstrate how the three assumptions discussed in this chapter can be utilized in therapeutic conversations.

After giving birth to her baby, Jody found she could not take off the unwanted pounds she had gained during pregnancy. She considered her "normal" weight to be about 175 pounds. She was now at 250 pounds.

JODY: This gastric bypass is pretty serious. I may never be able to have children again—women [who have this surgery] have children with an increased number of birth defects [later]. They would staple my stomach off and reduce it to the size of a golf ball.

TOM: So you're 250 pounds now, right? What would your life be like if you just said to yourself, "I'm just going to be 250 pounds"?

[My own inner conversation is that she is trying to fit into the current prevailing shape for women and seems very desperate to do this. I cringe inside as I listen to the lengths to which she may go in order to fit into the body shape that current cultural norms and medical science are voicing for her. I want to give voice to the notion of self-acceptance and invite her into dialogue with it and other voices in the therapeutic system that may have a perspective on the subject. I also want to check in with her to see if this voice of self-acceptance is already an inner voice that can be brought more into the conversation (Andersen, 1991).]

JODY: I can't—I'm just too fat. I know emotionally I have a problem with it. I'm tired. No energy . . . when I was thinner I had so much more energy. One hundred pounds more! The strain on my bones and joints— just getting up—it's a big effort, and I don't want to live at this weight.

TOM: So it's not so much motivated by wanting to just be attractive to men—like we talked about before—to please men . . .

JODY: Well, of course, you want to be appealing. But I want to be healthier—look and feel healthier. It's definitely an option for me to get this gastric bypass. I'm not losing any weight walking [she walks 3 miles a day at this time]. My mom thinks the bypass is a good option. "Phen-fen" [i.e., phentermine–fenfluramine drug therapy] won't work. The weight always comes back, I've heard.

TOM: So this gastric bypass is one of the best ideas so far, you're thinking now. . . .

[In terms of my assumptive framework, Jody's perceived obstacle to a happier and healthier life is "fat." Her attempts to contend with this obstacle have included walking, improved diet, contemplating medication, and considering this gastric bypass. In line with my assumptive framework, I intend to follow this question with more questions that may invite Jody into evaluating the possible effects of this operation on her life, but her next comment takes us there immediately.]

JODY: It's scary to me. It is. Like, I wouldn't want to be the one to be disabled by it or something. . . . Like, "I'm not fat any more, but I'm disabled!" (*Laughing*)

TOM: Do you see this fear as something to be listened to or as an obstacle to be overcome—or a little of both . . . ?

[I am wondering if the voice that is telling her that she is "too fat" is also telling her that fear of the surgery is an obstacle to health and happiness and needs to be overcome. But, as seen below, Jody can hear another voice when she is invited to reflect upon what she is hearing herself say in the conversation. Note that "fear," or any experience, can usefully be conceptualized as a perspective or voice participating in the dialogue.[5] Also, Andersen (1991) has described dialogue as evolving as participants hear themselves speak and respond with an "inner conversation" about their own and others' "outer conversation."]

JODY: A little of both. Almost as more something to listen to because it's almost as though my whole life I haven't listened to my fear, and I always end up taking the hard road—ya know? Just like with Jill [her 8-month-old baby]—I knew she would end up being a brat, sort of, by my trying this attachment parenting I'm doing with her.

[Here Jody is reflecting upon an attempt to parent that ignores this inner

---

[5]For an excellent discussion on the concept of "voice" related to therapeutic change, see Penn and Frankfurt (1994).

voice of fear. But in this reflection she is speaking in a new voice, which is saying, "Listen to your fear."]

TOM: So the fear initially said, "Don't do this attachment parenting," and you didn't pay attention to that?

JODY: That's right.

TOM: Is it kind of like the fear is your intuition or something . . . ?

[The fear appears to be a newly identified resource that she can use in her attempts to deal with any obstacle in her life. I want to find words with her to further describe and develop this potentially useful resource or perspective.]

JODY: Yeah. Or intelligence (*laughing*). Because it's usually right—you know? I just usually go right against it.

TOM: Hmm. So learning to listen to yourself a little better, then?

JODY: Yeah. Give myself some credit for knowing more.

TOM: So is the idea that this fear or intelligence could be saying something you should listen to, and [is it saying] for you to go slowly in deciding about this gastric bypass? Try to weigh out what your fear or intelligence is saying . . . ? So is this your usual way of going about things to pay attention to this fear?

JODY: No! (*laughing*)

TOM: So that's different for you to do that?

JODY: Uh-huh. Just like when I got married, for example. I got pregnant. I thought, "My God, I need prenatal care. I better get married." That's my mindset. Duh. Duh. So stupid!

TOM: Kind of like an impulse . . .

JODY: Exactly—that's what my whole life has been—one big impulse (*laughing*).

TOM: So rushing into this gastric bypass would be like . . .

JODY: Rushing into life is Jody. Rushing into life. . . . I have the ability to sit there and figure this out, but I just rush into it, and so I said, "I gotta get married!" I didn't consider government aid or anything . . . just rushed in . . .

[Here she has clearly identified a voice/perspective that has informed her attempts to deal with obstacles in her life. The voice says "Rush!" Upon reflection here, she is realizing that her life gets worse instead of better when she listens to it and ignores her inner voice of fear/intelligence.]

TOM: Was this fear/intelligence telling you, "Don't rush into this"?

[I am beginning to sense that perhaps Jody's history can be thought of in terms of her not trusting her own inner voice to help guide her attempts to deal with obstacles. Like a faithful friend, it has been there trying to speak to her. It has been drowned out by the suggestions of outer, "authoritative" voices telling her that something about her is a deficit[6] and that she needs to "rush and fix yourself now!"]

JODY: Yeah. But that voice is so quiet, compared to "Rush! Rush! Rush!" When I was younger, guys would pull up in cars and I would get in—just go—every day!

TOM: I'll bet there was a little something that said, "Don't do this." Was there?

JODY: (*Imitating a voice saying:*) "Hello! Jody! You're so psycho. They could hurt you—kill you—rape you." But I was just "Whatever!" Just really impulsive.

TOM: To rush into this gastric bypass would be that same kind of impulsive stuff?

JODY: And I'm too scared of the consequences of something like this— you know?

TOM: (*Ending the session*) Well, it sounds like that voice inside you—of taking care of yourself is getting louder now? (*Laughter*)

JODY: Yeah, that's why I look at Jill and she needs a schedule, or she'll turn out like me! (*Laughing*)

TOM: Sounds like one of the big problems in your life has been this "rushing into things." But you're changing this now . . .

[In our next meeting I plan to share with Jody my own inner conversation about this gastric bypass. I will tell her that my sense is that somehow she is vulnerable to certain kinds of suggestions. Suggestions that she is in some way "not good enough" seem to trigger this voice of "Rush! Rush! Rush!," which can drown out her own inner voice of fear/intelligence. In terms of the framework presented, Jody's attempts to deal with her obstacles will be more informed and balanced and will produce more of the effects she desires as she develops her ability to listen not only to outer voices, but also to the voices within herself.]

---

[6]As Gergen (1991, p. 13) states regarding the rapid proliferation of "deficit discourse" in Western culture, "the vocabulary of human deficit has undergone enormous expansion within the present century. We have countless ways of locating faults within ourselves and others that were unavailable to even our great-grandfathers."

CONCLUSION

The assumptions described in this chapter for working with teens attempt to enlist them in a project of becoming self-reflective agents actively authoring their own lives. Primary obstacles standing in the way of such a project are ways of speaking about teens as objects to be described, rather than as subjects capable of generating self-reflective self-descriptions of the specific plans and purposes for their own lives. Therapists utilizing privileged sets of categorical descriptions that subordinate the teens' utterances to expert evaluation can result in the teens' losing their own voices. Therefore, therapists enlist teens in a project of agency by encouraging the teens to generate their own descriptions of their lives as answers to any "official," "all-knowing" discourse. This can help youth claim responsibility and find their own voices in ongoing conversations about their next steps in life.

EDITORIAL QUESTIONS

Q: *(CS) I really like the idea of helping teenagers develop a more adequate reply to dominant expectations for their lives! This seems to address two major concerns: helping youth to become more responsible, and also facilitating the blossoming of their unique preferences and abilities.*

You speak of assisting adolescents in gaining "more of a position of self-reflective agency in the discussions relating to their lives." This suggests to me an openness to considering many different voices or perspectives, including predominant expectations that they conform to certain social standards. You seem to be more attuned to helping clients sort out their reactions to these different perspectives than to encouraging them to challenge particular voices or stories. For example, you asked Jody, "Do you see the fear [about the gastric bypass] as something to be listened to, or as an obstacle to be overcome—or a little of both . . . ?" Does this "sorting out" fit with what you are saying?
A: Yes—sorting out and enriching the conversation about the subject being discussed through locating and generating additional perspectives or voices. I'm always trying to stimulate additional perspectives, while slowing down the conversation so that these more silent inner voices can be heard. The more perspectives there are interacting around the subject under discussion, the richer the attempts to deal with the obstacles can become. Also, the more voices there are in the conversation, the more perspectives there are to help discern whether or not something should even be considered an obstacle.

As far as "encouraging them to challenge particular voices or stories" is concerned, I'm very interested in the process of locating or generating more voices to participate in the conversation, which then often results in these voices challenging the dominant voices. I am very interested in clients locating any voices that give them the experience of personal agency.

Q: *(CS) Part of our goal in this book is to share a wide variety of approaches using a narrative metaphor, so that readers can sense the range of possibilities in doing this sort of work. I'd like to tease out some of the differences and similarities between your work and that of others, so that readers can distinguish relevant assumptions. You use externalizing conversations (e.g., the one about "the fear," mentioned above), and you also help teens evaluate the positive and negative effects of their attempts to cope with obstacles. In addition, you speak of eliciting the "purposes and plans for their own lives." These all seem consistent with the re-authoring approach that Michael White and David Epston have developed.*

On the other hand, you don't discuss problem-saturated stories and alternative stories, the relative influence each of these stories has, or unique outcomes that can be used to re-story lives. You seem to be emphasizing helping adolescents become more responsible, dialogic participants in life. From your perspective, does this differ from a deconstructive, re-authoring approach? How do you see your work as compared with other narratively oriented approaches?

A: My intent is to stimulate dialogue in a conversational context that was previously monologic. Identifying and naming dominant voices in the conversation enables them to be set apart from the person's identity and creates room for a reply to be generated. I'm not thinking about deconstructing dominant stories. I'm thinking about facilitating my client in hearing what the dominant voices in the conversation are saying, identifying them along with the client, and inviting the client to become curious about the effects of listening only to that voice while ignoring his/her own inner voices. If the client finds these effects not to his/her liking, then inner voices can be further developed to reply to the dominant voices. The overall outcome I would hope for in therapy would be that the client comes to regard his/her own experience with increasingly respectful curiosity.

I suppose this would differ from a re-authoring approach in that my aim is not the creation of new stories, but the facilitation of dialogue. When dialogue is achieved, new stories are the result. I would hope that one outcome of this way of working is to assist people in responding to future situations in their lives with respect for the richness of both their inner and their outer experiences.

Q: *(CS) As you are familiar with, there seem to be differing ideas within the narrative community about how therapists should position themselves toward sociocultural stories. What sorts of reactions do you have about this? I notice that you didn't seem to invite Jody directly to challenge stereotypical notions about the necessity for losing weight for women to be acceptable. You said in response to her (and her mother's) idea for this serious, irreversible operation, "So this gastric bypass is one of the best ideas so far, you're thinking now . . ." Can you share some of what informed this response? Why didn't you invite her to challenge the gender assumptions leading to consideration of this operation? How do you see your role in regard to sociocultural expectations?*

A: If I have a strong reaction to a client's attempting to alter her/his life or relationships to fit with dominant sociocultural expectations—because of issues of personal safety, for example—I will tell the client. I will tell the client in the spirit of creating dialogue with my idea, and, most importantly, I will be open to changing my reaction. I don't usually "take a stand" for or against sociocultural stories as much as share my own inner conversation tentatively while remaining open to changing it if the client feels it doesn't serve her/him. I believe this position is consistent with my intent to create a dialogic speech context as opposed to a dogmatic one.

Of course, in the case of life-threatening situations, I must take a stand to insure safety or I would risk negligence. But I state this stand and my limits in terms of my own needs to continue functioning as a therapist within the standards of the professional community in which I practice. I would contrast this to steering clients toward my preferred stories for their lives without openly stating that I am encouraging them to conform to my preferred values.

In saying to Jody, "So this gastric bypass is one of the best ideas so far, you're thinking now. . . .", I was stating it as "unfinalized" (i.e, "so far," "you're thinking now"). Right after this she said, "It's scary to me." Facilitating the full expression of the voice directing her to have this operation, rather than challenging it or "taking a stand" against it, helped her generate a reply to it within her. The reply was her fear/intelligence saying that she may be disabled by this operation. Her voice of fear/intelligence not only began to challenge this operation, but began to speak about other times in her life when she "rushed" into something that made her life worse. I don't think challenging sociocultural expectations would have produced such a highly personal and effective answer to this voice telling her to have the surgery.

I see my role regarding sociocultural expectations as one of encouraging this voice to speak openly, of clearly identifying it, and of creating a context in which responses to it can be generated. Once this voice and the effects it will produce are more obvious to the client, the client is in a position to evaluate whether or not he/she wants this for his/her life.

Q: *(CS) If Jody hadn't shared her fears, and had said she definitely wanted to go ahead with this life-changing operation, how might you have responded? Are there any circumstances in which you might be open and transparent with a client about your own concerns and biases?*
A: I usually am open about my biases and concerns, and speak openly about how I feel these might influence how I participate in therapy. So, if Jody had not shared her fears and had said she was going to have this surgery, I would have told her that I was not comfortable with it and that she should know that this feeling would steer me toward trying to talk her out of it. I could have talked with her about what it would be like for her to have me do this, and asked her to tell me if she wanted me to back off. My openness about my biases and willingness to stop pushing them when she asked would have let me know I had done what I could for her safety without interfering with her right to do as she wished.

REFERENCES

Andersen, T. (Ed.). (1991). *The reflecting team: Dialogues and dialogues about the dialogues.* New York: Norton.

Anderson, H., & Goolishian, H. (1988). Human systems as linguistic systems: Preliminary and evolving ideas about the implications for theory and practice. *Family Process, 27,* 371–393.

Gergen, K. (1991). *The saturated self.* New York: Basic Books.

Hitchcock, P. (1993). *Dialogics of the oppressed.* Minneapolis: University of Minnesota Press.

Penn, P., & Frankfurt, M. (1994). Creating a participant text: Writing, multiple voices, narrative multiplicity. *Family Process, 33(3),* 217–232.

Rorty, R. (1979). *Philosophy and the mirror of nature.* Princeton, NJ: Princeton University Press.

Warnke, G. (1987). *Gadamer: Hermeneutics, tradition, and reason.* Stanford, CA: Stanford University Press.

16

Re-Authoring Problem Identities

SMALL VICTORIES WITH
YOUNG PERSONS CAPTURED
BY SUBSTANCE MISUSE

COLIN SANDERS

Peak House is a program of the Pacific Youth and Family Services Society, Vancouver, British Columbia, Canada. Peak House is a nonprofit, government-funded program. It was started in 1988 as a traditional chemical dependence treatment program, and has evolved in a narrative direction since that time. The program is voluntary, coed, and residential; lasts for 8 weeks; and takes clients aged 13–19.

In my work at Peak House, all too often I find that young persons and family members enter the program under the influence of a variety of problem discourses. In effect, their experience and relationships, and their dreams of future possibilities, have been colonized by the problems. Commensurate with this is a kind of overwhelming of their lives by a cadre of well-meaning problem solvers, consisting of various members of the helping professions (be they therapists, psychologists, psychiatrists, social workers, or teachers). Among the problem discourses that have successfully entered into the lives and relationships of many of these young persons, I would include such descriptions as "addict," "alcoholic," "manic–depressive," "depressed," and "anorexic/bulimic." In addition, many families describe themselves as being "dysfunctional" and "multiproblemed." Within the predominant sociopolitical context, the presenting problem has become identified as one of "substance abuse." Accordingly, many of the young persons have a sense of their identity as being represented by the label "addict/alcoholic."

Within the lived experience of most of the young persons with whom I have collaborated, substance misuse becomes problematic within the context of their lives and relationships. At Peak House, we imagine our work with young persons and their families as entailing a collaborative adventure intent upon dissolving the impoverishment that occurs when people are oppressed or overwhelmed by difficulties, dilemmas, and discord within their lives.

I have written elsewhere (Sanders & Thomson, 1994; Sanders, 1994, 1995) of the evolution of our ongoing attempts to co-create with clients counterpractices to traditional drug and alcohol interventions within the lives of young persons and families. Significantly, the practices we engage in and utilize are practices young persons themselves have had a hand in creating. We consider these practices to be more effective than practices that omit such collaboration. Our practices are not imposed from above, but instead reflect ideas, solution knowledges, and wisdom evolving out of consultation with those seeking our services. Increasingly, this way of working has made more sense, has been less coercive, and has assisted many more clients in becoming liberated from the oppression of substance misuse and the restraints associated with particular diagnoses and labels.

For the purposes of this chapter, it may be useful to be aware of the following points, as contained within our program brochure:

Peak House Program Philosophy:

- We believe that *the problem* of substance misuse can disappear when young persons, together with their families and other concerned persons, join in creating solutions.
- We believe that young persons can rediscover stories about their lives that challenge the story that they have defective identities.
- We believe that change is inevitable, and that making change to create a difference in one's life is hard work.

Our Approach:

- We collaborate with young persons, families, and other concerned persons in assisting to separate clients from *the problem of substance misuse.*
- How we assist depends upon the uniqueness of the young per-

son, but our focus is always on moving forward with wisdom, knowledge, abilities, and strengths the young person has.

• In consulting with former clients, we have learned that working toward change with young persons without regard to family, care providers, and other community support is most often ineffective.

DEFICIT IDENTITIES AND THERAPEUTIC VIOLENCE[1]

For many of the young persons with whom we consult, there are innumerable pressures, expectations, and desires contending for, and shaping, their attention. In addition to family members', educators', and peers' expectations, there are complex sociocultural discourses. For example, a predominant psychological discourse insists that young persons should have achieved certain milestones at specific points or stages in their lives. This thinking is perhaps best exemplified in the work of Erik Erikson (1963). Based upon conversations with many young persons and families, my own thought is that this kind of sociocultural discourse can create a sense of inadequacy within a young person, and that this sense may hook up with all kinds of other problems to influence the young person into thinking of herself/himself as incompetent, unworthy, less than others, and so on. The sense of inadequacy can also have an enormous impact upon the thinking and behavior of the young person's mother and father, who may start to doubt their parenting abilities, or become convinced by the problem that they should come down hard on the young person.

Another example of this occurs with many clients (young persons and adults alike) who have informed me that they have "addictive personalities."[2] Having been entered into by this sort of identity descrip-

---

[1] For the importance of an ethical therapeutic practice, see the distinction between therapeutic violence and therapeutic love—an original idea of Maturana and Varela (1987), as developed by Tomm (1990a).

[2] Rachel T. Hare-Mustin and Jeanne Marecek (1996) have recently added their voices to those critiquing formal diagnostic labels as debilitating of persons' purposes in life, and as serving "to mystify everyday experience." The "anti-psychiatrist" Thomas Szasz (1970, p. 203) was one of the first to speak against these practices of therapeutic violence, when he wrote: "The diagnostic label imparts a defective personal identity to the patient; it will henceforth identify him [sic] to others and will govern their conduct toward him, and his toward them. The psychiatric nosologist thus not only describes his [sic] patient's so-called illness, but also prescribes his future conduct." The ramifications of this kind of therapeutic violence have been horrifying for many persons who have experienced the debilitating and totalizing effects of diagnostic labels in terms of self-blame, self-loathing, and intense self-monitoring. See also Tomm (1990b).

tion, many people experience a kind of paralysis or immobilization when considering alternative possibilities for making a difference in their lives. Many people begin to think that there are biological reasons why they cannot make changes in their lives, and that their "personalities" have been predetermined genetically. In such situations, personal agency becomes subjugated and oppressed. Self-doubt often becomes a lingering presence within these persons' experience, casting aspersions on their ability to evade or ignore denigrating voices.

For a young person captured by the lifestyle substances offer, there is always a possibility that in seeking assistance against the influence of substances, the young person (and the family) may become pathologized. Although this is not always the case, it is a situation that occurs often enough. I recall a conversation with a young woman who at 17 years of age had experienced a number of candidate identities. At certain points in time, influenced by experiences of violence and by engendered and internalized "bad girl" and "unworthy person" thoughts, she was often overtaken by the thought that she could never be anything but an "alcoholic/addict." In the course of several conversations with her, I expressed an interest in how she accounted for her ability sometimes to step outside of this identity, and to speak out and stand up to the "negative voices" that attempted to confuse her and convince her she was condemned. Within the narrative of her life at a certain point in time, this identity became the totality of her experience; yet there persisted a barely audible[3] voice within her that persevered in its attempt to keep alive the possibility that there were alternative, and preferred, ways to be in the world. Within the collaborative context of Peak House, she rediscovered a safe, trustworthy space in which she could enter into dialogue with this other, barely audible voice, imagining aloud *worthy* ways of being, and making meaningful connections with others in the world.

I often find that when a young person enters Peak House, there exists a monologic relationship between the person and the problem. That is, the problem's voice and influence have come to dominate and oppress the person, placing severe constraints upon the person's ability to relate to others and to access his/her own knowledge and wisdom. The

---

[3]Mary Catherine Bateson (1994, p. 64) writes,

> Within the framework of Western assumptions, we begin to know a little about how the self is differentiated from others, how it takes shape for males and females, the kind of resilience associated with it. A wide range of pathologies have been associated with flawed attitudes toward the self: lack of self-esteem on the one hand and narcissism on the other. Physical violence and sexual abuse deform the sense of self, or split it into multiples. So do insult and bigotry. *So does invisibility or the realization that in a given context one is inaudible.* (Emphasis added)

problem has left no space for the possibility of alternative, barely audible voices to break through. This monologic relationship is hierarchical and imposing, and is representative of the problem's power over the person. This way of being is both subjugating[4] and disqualifying of the person's courage, determination, commitment, and solution knowledges. If the problem is substance misuse, and the person has become subjugated to the intentions of the problem, the effects are often detrimental and sometimes lethal.

RESTRAINING BELIEFS AND LIBERATING EXPERIENCES

As mentioned above, at Peak House many young persons enter into the program heavily influenced with previously constructed identities as "alcoholics" or "addicts." Often enough, these diagnoses have served to provide a form of identity to them, complete with a belief system and guidelines for personal conduct (e.g., the Twelve Steps of Alcoholics Anonymous [AA]). In a respectful fashion, our practice is to wonder how the persons were initially invited or recruited into such an identity, and whether or not this particular way of understanding themselves works for or against their purposes in life. In conversation with the young persons and their families, I will wonder who initiated or assisted in the composition and storying of such an identity, and just what the real effects of this identity have been upon the persons relative to actions they can or cannot accept as their own, thoughts they can or cannot accept as their own, and so on. I am always curious regarding the rules or guidelines associated with these manufactured identities, and will ask questions such as these: "With whose authority do these rules speak? How is it that you have sometimes questioned the authority of these rules in reclaiming your life from substance misuse? When you have re-

---

[4]Michel Foucault (1980, p. 81) wrote of the liberating re-visioning of the histories of medical and penal practices that occurred with the *"insurrection of subjugated knowledges"* (emphasis in original). He referred to these knowledges and histories as "disqualified," "marginal," "low-ranking knowledges" (1980, p. 82). Inspired by the work of Epston and White in this area (see Madigan, 1992, for an explication of White's utilization of Foucault's ideas), many of us have taken to referring to aspects of our work as involving the documentation of alternative, "subjugated" knowledges and wisdoms, as witnessed through the conversations and actions of clients. Recently, consumers of substance misuse services in British Columbia have compiled documentation from their own youth-initiated project as to what kinds of services are effective and what sorts of services are required (see Caputi & Mullins, 1995).

claimed moments of your life, and have a sense of increased confidence in yourself, do drugs start a more intensive campaign to get you back again?"

My intention in such conversations is to bring forth an externalization of the restraining aspects of the identity, while at the same time internalizing a sense of personal agency (Tomm, 1989). In other words, what is it the persons have done for themselves—alone or in conjunction with others—that has liberated them from restraining thoughts and behavioral patterns, and has expanded the horizon of their experience in the world? In my experience, I encounter many young persons for whom the AA philosophy has become unacceptable as an effective way of addressing the problem of substance misuse. For such persons, we have found the following questions to be useful in testing the authority and truth claims offered up by acceptance of such opinions, and in opening entry points for alternative stories involving intentionality, empowerment, and personal agency.

- Who helped you begin to think of yourself as an "alcoholic" and/or "addict"?
- What meaning is there in these words for an understanding of your life?
- Do you imagine this to be hereditary identity, or did some members of your (extended) family refuse this identity?
- Do others in your life know you as an "alcoholic/addict," or as someone else?
- Does this identity hold you back from certain thoughts, desires, values, and actions?
- What intentions does this identity have for your life?
- Do you have other intentions for the paths your life could take?
- Do your own intentions sometimes get clouded or overshadowed by the intentions that follow from this identity?

Many young persons believe that being an "alcoholic" or an "addict" involves a lifelong experience of being "in recovery." This can be an overwhelming prospect, suggesting that no matter what else changes within the context of their lives, they will never be in a position to practice moderation in their substance use. This prospect makes no sense to the majority of young persons with whom I have worked.

Many young persons do not have their lives and relations taken over by substances because they are possessed by so-called "addictive personalities"; nor is such colonization explained by theoretical perspectives arguing for a genetic predisposition or for family-of-origin transmission. Increasingly, in conversation with young persons, I am informed that substances have infiltrated their lives in contexts where there has been a history of exploitation, whether emotional, physical, or sexual; where there has been a history of oppression relative to the effects of racism and ethnic bigotry; and where there has been a struggle against homophobia. In such instances, chronic and severe substance misuse arises not out of a biological and genetic etiology, but out of a sociocultural and sociopolitical context of human relations. The desire to misuse substances to obliterate pain and suffering associated with exploitative lived experiences is a comprehensible one.

SITUATING THE "ALCOHOLIC/ADDICT" SELF WITHIN THE SOCIOPOLITICAL CONTEXT OF ADDICTION MYTHOLOGY

Acceptance of the dominant identity "alcoholic/addict" becomes problematic for some young persons, in that it limits the range of alternative possibilities in their lives. For some, it situates them as victims of an illness or disease. As such, this may restrain not only their thinking in relation to themselves, but the ways they are viewed by others, such as peers and family members. For example, Kaminer (1992, p. 28), in her investigation of the recovery movement, found a "pervasive fascination with victimhood as a primary source of identity"; she suggests that the recovery movement is yet another example of that peculiarly North American penchant for "personal development fashions" (p. 27). Delving into psychology's wealth of "developmental" theories[5] providing the intellectual presuppositions behind such fashions, Kaminer (1992, p. 59) especially highlights Maslow's "rhetoric about individual wholeness and autonomy," and the effects this ideology has upon persons as they struggle in pursuit of culturally manufactured ideals specifying current norms representative of "perfection," "beauty," "status," "intelligence," and so on.[6]

Situating this rhetoric historically, Cushman (1995, p. 224) writes

---

[5]Examples include theories such as Erik Erikson's (1963) psychosocial stages of human development, and Kohlberg's (1969) stages of moral development. For engaging critiques of these and other theories, see Gilligan (1982), Flax (1990), Dickerson, Zimmerman, and Berndt (1994), Weingarten (1992), and Hare-Mustin and Marecek (1994, 1996).

[6]David Epston has done much to deconstruct the often harmful and destructive thoughts that enter into young persons' lives as they attempt to "measure up" to great sociocultural expectations and ambitions. Questions David has asked that I find particularly useful are ones like these: "How long have you lived under the curse of perfection?" and "What ef-

that in the United States, "Youthfulness, expressiveness, personal entitlement, self-centeredness, acquisitiveness, self-confidence, optimism
[were] some of the qualities that describe[d] the new developing spirit of
the postwar era." Cushman suggests that humanistic psychology promoted "a preoccupation with 'the self,' its natural qualities, its growth,
its 'potential,' *abstracted out of and removed from the sociopolitical*"
(p. 240 emphasis added). Accordingly, "the self of humanistic psychology was subjective, often antitraditional, ahistorical, and preoccupied
with individualist concerns such as personal choice, self-realization, and
the apolitical development of personal potential" (p. 243).

For many young persons, substance misuse is not the problem; the
problem has much to do with socially constructed contexts related to
experiences surrounding their gender, race, class, culture, sexuality,[7] and
so on. Based upon this shared knowledge, I propose that serious, chronic substance misuse arises as an effect of socioeconomic, sociocultural
politics of experience, often compounded by existentialist dilemmas[8]
contributing to impoverished lives. As such, the suffering associated
with substance misuse does not arise, or continue to exist, within a vacuum; it is founded upon lived experiences and relations with others.

SITES OF COLLABORATIVE ENGAGEMENT

This more collaborative way of engaging with young persons and families against the problem's influence represents a respectful, compassion-
ate way of being with others. This is counter to traditional, coercive,
confrontative approaches that couch their practices in language that
speaks with so-called "scientific" validity and authority—a language
suggesting "truthful" expert opinion and assuming theoretical impar-

fects have you suffered in life under this curse?" Michael White (1995b) has also critiqued
humanistic psychologies that suggest we can always achieve more: "Many of us are relatively successful at torturing ourselves into a state of 'authenticity' and, in so doing, reproducing the 'individuality' that is so venerated in this culture" (p. 140).

[7]See Michael White (1995a, p. 4): "The culture of therapy is not exempt from the politics
of gender, race, class, age, ethnicity, sexual preference, etc.,"; "The culture of therapy is
not exempt from the structures and ideologies of dominant culture."

[8]In a future paper, I would like to further develop Levinas's (1995) accounting of Heidegger's "analysis of 'anguish' as the fundamental mood of our existence. Heidegger brilliantly described how this existential mood . . . revealed the way in which we were attuned to
Being. Human moods, such as guilt, fear, anxiety, joy or dread, are no longer considered
as mere physiological sensations or psychological emotions, but are now recognized as the
ontological ways in which we feel and find our being-in-the-world, our being-there" (p.
181).

tiality. Michael White (1995b) has been specific regarding the narrative metaphor's position on the dangerous myth of therapeutic neutrality. He writes:

> Rather than trafficking in those metaphors that encourage therapists to assume objectivity, and to step into a formal vocabulary of language that emphasises a posture of therapist spectatorship and impartiality, the metaphor of narrative emphasises the constitutive nature, or the life-shaping nature, of all interactions. This discourages us from entertaining the illusion of neutrality, and from proposing an innocent bystander status for ourselves. (P. 218)

In addition to the kinds of conversations and questions outlined above, such collaboration can take a variety of other forms. For example, in a recent teaching experience, I invited a number of young persons to come and share their thoughts in regard to ways they had come to "escape" problem identities in their own lives. Following the consultation, one of the participant therapists, also a university professor of family therapy, exclaimed, "Wow! It's never occurred to me to have some young persons come into class and assist in teaching. I always deferred to the parents in terms of whether the therapy was useful or not."

In other public contexts, I continue to learn from young persons about ways in which their experiences have been disqualified, minimized, and marginalized. Recently Sarah, 19 years old, who had escaped a problem lifestyle ("junkie" and "slut"), co-presented a narrative therapy and substance misuse workshop with myself and other counselors from Peak House. According to Sarah, age has much to do with ways in which youth knowledge becomes disqualified by experts. In Sarah's experience with some professionals, there had been an unspoken yet distinct hierarchical relationship. During one such encounter, the counselor (a psychiatrist), following 20 minutes of questioning, had labeled Sarah with a diagnosis of "borderline."

Jana, also 19, co-presenting at the same workshop, spoke of her experiences of being "patronized" by various professionals because of her age, but also described how she had been affected by their "judgmental" attitudes toward her use of narcotic drugs. For Jana, the marginalization she experienced in the therapy was explained by a professional attitude that "there must be something wrong" with her, in order to explain why substances had infiltrated her life. For Jana, her misuse of substances had more to do with wanting to erase the memories of sexual exploitation and violence she had experienced within her family. Jana, whose father was East Indian (i.e., *from India*) and whose mother was First Nations, also spoke of racism's effects on her as she was growing up in an isolated rural community of British Columbia.

IN MEMORY OF EDWIN[9]

Edwin was a Chinese man whose parents had immigrated to Canada; he entered Peak House struggling with a variety of complex dilemmas, which included serious heroin misuse. The first time I spoke with Edwin, he had come for a visit to Peak House to gain some understanding of the program and to see whether it was the kind of place he might be comfortable talking about the "troubles" affecting him. That first afternoon Edwin came with his mother, and as he and I spoke he translated from English into Cantonese, as neither his mother nor his father spoke English.

A significant part of Edwin's struggle to exist was bound up with his attempt to straddle two very different cultural landscapes—his parents' strong traditional Chinese values and beliefs, and the norms of Vancouver's predominant (white, middle-class) culture. In a number of conversations, Edwin spoke of the distress (and sometimes despair) he suffered in attempting to combine and reconcile these two diverse cultures within his life. Edwin spoke of the racist attitudes, and lack of knowledge regarding other cultures, that he often encountered within the predominant culture. Edwin also spoke of the hostility he sometimes faced from members of this culture, especially peers.

Edwin spoke eloquently regarding the effects of "loneliness" within his life. According to Edwin, loneliness spoke the loudest when "misunderstanding" infiltrated his life, driving a wedge between himself and his parents and siblings. The effects arising from misunderstanding were particularly disconcerting and confusing for Edwin.

Approximately 1 year following this conversation, Edwin died. For those of us who were inspired by his courage and humor, we will never know exactly what forces conspired against him. From the fragments we have been able to learn about his final few weeks, we understand that heroin did make an intense comeback in his life. It is entirely possible that heroin successfully recruited misunderstanding and loneliness in its efforts to erase Edwin's commitment to life.

---

[9]Edwin, (a pseudonym), was an integral part of, and one of the principal organizers of, Vancouver's Drug Awareness Week in 1995. Edwin worked tirelessly on this project, bringing his enthusiasm and humor into a hectic organizing schedule. Edwin was known, well liked, and respected by many. The 1996 Drug Awareness Week in Vancouver was dedicated to his memory.

COLIN: Edwin, what were some of the promises that heroin made to you?

EDWIN: Heroin promised me, "No pain, no loneliness, no frustration."

COLIN: Was heroin able to keep any of these promises?

EDWIN: Not after a while. After a while, heroin seemed to have fooled me.

COLIN: At that point, how did you begin to think about heroin's promises to you?

EDWIN: I began to think that heroin had tricked me into a lifestyle that could end with death.

COLIN: What is different for you these days?

EDWIN: I seem more capable of resisting heroin's influence in my life. There is a mutual trust and honesty between my parents and myself. Now we talk more openly and honestly with one another. Before, under heroin's influence, I could be in the house with everyone home, and I would feel so lonely. That's when heroin would call.[10]

COLIN: Where is heroin today? Is it close by?

EDWIN: No. Today it's far away! (*Laughing, looking outside the window*)

COLIN: If heroin could hear our conversation—if heroin were to listen to and experience your resistance, and witness our celebration of your escape from its grasp—what do you imagine heroin would say?

EDWIN: (*Long, thoughtful pause*) I don't think heroin would be too happy. Heroin would probably be thinking of sneakier ways to get me back.[11]

COLIN: So it's not really going to give up, and you have to be mindful of its vigilance and trickery?

EDWIN: Yes.

---

[10]Edwin adopted this way of externalizing heroin's influence as a result of being initiated into a new vocabulary—an "anti-language," as David Epston might say—countering other theoretical perspectives tending to locate problems within persons.

[11]Quite often, young persons with whom I work have informed us that in their experience substances are always "waiting in the wings" for moments where they can "move in" and take advantage of contexts of vulnerability and confusion. I think it is useful to ask this kind of question in order to evoke or imagine an understanding of the extent to which the problem may exert its presence, in order once again to become the dominant narrative within a person's life.

SHELLEY'S STANCE AGAINST
LONELINESS AND DEPRESSION

In the following conversation, Shelley,[12] a 14-year-old First Nations woman, recounted some of the ways in which her experience in the world had been entered into by the problem of substance misuse. Shelley spoke of ways she discovered to diminish alcohol's influence within her life and relationships. In the larger sociocultural landscape of Shelley's experience, her identity was also being informed by conditions of abject poverty, crowded living conditions, and a lack of safety and protection from male violence, including sexual exploitation.

Before I relate her conversation, it is important to note that the Peak House program accepts clients from all areas of British Columbia, and that Shelley lived (and continues to live) in a small town in the interior of the province. Her community is severely socioeconomically affected by a lack of employment opportunities, particularly for young persons. For First Nations persons, regardless of age, the lack of employment opportunities is even more pronounced. This situation has its roots in the history of colonization and the way in which "Indian reserves" were established as isolated communities. In the reserves, a paternalistic dependence upon the Canadian state was fostered, with reliance upon social assistance and with forced re-education of young native persons in residential schools, totally disconnected from their extended families and communities of origin. Today, considerable racial tension exists between the white, dominant culture and the First Nations people in Shelley's community. In other conversations, Shelley spoke of how she experienced this tension through being verbally abused, shunned at school, and monitored by shopkeepers.

COLIN: Shelley, if you were alcohol, would you take particular advantage of certain situations within a person's life?[13]

SHELLEY: Mostly when they are lonely, or when someone is feeling hopeless. Like, that's what it does to them.

COLIN: Uh-huh.

SHELLEY: And once you're addicted, you lose your self-respect.

---

[12]This and all other client names used in this chapter are pseudonyms.

[13]In my work, I often ask persons to imagine what the problem's intentions for their lives are, and to adopt the problem's perspective in accounting for ways to undermine the intentions they may have for their own lives (cf. Roth & Epston, 1996; Dickerson & Zimmerman, 1996).

COLIN: So then, a heavy-drinking lifestyle involves a loss of self-respect, and alcohol would continue to take advantage of that . . . and so would hopelessness?

SHELLEY: Yup . . . and also depression.[14]

COLIN: Yeah . . . could you say something about that, the relationship between hopelessness and depression?

SHELLEY: Well, when I felt alone, and all my friends were out doing something else, I would have a drink; and when I felt bad, because I was just so used to taking it [alcohol], that brought me up. . . . You'd have a good time, and you'd try to get that feeling again, and you'd keep taking it and taking it.

COLIN: What kinds of things did alcohol suggest it could help you with, in terms of those feelings or situations involving loneliness and depression?

SHELLEY: (*Brief laugh*) It seemed like it thought that alcohol could take all the loneliness and depression away, and bring you into a whole different world, away from reality.

Voice from the group: Did it?

SHELLEY: Never! Like, as much as it may seem it could have, or would have, it brought you down lower.

COLIN: It just took further advantage of you?

SHELLEY: Yeah, like your self-respect—when you're drinking, it [alcohol] chips away at your self-respect!

COLIN: What kinds of things did you do to challenge alcohol . . . apart from coming to Peak House, which was a very courageous thing to do? What other little things did you do to challenge alcohol?[15]

---

[14]Shelley had been diagnosed by a mental health counselor as being "depressed." For me, this diagnosis ignored the sociopolitical and socioeconomic conditions of Shelley's lived experience; it represented a point at which a label entered into her experience. When the diagnosis was made, she commenced to understand herself through "depression's" eyes and mind, with the problem now officially situated within herself. This may be viewed as yet another example of therapeutic violence. An alternative way of understanding Shelley's despair would be related to the impoverished material and spiritual conditions in which she was attempting to survive and struggle toward a sense of connection and belonging (Waldegrave, 1990; Waldegrave & Tamasese, 1993).

[15]I said "little things" because, at times, the small victories against the problem's influence may not be realized or acknowledged; yet these unique moments (White & Epston, 1990) can become pathways to re-authoring accounts of one's life. From a solution-focused perspective, Berg and Miller (1992) have discussed the importance of punctuating the small initial actions persons take toward dissolving seemingly enormous dilemmas, especially in the domain of substance misuse.

SHELLEY: Like, I started out with just staying away from it as much as I could; then it started getting harder and harder to stay away. So I talked to a friend of mine, and she suggested going to AA with her.[16]

COLIN: Yeah.

SHELLEY: I was ready to go out and have a drink, and she said, "There's an AA meeting tonight," and I walked in, and it just blew me away! What they were all talking about was *exactly* what I was going through.

COLIN: So then, having that community of others around you of people who'd experienced what you had also experienced enabled you to . . .

SHELLEY: Yeah, like I thought I was the only one going through all this . . .

COLIN: You're kidding!

SHELLEY: . . . but it turns out I wasn't alone at all (*smiles*).

COLIN: Do you think alcohol wanted you to feel isolated and alone, so that it could "get you"?

SHELLEY: (*Pause*) Yeah.

COLIN: Do you think that's a common strategy with all drugs? The drug wants you to think you're alone, and has you compare yourself with others, suggesting, "I'm not a worthy person, I'm less than others"?

SHELLEY: Yeah, probably.

Voices in the group: Yeah . . .

COLIN: So you took that experience of being involved in the AA group, and how did that experience work for you when you went back into your life again?

SHELLEY: Oh, it was scary. Like, the last meeting I went to, I found that

---

[16]Our program philosophy and practices do not negate the useful fit with a person's experience of AA. As mentioned above, only when persons feel further impoverished, or restrained, by their experiences with the AA program do we pursue a line of inquiry as reflected in some questions described earlier in this chapter. For example, some clients have suggested that, for them, it is oppressive to think that they have "defects of character" or that they are "powerless" over certain areas of their lives. In remaining respectful and honoring of each client's point of view in this regard, we choose to accept Erickson's (1954) notion of "utilization"—a notion that promotes listening to, and carefully attending to, an understanding of the words and worldview that make sense and provide meaning to the client.

AA helped me. I went uptown, and noticed myself standing up to my friends. . . . Like, they looked down [at me] and said, "Oh, do you want to go and have a couple of drinks . . ."

COLIN: (*Interrupting*) Sorry, you were *standing up* to them?!!

SHELLEY: Yeah. I said, "No, I'm not really that interested right now."

COLIN: Good for you . . . was that tough?

SHELLEY: Yeah. It *was* tough!

COLIN: Shelley, do you think that alcohol is quite a weak thing, given that it wants to take from people like yourself, who are quite strong?

SHELLEY: Yeah, in a way . . .

COLIN: You know what I mean—that it would take advantage of your sadness and loneliness, and try to keep you isolated . . . that's not very fair . . .

SHELLEY: Not at all.

COLIN: Alcohol wasn't being very fair, or cooperative.

SHELLEY: Like, all the other drugs basically make you feel great, right? Alcohol just takes you down the hill, and you'll never be the same after that one drink.

COLIN: How do you, or how did you, get back up the hill?

SHELLEY: Yeah, I spent some time by myself and all that. I'd be depressed, and I would see if I could stand up to it [alcohol]. It was a risky thing to do. It was a scary thing to try. But I was strong enough to do it.

COLIN: And what does that tell you about yourself as a person, that you were strong enough to do all that?

SHELLEY: Well . . . basically . . .

COLIN: Yeah, what is it you know about yourself now?

SHELLEY: That if I put my mind to something, I can, if I really want to, follow through with it.

COLIN: So then, if you're mindful, and aware of what you are up to, you can stay on that other sort of path you've discovered for yourself?

SHELLEY: Yeah.

COLIN: (*Smiling*) How old are you now?

SHELLEY: (*Smiling*) I'm turning 15.

COLIN: Shelley, I wondering what's it like in terms of being in your particular community. Are there lots of opportunities for alcohol to make a comeback in your life?

SHELLEY: Oh, yeah. Most of the adults are already sober, but there are a few who aren't. Most of the young people drink. There's not a lot to do. Most adults don't find work all the time; it's seasonal.

COLIN: What are some of the solutions that you've thought of to get young people away from alcohol's influence?

SHELLEY: Oh, basically, focus on other interests, like playing pool. I was very athletic before I got into alcohol, and when I was in it I didn't want to do anything. Now that I'm out of it, I feel kind of energetic all the time!

COLIN: So alcohol robbed you of your athleticism?

SHELLEY: Oh, yeah!

COLIN: Seems it's a real ripoff, doesn't it?

SHELLEY: Yeah, even though it didn't [originally] feel like it, though.

COLIN: And yet, when you get some distance from its grasp, it seems exploitative of you?

SHELLEY: Yeah.

COLIN: Do you think alcohol is only happy when people are kept down, oppressed?

SHELLEY: Oh, yeah!

ALLY'S STORY OF DETERMINATION

My final illustration of a re-storying conversation involves a young woman who, after a time, reclaimed her desire to live and to move forward toward a career that held meaning and purpose. Ally has also co-presented at workshops with me. Most recently she gave birth to her second child, a son, and is raising him with her partner of the past couple of years. These new developments contradict the old, dominant story that others had created about her.

Ally had been living in an abandoned downtown Vancouver "squat" with some "punks." She and her acquaintances were living off social assistance and misusing a variety of substances, including "angel dust" (phencyclidine, or PCP) and "acid" (LSD).

At some point in her career as a street person, Ally formed a connection with a street youth worker from a substance misuse day program. Over time, as their connection became established, he suggested Peak House to her. Ally came for a brief visit one day, and several months later decided to enter the program.

The dominant story in Ally's life represented her as an "uncaring, selfish person," an "irresponsible person," an "unfit mother" to her first child, a "slut," and a "person who would never love anyone." This dominant story had been co-authored by various professionals, including teachers, social workers, court mediators, judges, and others.

In an early conversation, I asked Ally (then aged 17) what her dream for a preferred future life would be. Her response to this question spoke against the version of her life created by others.

COLIN: Ally, could you tell me about your dream for the future?

ALLY: Yeah. I want to work overseas, maybe with CUSO [Canadian University Services Overseas].

COLIN: Great! What type of work would this involve you in?

ALLY: Working with people who have less. Maybe working especially with children.

COLIN: Has this possibility been a dream of yours for some time?

ALLY: Yeah. For a couple of years now.

COLIN: With everything that has gone on during the rough moments of the past year, how is it you've been able to hang onto this dream?

ALLY: I don't know . . . I just have.

COLIN: Sounds to me like an extremely caring, giving thing to want to do. Who else do you think is aware of this quality you have, this caring, giving quality?

ALLY: (*Pause*) I think my mother knows this about me, even though right now she thinks that I'm selfish and irresponsible. That's why she has Teresa [Ally's 2-year-old daughter, entrusted to her mother's care, through a legal agreement in which the courts had deemed Ally "not responsible enough" to care for Teresa].

COLIN: Is it possible this aspect of yourself—this caring, giving quality—is merely something that your mother has lost sight of in the past year?

ALLY: Yeah, but I never thought about it like that before.[17]

---

[17]I think that Ally's reflection, "I never thought about it like that before," is indicative of how therapy might offer a client a new understanding of how there are times when the problem's intentions for the person conspire against others' seeing, or realizing, the abili-

COLIN: With some of the confusion that's been coming between yourself and your mom, do you imagine it's possible confusion was successful in "disappearing" these other qualities of yours?

ALLY: Yeah. With everything that was going on, I think she could have easily forgotten.

COLIN: Your mom described you, at various times over the past couple of years, as being dominated by a pathetic confusion; is this a description with which you would agree?

ALLY: At times, yeah.

COLIN: Is it possible, then, that pathetic confusion was directing your life toward demeaning behaviors and practices? Do you think that pathetic confusion was on a campaign to have you hurt yourself, or for some harm to come your way?

ALLY: Yeah. I felt scared to change, scared to leave. I thought I was comfortable with Teresa's dad, even though he used "roids" [anabolic steroids], and we would fight. It was pathetic, especially for Teresa to hear.[18]

COLIN: With your situation being influenced by pathetic confusion, I wonder how you became able to challenge or resist its influence in your life?

ALLY: Well (*laughing*), I got pretty fucked up!

COLIN: Yet you never gave up.

ALLY: Well . . . (*pause*) . . . I had faith, I guess.

COLIN: What kind of faith? Faith in yourself, in your courage?

---

ties and qualities that are immanent within the "troubled" person. In this sense, others become "blinded" to "peripheral vision," as Mary Catherine Bateson (1994) might put it. Yet this "blinding" also has the effect of causing important persons to "disappear" from the wider audience within the client's life, thereby contributing to the strengthening of the problem's grasp on the person through further isolation, comparison against others' expectations and achievements, and so on. Unfortunately, in scenarios such as this, substances are always "waiting in the wings," preparing to misguide the person's life.

[18]In other conversations, Ally described the history of her relationship with Teresa's father. His misuse of various substances, especially steroids, had exacerbated conflict within their relationship and eventually resulted in his violence against her. As is the situation for many women in this culture, Ally had been reluctant to leave for socioeconomic reasons. At the time Ally entered Peak House, her former partner was in jail. Ally maintained some contact with him through letters and phone calls. Ultimately, Ally considered that it might be a good idea to have her mother provide the primary care for Teresa. This reasonable decision was not arrived at in a carefree manner, and for Ally there was considerable anguish involved. For Ally, making this decision amounted to a re-visioning of many of the values within which she had been socialized.

ALLY: Yeah, in myself. I knew I could be strong-willed, stubborn! I knew I was a rebel.[19]

COLIN: Was this part of that fierce Irish determination we've spoken of before?

ALLY: Probably. Also, conformity. There came a time when I knew I didn't want to conform.

COLIN: Conform to what, or to whom?

ALLY: Conform to the way some people wanted me to act. The way Ryan [her stepfather] wanted me to act, and the way some teachers wanted me to act.

COLIN: How did Ryan want you to act?

ALLY: Like his little girl![20]

At this point there ensued some discussion of male, patriarchal attitudes toward women, particularly in regard to some men's struggles concerning entitlement when their daughters begin to develop interest in males outside of the family.

SUMMARY

In this chapter, I have discussed some of the ways young persons find themselves entered into or captured by problem identities, especially those relating to the problem of substance misuse. It has been mentioned that young persons in North American culture face a complex of demands, expectations, and contending "voices" vying for their attention. Some discussion has taken place into ways in which young persons may construe themselves as representing the problem, and ways in which members of the helping professions may assist in constructing such an identification.

A narrative, re-storying way of collaborating with young persons and families has been introduced as a means of engaging with clients

---

[19]At this juncture, I remembered an even earlier conversation between myself, Ally, and Mary (Ally's mother) regarding the important relationship between Ally and her maternal grandfather. Ally spoke affectionately and respectfully of her consideration for her grandfather. There had developed within their family mythology considerable mystery related to the grandfather's activities as an Irish Catholic volunteer against the occupation of Northern Ireland by the British army. Mary was active in British Columbian labor union political activities, and was shop steward in her own local. The thread of "rebellion" was a powerful alternative story to obedience and submission.

[20]See Elliott (1996) for a feminist, narrative account of ways of situating oneself as a therapist in a deconstruction of engendered relations.

against the negative influence and often oppressive reign of the problem. This particular way of thinking about problems, problem discourse, and the ways identity is shaped and constructed is a heartening therapy that works with clients toward evoking future possibilities.

EDITORIAL QUESTIONS

Q: *(DN) Colin, your work with young persons captured by substance misuse is impressive! I see your work as quite revolutionary and in stark contrast with traditional recovery models. To offer an alternative framework in the area of substance misuse is challenging, given the hegemony of the medical/recovery model. Bravo on introducing these ideas at Peak House! It must have taken a great deal of passion, commitment, and energy to influence Peak House to adopt narratively informed ideas. I imagine that in your journey, Colin, you have had to interface with professionals who are informed by traditional recovery models of substance misuse. Do you have any guidance for therapists who are interested in practicing narratively in traditional recovery models?*

A: I am not entirely convinced that it *is* possible to practice narratively within the domain of traditional recovery facilities. The so-called narrative metaphor in therapy represents a radical break with traditional chemical dependence approaches to working with persons suffering from substance misuse; it promotes a language of personal agency and empowerment, not one of dependence and powerlessness.

Having stated this, I do think that therapists within traditional facilities can begin to speak with clients about areas of their lives over which they think they *do* have some personal agency, even if they acknowledge that substance use is not one of these areas. In this case, it is still possible to arrive at new understandings of conditions and experiences that eventuated in substance misuse's becoming a predominant narrative in the clients' lives, and in continuing a search for alternative and preferred future paths.

Q: *(DN) In your chapter, you argue that narrative practices help counter traditional, internalizing language that subjects persons to professional substance abuse discourse. Instead, narrative work encourages the persons to reclaim their own local knowledges to defeat substance misuse. Do you ever work with persons who find AA helpful? If so, how do you integrate such tenets of AA as "I am powerless over alcohol" with narrative ideas about personal agency?*

A: I have worked with a considerable number of persons of all ages who have found both AA and Narcotics Anonymous (NA) useful to their purposes. What many people tell me is that they have come to utilize the fellowship of these support programs to assist them in maintaining drug-free, abstinent lifestyles. Many of these people have informed me that they do not, or no longer, believe that they "have a disease"; they caution others not to develop "too strong" a reliance upon AA or NA, and stress the importance of "getting a life!" Speaking narratively, it is possible to envisage these kinds of groups as communities of concern.

With persons who have some sort of absolute belief in the efficacy of AA or NA, I will respectfully support this choice in their lives, and speak with them of new developments and futures they imagine for themselves within the realm of substance-free possibilities.

ACKNOWLEDGMENTS

I want to thank all the individuals whose voices speak out in the transcripts, and the many young people and family members whose lives have been of inspiration and assistance in writing up some of this work. I also want to thank everyone with whom I "keep on trucking" at Peak House and at Yaletown Family Therapy, especially those who took time to read and comment on earlier versions of this chapter. Finally, a warm thanks to my companion, Gail Marie Boivin, and to my children, Maya and Adrian.

REFERENCES

Bateson, M. C. (1994). *Peripheral visions: Learning along the way.* New York: HarperCollins.

Berg, I. K., & Miller, S. (1992). *Working with the problem drinker.* New York: Norton.

Caputi, M., & Mullins, J. (1995). *Teens in recovery: Consumer feedback.* New Westminster, B.C.: Nisha Children's Society (Astra Program).

Cushman, P. (1995). *Constructing the self, constructing America: A cultural history of psychotherapy.* Reading, MA: Addison-Wesley.

Dickerson, V., Zimmerman, J., & Berndt, L. (1994). Challenging developmental truths: Separating from separation. *Dulwich Centre Newsletter,* No. 4, 2–12.

Elliot, H. (1997). Engendering distinctions: Postmodernism, narrative, and feminism in the practice of family therapy. *Gecko: A Journal of Deconstruction of Narrative Ideas in Therapeutic Practice,* 1, 52–71.

Erickson, M. H. (1954). Special techniques of brief hypnotherapy. *Journal of Clinical and Experimental Hypnosis,* 2, 109–129.

Erikson, E. H. (1963). *Childhood and society* (2nd ed.). New York: Norton.

Flax, J. (1990). *Thinking fragments: Psychoanalysis, feminism, and postmodernism in the contemporary West.* Berkeley: University of California Press.

Foucault, M. (1980). *Power/knowledge: Selected interviews and other writings, 1972–1977.* New York: Pantheon Books.

Gilligan, C. (1982). *In a different voice.* Cambridge, MA: Harvard University Press.

Hare-Mustin, R. T., & Marecek, J. (1994). Feminism and postmodernism: Dilemmas and points of resistance. *Dulwich Centre Newsletter,* No. 4, 13–19.

Hare-Mustin, R. T., & Marecek, J. (1996). Abnormal and clinical psychology: The politics of madness. In D. Fox & I. Prilleltensky (Eds.), *Critical psychology: An introductory handbook.*

Kaminer, W. (1992). *I'm dysfunctional, you're dysfunctional: The recovery movement and other self-help fashions.* Reading, MA: Addison-Wesley.

Kohlberg, L. (1969). *Stages in the development of moral thought.* New York: Holt, Rinehart, and Winston.

Levinas, E. (1995). Ethics of the infinite. In R. Kearney (Ed.), *States of mind: Dialogues with contemporary thinkers.* New York: New York University Press.

Madigan, S. (1992). The application of Michel Foucault's philosophy in the problem externalizing discourse of Michael White. *Journal of Family Therapy, 14,* 265–279.

Maturana, H. R., & Varela, F. J. (1992). *The tree of "Knowledge": The biological roots of human understanding* (rev. ed.). Boston: Shambhala.

Roth, S., & Epston, D. (1996). Developing externalizing conversations: An exercise. *Journal of Systemic Therapies, 15*(1), 5–12.

Sanders, C. (1994). Workshop notes: Deconstructing addiction mythology. *The Calgary Participator, 4*(1), 25–28.

Sanders, C. (1995). Narrative imagination in evoking a language of mind. *The Calgary Participator, 5*(2), 44–49.

Sanders, C., & Thomson, G. (1994). Opening space: Towards dialogue and discovery. *Journal of Child and Youth Care, 9*(2), 1–11.

Szasz, T. (1970). *Ideology and insanity.* Garden City, NY: Doubleday/Anchor.

Tomm, K. (1989). Externalizing the problem and internalizing personal agency. *Journal of Strategic and Systemic Therapies, 8*(1), 54–59.

Tomm, K. (1990a, June). *Ethical postures in family therapy.* Paper presented at the annual meeting of the American Association for Marriage and Family Therapy, Philadelphia.

Tomm, K. (1990b). A critique of the DSM. *Dulwich Centre Newsletter,* No. 3, 5–8.

Waldegrave, C. (1990). Just therapy. *Dulwich Centre Newsletter,* No. 1, pp. 5–46.

Waldegrave, C., & Tamasese, K. (1993). Some central ideas in the "just therapy" approach. *Australian and New Zealand Journal of Family Therapy, 14*(1), 1–8.

Weingarten, K. (1992). A consideration of intimate and non-intimate interactions in therapy. *Family Process, 31,* 45–59.

White, M. (1995a, September). Workshop handout, "Power and culture of therapy." Seattle, WA.

White, M. (1995b). *Re-authoring lives: Interviews and essays*. Adelaide: Dulwich Centre Publications.

White, M., & Epston, D. (1990). *Narrative means to therapeutic ends*. New York: Norton.

Zimmerman, J. L. & Dickerson, V. C. (1996). *If problems talked-Narrative Therapy in Action*. New York-Guilford.

17

Tales Told Out of School

LISA BERNDT
VICTORIA C. DICKERSON
JEFFREY L. ZIMMERMAN

Remember school? How it looked? The smell of the chalk and the cleanser, the look of the hallways, the metal chairs, the desktops that looked like wood but weren't, the hollow sound when you put your head on your desk? Was that desk your territory or was it a confinement? What did the windows look out on? What about the clocks? At what speed did the hands move—too fast or too slow? Was the schoolyard a place of acceptance, or was it a field of social tests and physical ordeals?

Remember the sound of the steps in the hall? Could you tell who was coming and what mood they were in? Was it a welcoming place? How did you know? What were the cues that let you know you were welcome or not? What about people's faces? Did they look like yours? Who seemed to be in charge? Who worked in the office? Who worked in the cafeteria? What did that tell you about power and possibilities?

Memories of school can be uplifting, but they can also be quite painful. How can we reduce the pain and enhance young people's sense of engagement in their learning in schools? Sometimes it's hard to remember how disorienting and alienating school can be from the moment one first arrives. This experience of alienation can be so powerful as to crowd out the other lessons that schools might want to convey. These effects can be magnified several times when the school environment is notably different from that to which one is accustomed. I (LB) recently had a "strange context" experience when I ran an errand at a swank financial institution. The building was not marked, but I had a vague idea of where it was supposed to be. I asked at three different stores for directions and was directed to a public phone a block and a half down. When I found no phone booth and no phone book, I started to wonder, "Is this a secret?" At last a man gave me directions. I felt a surge of relief and hope. Sure enough, there was the building. "I'm in," I thought. But no: What looked like a door was actually a window, and what looked like a wall was actually an exit. My temperature rose. I could see in but could not get in. It occurred to me to break in; it occurred to me to give up. I finally found a door concealed in edifice number four. When I finally got in, I saw that the walls were dark wood with brass, and hanging on them were 19th-century prints of white men in waistcoats doing business. Although I knew where the elevators should be according to custom and experience, I saw nothing that looked like doors or buttons. Fortunately, a woman came along who knew the part of the wall to push. As we boarded the elevator (wood-paneled, reflecting ceiling, plush white carpet), I looked at my blue jeans and running shoes, started wondering about my presentability, and glanced at the woman. Looking for some kind of validation, I asked her, "Is this a difficult building?" She beamed and responded, "Isn't it beautiful?" I sighed.

This experience makes me think of young people and their possible experience of another kind of institution—school, an institution that reflects and represents so many institutions. What does the physical layout tell them about their welcome and what might be in store for them? Whose pictures hang in the hallways? And how might this story help us think about staying aware of the effects of our actions? How can we make what we are doing consistent with our intentions? Even more, how do we see where we are when we're in it?

My early memories of school were a blending of moving from the culture of my home, where people still had time to read and intellectual curiosity was rewarded, to a new setting, where I remember the smell of Pogo paste and the fat crayons in five colors. Because I came from a home that was white, middle-class, professional, English-speaking, and school-centered, the entry into school was not that big a step. My mother had a new job teaching kindergarten, and it seemed like a good idea that I start first grade where she worked. My brother was in the fourth grade, and I was impressed with what he knew. Schoolwork seemed like just one of his many activities for me to covet and emulate. Even then, as I looked around at my neighborhood, the toys scattered on the sidewalk of my suburban subdivision, I sensed that my childhood was ending.

I was hopeful. I felt secure in my coloring skills, and even though I wasn't sure about math, I was being asked about things with which I was still comfortable. But then came the day of the triangle problem. We were given a handout depicting a big triangle divided by lines into several smaller triangles, and we were told to count all the triangles. I got the big one. I got the little one. But when I caught on that there might be overlapping triangles, I was overwhelmed. I started to cry. "It's too hard," I sniffed. The next thing I knew, I was being taken to the kindergarten class and told to sit with my head on the desk.

I'm sure that this was a gesture of compassion on the adult's part. I'm sure the intention was to take some pressure off me and to put me in an environment that was less demanding, more soothing. However, the meaning I carried was one of failure, humiliation, and no help available. I felt I had let someone down. I was ashamed. I was sure that my failure reflected not only on my current but also my future abilities.

In my mind and fantasies, adults come and acknowledge that it is sometimes hard to be only 5 years old and in the first grade. In my mind, someone comes and takes me for a walk, talks and laughs with me, and reminds me that my life does not depend on mastering the triangle problem. This person reminds me—not by saying it, but by being with me in a way that I just know it—that I'm a competent person with unique knowledges, interests, and talents. In my imagination (and possibly even in my lived experience), the companion accompanies me when I'm ready, and only when I'm ready, back to the class and offers to help me with the problem. She doesn't assume she knows how to help, but lets me instruct her on what I need. In this case, I can find the triangles. It's the overlaps that get confusing. If she can make a mark as I outline the triangles when I find them, I can count the marks.

I tell this story for at least two reasons. To this day, that memory is strong and filled with meanings: about myself, my competence, what kind of help is available, and also some sort of problem-solving deficit that must be about me and the world and my job in it (i.e., you figure it out by yourself or you lose your chance to try). I also tell it because the task of writing about work in the schools is very much like counting triangles. There are so many things to consider when entering such an institution. There are so many lives and stories that weave together. In pursuing one outline, I lose track of several others, only to find them later and wonder if they have already been counted. Moving back and forth between background and foreground, I forget which is which and resort to stories that recount learnings, mistakes, and impressions; these may be the seeds of future learnings, or they may suggest things that readers learned long ago.

Schools provide a wonderful, humbling opportunity to watch power/knowledge at work, because we all run smack dab into the dominant culture there. We can see techniques of power at work in what is presented as curriculum and what is not, as well as in what is conveyed by the arrangement of physical space and bodies. We can see technologies of management of persons through discipline, classification, and surveillance. We can see the legitimization of certain groups, and the exclusion or erasure of others by rendering them invisible or portraying them as inferior or dangerous.

ENTERING SCHOOLS TO WORK

We were given the opportunity to work in schools when, in 1990, Bay Area Family Therapy Training Associates (BAFTTA)[1] was invited to provide mental health services for a high school district in the Silicon Valley area of California.[2] The invitation arose as a late consequence of school policy changes in the 1970s, when counseling time and personnel in schools were eliminated because they were seen as superfluous to teaching and learning. Increasingly, the perceived emotional and behavioral problems of children in schools were seen to arise from stress outside the school system. In popular parlance, schools were "besieged by social problems," and extra "reinforcements" were expected to come from outside in the form of standardized programs, packages, and projects. In times of scarce resources (i.e., always), different programs and agencies vie for school contracts. They often feel a need to present themselves as efficient in order to win the few contracts that are available, and sometimes do so by claiming that a problem lies with a student's family, in which they propose to intervene to solve the problem. There is not much time or space granted to examine their definitions of "efficiency."

Those of us working at BAFTTA in 1990 were excited about the possibility we felt had been handed to us with the invitation to provide counseling services in five high schools. Many of the BAFTTA staff were

[1]LB was at BAFTTA in Cupertino, California, from its beginning in 1990 until mid-1996. She was the school coordinator from 1993 to 1996, and director of training from 1995 to 1996. She is currently at Project Respect in San Francisco. VD and JZ started BAFTTA in 1990 and did the initial groundwork in creating the possibility for work in three different school districts in the South Bay. The three of us provided the training and supervision for the counselors (most of whom were working as pre- or postdoctoral or postmasters' interns). Persons who wish to contact anyone at BAFTTA can call (408) 257-6881 or fax (408) 257-0689. The counselors at Project Respect can be reached at (415) 824-1734.

[2]Fremont Union High School District, with which BAFTTA has its longest-standing contract.

new to narrative ideas, but we had an idea that we could challenge some of the taken-for-granted assumptions and practices. When we actually arrived at the schools, we were greeted warmly by administrators and introduced to staff members who were sympathetic to the idea of counseling for students and families. Their eyes would soften and widen, and they would say in various ways, "Oh, do we have a case [or a whole batch of cases] for *you*." It was easy to feel useful, but we had to wonder: What ideas shaped these expectations of us? What discourses about young people, adults, problems, counseling, and help informed these referrals? What was happening in school culture, in Silicon Valley cultures, and in the wider society to account for the stack of files in the counseling office, and what was telling the school staffs that students needed the kind of "professional" help that they themselves could not provide? And what about the staff members for whom counseling was just "touchy-feely stuff," performed by gullible "bleeding hearts" who took students out of classes and gave them excuses for shirking responsibility? What if we actually shared some of their criticisms and concerns? All of these attitudes and positions reflected (and often still reflect) distinct worldviews and ideas about the purpose and best functioning of schools. These and other discourses form a backdrop against which young people, their families, staff members, and the wider community relate to schools.

Some of these attitudes and positions are the effects of mental health discourses at work on us and on school personnel, and they lead to certain expectations. One discourse at work is that there is such a thing as "mental health," and that we know what that is and can cure "dis-ease." Another is a strong belief in the descriptive and predictive power of test scores. These lead to a vigilance for "warning signs" and to therapists' marketing themselves by giving workshops to school staffs and parents, which talk about the latest in problem identification technology and offer therapy (usually by the workshop presenters) as the only responsible solution. This then leads to concerns for students "at risk." (At risk of what? And what does this say more about, students or theories?) Another discourse leads to a belief in "container" models, which posit that people need to discharge anger and to fuel up on self-esteem. An effect of this discourse is a belief in the literature that has invented dysfunctional families, denial, repression, and interpretation. All of these ideas intersect in the content and process of referral—how school staff members are thinking about themselves and about students, and where hope and help lie. In the mass media and in public conversation, youth blaming, parent blaming, and school blaming are alternatively put forward as explanations for troubled times. Mental health workers are invited in at any of the three points to intervene in ways that can actually keep the "pitting against" going and can keep considerations of power and politics unexamined (e.g., who gets to decide what point of view to hold, how does that represent dominant ideas, and what effect does this have on what groups?).

Given all this, how did we at BAFTTA want to position ourselves in an institution, and what kinds of choices did we have? What invitations were there in people's expectations and ideas about what was helpful, and how did we want to respond to these invitations? Which ones did we want to accept? Which ones could we turn down or deconstruct? How might we use our position to assure that local knowledges and talents were valued?

Narrative ideas gave us a place to start (even though when I [LB] was first learning about them, I felt the floor had disappeared). We looked at problems as existing outside of persons, and this is how we talked about them with school staffers, students, families, and each other. We were aware that problems have partial but not complete influence in people's lives, and that although they can get in the way of people's own wisdom and interfere with relationships in such a way that people forget their fondness for one another and their confidence in themselves and the values they hold dear, there is always resistance to this. In other words, there are always points of brilliance and inspiration, stories of perseverance toward dreams and commitments, and examples of interactions that defy the constraints of the problems. We saw it as our job to hold out for these experiences and to do what we could—through questioning, openly wondering, and noticing aloud—to contribute to building structures for the stories of these experiences to be told. Believing as we do that meaning is made narratively, through stories, our questions would be ones that would invite people to relate their lived experiences through time, as we have noticed them, and thus become alternative stories. We also believe that meaning is made in community, so we looked for opportunities to invite others into hearing and co-creating the stories. As they recount previously undertold stories, and as people hear them and participate in their meaning, it can become more and more a story of their own competencies, knowledges, values, and desires. (See Freedman & Combs, 1996; White & Epston, 1990; and Zimmerman & Dickerson, 1996, for a thorough description of the development of narrative ideas and practices.)

Most of our "work" with school staff members involved informal time, which occurred in the teachers' lounge, by the mailboxes, in the office, in the hallways, and in classrooms after school. Since almost every moment on campus is spoken for by tasks, these moments of casualness and friendliness that school staffers still managed to seize or create were in themselves unique outcomes; being able to stop and share a smile or a story about the weekend allowed us to know them and them to know us in territories where school-related problems did not have so much influence. It was important for us to keep in mind that we were entering schools with long and rich histories, and that the adults there had considerable life experience of being and working with young people. It was not for us to proselytize or come up with new and better ways to do their jobs. (This already happens at least twice a year in in-service training programs extolling some new teaching technology, learning theory, or behavioral management package.) We believed in people's wisdom, good sense, and commitment to help young people, and we saw how problems located in discourses of schooling and in wider social discourses could interfere with the expression of these things. We wanted to hear about the ways problems had interfered in people's lives, and we listened and watched for areas of freedom from problems—areas where the persons had acted according to story lines more consistent with their values and intentions. If we were aware of the adults' hopes, and the conscious purposes that led them to choose to work with young people, we could help them notice when they were managing to act on these hopes and purposes, and to contrast these times when problems had them persuaded of their inadequacy or of the hopelessness of "these kids." We were also always on the lookout for ways to "thicken" these preferred stories; thus, we would often be curious about what someone had done to make something wonderful happen, who they thought might want to participate further, what it told students about them and about themselves, and what obstacles they might have had to overcome to make the preferred events happen.

With time, too, we came to be more mindful of how our questions or comments about students could bring forth different stories. For example, asking "How's Jack doing?" was usually heard as an invitation for evaluation and a report on the problem. Then we would be in a bind—wanting to acknowledge the adult's experience without joining in the problem-dominated description. It seemed to go better when staffers were invited up front to join in the "outsmarting" of the problem. Isobel Sher[3] has found that including referring staff members in first interviews lets everyone participate in anti-problem efforts. Then the conversation could go more like this: "Jack noticed the other day that he was able to

---

[3]Isobel currently works for BAFTTA as a student advocate in an alternative school program in the Fremont Union High School District in Cupertino, California. She came to the program from South Africa, via the Mental Research Institute in Palo Alto, where she did a narrative therapy externship. All therapists, counselors, and other professionals named in this chapter, as well as the schools or places where they work, have given permission to be included.

get involved in the group project. Was that a private noticing, or did you see it too? Would you have anticipated that? Why? Why not?"

We also learned from what the students taught us—learnings that allowed us to gather further information to challenge dominant discourses about schools. So . . . let the students speak.

ENGAGEMENT AS A STARTING POINT

Sid

Sid,[4] age 15, was referred by a group of concerned teachers. His name kept coming up in conversations. People would shake their heads. Sid, they said, had "attitude problems"; he was "trouble, "aggressive," "surly," "oppositional," "defiant," and "truant." These were the words on which his file rode to the Student Assistance Team[5] and then to my (LB's) desk. It seemed that when there was trouble on campus, Sid's name always came up. Indications from the assistant principal were that "his days were numbered" at this particular high school. Such notoriety had me fascinated. I was eager to meet Sid, but also doubtful about his interest in talking to me. He was amiable, though, and after a period of checking each other out, we found some ways to laugh together and to enjoy our conversations. One teacher attributed this to Sid's being a "con artist." Since con artist skills can lead to great success in U.S. society, I was interested in whether he recognized his talents with people or whether the teacher was mistaken. He grinned at the question and told me about some of the ways he had developed skills with people.

Together, we puzzled over what we might call the problem that had people so concerned and aggravated. Using some of the teachers' words, we tried talking about "attitude," but that was not different enough from the "bad attitude problem" description that was so pathologizing. What did he think had people interpreting his actions as "attitude" and writing him off for it? "They're tripping," he said. So what did this "tripping" get them to think about him? How did it get them to act toward him? What did the "tripping" tell them about their job in relation to him? Did he like that? What got the "tripping" directed at him? What did he know about what brought it on? What kinds of things were influencing people to hang this "attitude thing" on him? What did

---

[4]Sid is a pseudonym, as are all the names of students in this chapter. The students have given their permission for these stories to be told.

[5]Student Assistance Teams were created to facilitate a triage process for getting help to students that is appropriate to their needs. Discussions about mental health discourses and school metaphors in this chapter are also applicable to the workings of these teams.

it keep people from knowing about him? Did he like it that way? Why or why not? What was it like when teachers looked at him? Did they only see this "attitude thing" and not see anything else? Was it like a "reputation?" How did the "reputation" actually affect his life? How did it get people to see his actions as self-destructive? Was it the same as how he liked to see himself, or were there differences? He explained that a "hard guy reputation" was important in some settings, for respect. When I wondered what it kept people from understanding about him, we talked more about his values, his caring for his family, and his hopes for the future. He had moved away from his home neighborhood to avoid trouble, and of all his family members, he felt closest to an uncle in prison. He explained that every day was a struggle to stay true to himself. It was hard to come to a school where his hopes, his loves, and his Filipino culture were dishonored. Adults were interpreting his behavior as self-destructive and death-directed, but Sid's experience was a protesting of the deadening effects of classroom practices that ignored or demeaned his culture and identity.

I asked if there were any people on campus who knew these positive things about him. Fortunately, there were. We talked about how he could invite them to join us in spreading richer versions of Sid around campus. He began to take active charge of his "reputation." One of the teachers he wanted to include in this project was an art teacher. We asked the teacher to be part of a videotaped interview with Sid about his hopes and dreams, and we also recorded a reflecting team process, in which the teacher and Sid's friends responded to the interview with respect and curiosity. Sid shared this video with his family, and then later he, along with his friends and his teacher, were involved in training the Student Assistance Team in the use of reflecting team processes (White, 1995).

I speak of Sid not to suggest that this "therapy" did wonderful things for him, but to pass on what he taught me. He agreed to talk with me and to grant me a small degree of trust, because, he said, I was funny and didn't try to tell him how to be. Narrative techniques didn't change his life. The questions described above didn't come in a torrent, but emerged gradually and within a context of mutual affection. They came out of my view of Sid as separate from the problem descriptions that had followed him and that were beginning to precede him. "Effects questions" checked on the extent and power of the problem description and on whether and how it interfered in what was important to him. Talking about these values and hopes opened up wonderful narratives weaving together past, present, and future, and honoring traditions that kept his community strong through many trials. Inviting friends to bear witness and bring in their stories further brought that community into our room, and allowing teachers to participate in the performance of new stories helped expand the circle of preferred accounts. (See White's [1996] current work about "re-membering.")

Sid and some of the Latino students on campus continued to meet the following year. With the assistance of Susan Sandler,[6] a colleague who had worked extensively to understand issues of social justice and to bring them to the forefront of our work, the students named some of the effects of racism and classism on campus, and invited some of the teachers into conversations on these issues. Their consultation contributed to Susan's thinking as she went on to create Project Respect in San Francisco, an anti-violence program working for school equity.

From Susan and from the Latino, African-American, and Asian students, I learned the importance of an awareness of the real world and of the sociopolitical context in allowing for meaningful inquiry. My externalizing of "attitude" or "reputation" actually missed Sid's daily experience of overt and covert racism on campus, and by missing it I inadvertently colluded in it. I didn't know yet about the racist overtones in the words that white professionals often use. For instance, words like "threatening," "menace," "gang activity," and "con artist" are interpretations that masquerade as descriptors for youth of color far more often than they would for white middle class-looking youth. If I were to meet with Sid now, I might ask directly about effects of racism. I could acknowledge my whiteness and his Filipino heritage. Instead, I participated in glossing over or denying it. And I missed opportunities to open conversations with staff members on better understanding racism's effect on all of us, and on what it means for different ones of us to be working in white middle-class institutions.

Amy

Everyone loved 15-year-old Amy, and everyone worried about her. "A matter of dysfunctional families," said some of the teachers who knew her. "Laziness," said others. Or just "not living up to her potential." Or "not knowing what was good for her." Amy believed and lived all of these, along with vivacity and a great hunger to learn about life through experience. She was referred to me because she was part of a group of six students described as "children of alcoholics"—an existing group held over from the previous year (1989–1990), when counseling services had been provided according to a substance abuse recovery model.

---

[6]Susan was at BAFTTA from 1993 to 1995 as part of her postmaster's internship.

Through Amy, I began some conversations with these "children of alcoholics." I was curious about the effects the definition of the group had upon them. As we checked with each other on the effects of its identity on them, we recognized separation from their families; a sense of inadequacy about how to create families of their own; and a pervasive sense of woundedness and incompleteness, which persuaded them that they were hobbled in life. There was a hopelessness about the future and a distrust of existing templates for adulthood, as well as a distrust of parents and a scanning for personality defects in themselves and significant others. It persuaded them that they had large "deficits." It had them both doubting their own minds and fighting for their own reality in ways that looked destructive. It persuaded these students that they had to have an all-or-nothing relationship with drugs and alcohol, and convinced them of the inevitability of drug- and alcohol-dominated futures for themselves. All of these undermined their confidence. The label also undermined their teachers' and administrators' confidence in these students. For example, when Amy helped other students or took leadership in the peer counseling program, adults saw it through the "children of alcoholics" lens, storied it as "co-dependent," and looked upon these activities with concern. Nevertheless, coming together as a group had been a powerful experience for all of these students, and we decided to continue our discussions. (See Epstein, 1996, for a series of articles challenging traditional alcohol and drug discourses.)

Amy dived headlong into the deficit definition of herself, but was willing to join with others in the group in exploring the limitations of this definition. We decided as a group to spend less time on recounting family disappointments and more on exploring the group's knowledges about relationships, at different times externalizing and investigating the nature and effects of rumors on campus. We did a study of reputation, and recruited audiences among teachers and administrators for stories of competence and responsibility. At times members of the group would invite other students or teachers in to talk through conflicts, or to expose the effects of rumors (Lobovits, Maisel, & Freeman, 1995).

Amy and I continued to meet for mutual consultation for 2 years after the rest of the group had graduated or left school, so I got to witness the direction and firmness of her steps. School staff members were very open about their fondness for Amy and their belief in her. Through "experience-of-experience questions," she could see herself through their eyes, and came more and more to identify things she liked and enjoyed about herself. In tracing the history of these qualities, we found that Amy remembered living strength, confidence, fun, and boldness as a younger child. She was also aware of the absence of context for this energy and enthusiasm in her present life, and how the only contexts she could have from the age of 12 were fights or stating her case in the ways called "talking back." Her expectations and hopes for herself had diminished when she arrived at middle school, and she found the possibilities for enacting her smartness and her love of people very limited. She felt she had to choose between relationships and academics, and she pursued relationships, being there for others to the point of losing sight of her own smartness. In mapping the domains taken over by these habits of "everybody-else-ness," we discovered some infiltrations into several relationships. She had managed to keep some time, energy, and ideas for herself, but "guilt," "self-doubt," and "prescriptions for young womanhood" kept trying to steal her rights to these experiences from her, all the while trying to convince her that it was she who was stealing. For example, they had persuaded her that cutting classes was the only way she could maintain relationships and still have time for herself. However, on the basketball court Amy had managed to keep her confidence and enthusiasm. This proved to be an important point of entry, as was her consistent participation in the group. In these arenas she had maintained trust in her perceptions, reflexes, and skills. She knew how to participate and facilitate teamwork, and to experience herself as flexible, strong, graceful, and determined.

Amy's account of her experience as a young woman resonated with my own, and we became more and more interested in the experience of other young women. Inspired by the work of Carol Gilligan (Brown & Gilligan, 1992; Gilligan, 1990), we began to research together what happens to young women's voices. An important step in clarifying our thinking and coalescing as a community of women came when we decided to invite speakers from the battered-women's movement to speak to some classes. The way they talked about power, intimidation, and male dominance rang true with several young women, who decided to continue to meet to support one another and expose the "dominance thing" in their relationships. Informed by the collective knowledges of Amy and the other young women we consulted, we started noticing the effects of male dominance in other schools. Young men, one or two at a time, became involved in talking about resistance to how male culture stigmatizes creativity, sensitivity, and identification with women's issues. These young men were brutalized for their resistance, yet continued to critique violence. I think with pain and regret of what I missed of their struggle and resistance, and how I wish we had thought through how to support them more for the stand they were taking, as well as how we might have included men across cultures and generations to stand together. This is work still to be done (Denborough, 1994; Hall, 1994; McLean, 1994).

Date Rape

When four young women at another campus came to us with experiences of date rape, the experiences at Amy's school helped us as workers to respond with more awareness of the gender politics involved. The young women knew that they wanted help with the issue, but they weren't sure what would be helpful, It was extremely important that the young women had a forum for speaking of their experience in ways that named the injustice. We (Rita Giacalone, Tamara Hicks,[7] and LB) started asking questions like these: "What do you make of the fact that so many women have been through similar experiences? Do you have ideas about why it's not talked about very much? What kinds of things make it possible, even prestigious, for young men to assault women they know? What does it say about you that you're here speaking out about this?" What started as a support group for young women became a movement on campus to expose male dominance and sexual harassment. As the girls spoke of their experience, they noticed the ways that they were often persuaded to participate in activities that helped keep male dominance in place—activities such as spreading and acting on rumors, competing with other women for male attention, defining themselves by male standards, cooperating with practices of exclusion, and yielding to the tyranny of being "cool." These forces beset the group from week to week, but naming them helped us stand against them. We tried to keep track of what kept us on course and to predict the tricks that patterns of dominance might play on us. Among the most powerful undermining forces were shame, secrecy, the lure of popularity, the threat of aloneness, the myth of scarcity, and the competition accompanying these things.

Once the young women saw the effects of silence in protecting the status quo, they decided to take action by inviting administrators to listen to their reflections on sexism on campus. This led to invitations to run class discussions in the high school. They thought it especially important to go back to the middle school they'd attended and talk to young women there, as well as to the staff and administrators, about how to make "sex education" more relevant to young people. For example, they said, "First they should consult with us about what we really know and don't know and what's really important to us." They invited male staff members to join them in standing against sexual harassment; they also invited influential male students to listen to their experience, to respond to them, and to try to influence their peers.

[7]These were women doing their graduate school internships with us. Rita came from the Wright Institute in Berkeley, and Tamara was a student at California School of Professional Psychology in Alameda. Both worked for BAFTTA for 1 year.

The way they were received taught me about the importance of working with the dominant group on dominance. There are so many invitations to defend time-honored positions. Even those who consciously want to change experience much confusion and helplessness about alternatives. The young women were inviting men to be their allies, and this presented much more of a challenge to the men than we anticipated. We were asking them to separate from the abusive practices (on women and on each other) that kept male dominance in place. I realize now that asking men to acknowledge dominance, much less do something about it, is a huge and vital task. The young women experienced their own agency and ability to affect the environment by speaking out and negotiating new ways of relating to sexism, but the backlash was (and is) real and powerful. We encountered judgmental statements (e.g., "People are overreacting with all this fuss about sexual harassment") and guilt-inducing questions (e.g., "Can't we even flirt any more?"). This taught us that what we were trying for was the transformation of a culture of dominance, and that it would be important to implement partnership accountability processes between adults and students and between men and women on campus (Hall, 1994; Frank, 1996).

Al

Another "teacher" in standing up to dominance was Al. Al, aged 17, was a junior in high school when I met him; words like "school phobia" and "depression" accompanied his referral. Although academics came easily for him, and he liked many things about school, he found himself increasingly allergic to going to school. Talking about his situation in externalizing ways, and detailing the effects of "panic" on his life, his friendships, his aspirations, his confidence, and his interest in living, freed us from a nonproductive quest for causes—which we found actually fueled the anxiety. This practice allowed us to appreciate the scope of the problem and to understand how formidable it was. Al's coming to see me was in itself a unique outcome, a point of entry into realms not frozen out by "panic." Standing in those realms, we could see that the exquisite sensitivity and the keen awareness he had developed through the years enabled him to identify some of the harshness and injustice that many of us did not notice.

The more Al was able to shake off the "sick" and "wounded" stories of himself and to embrace and enjoy his talents and insights, the more he valued his ideas and plans for himself. He instructed his family, his friends, certain teachers, and me on how best to help him. For example, he let us know that our worry and our checking on him actually diminished his confidence in himself. He also told us that he would let us know when to get excited and hopeful with him, but he did find it helpful to look together at steps he identified as desirable, and to figure out how he had taken them. At his own pace and in his own way, he met the conditions of an alternative education program provided by the district, and he graduated. (The alternative programs have made a huge difference for many of the students I have known. Students choose these programs as contexts where they can continue to value and cultivate their uniqueness in ways that they cannot in traditional classrooms.)

Along the way, as we looked at the ways "panic" assaulted Al as he faced the idea of a new day, I thought I recognized some of the voices of popular male culture. We talked about this, and Al agreed. For him, the "between-the-lines" aspects of school culture had been most painful. These had had him second-guessing himself and had terrorized him with the fear of rejection, ridicule, humiliation, and even violence that might come with one false move, one deviation from the norm. It was 2 years into our relationship that Al told me he had reached the point of being able to acknowledge his gay sexuality. I was honored that he told me, but very sad that I might have contributed to his aloneness by not making room for that realm of his experience. I had considered the effects of patriarchy and male dominance, and I had thought that a theoretical understanding of heterosexual dominance and how it works together with sexism put me above them. But here they were, and here I was.

I asked Al about this later. He said, "I thought you would be cool with it, but some kind of sign from you—some positive words naming it—could have helped me talk about it sooner."

Al taught me about my complicity in heterosexual dominance and about its effects on my relationships. His words have helped me look back at my own high school experiences as I've begun to re-story my love for women. Al has also been with me in my mind as I've asked at staff meetings what kind of welcome gay, lesbian, and bisexual students and staff members feel on campus, and what might be the implications for adult responsibility in the high suicide rate of young gay persons.

When I asked Al whether he would like to add anything more to this chapter, he offered the following story to illustrate the power of heterosexual dominance in his school experience. "When I was in the eighth grade I hadn't come close to putting it together about being gay, but I could tell there was something. I remember I really wanted to take art, but I thought that if I did, I'd be there with mostly girls and everyone would think I was gay. So I signed up for a boring drafting class." Al saw this as a significant moment in his experience of alienation from school and from his desires.

Matthew

At age 16, Matthew had an exquisite talent for bullshit detection. He'd been identified early on with various learning disabilities, and he was angry about those labels. "All they see is what is wrong with me," he protested. He was almost finished with high school and had been in special education classes since the third grade. His parents were in a bind. What they wanted most was his happiness and success; they wanted to listen to him and to believe in him. Yet the professionals seemed intent on having them adopt a different point of view. "The doctor says there's a new medication. It's our duty to do everything we can to help." The parents were caught in popular discourses about parenting and the power of so-called "scientific" knowledge. The real effects were that Matthew's actual experience was eclipsed, and that their happiness and joy as a family were eroded. (See Nylund & Corsiglia, 1996, for more information on the effects on families of these designations.)

Matthew's contempt for and frustration about the world grew. Without his consent, he was referred for therapy as part of the special education program. He knew what we were about and wanted no part of it. He recognized every narrative "technique" we used. We externalized. We pointed to unique outcomes. We recruited audience. We interviewed his parents about cherished moments in their relationship with Matthew and as a family. We made room for alternative accounts. Yet we still didn't get it. "Patronizing!" he'd say. "Manipulative! What do you take me for?!" He was furious. Ten years of help from people like us had convinced him that he was better off making his own way in the world. He saw all the efforts to help him as demands for change. He was emphatically not interested in and, indeed, was appropriately insulted and outraged by—attempts to shape him. Our ideas of adult power, responsibility, and rightness had co-opted our good intentions and led us right off the rails. This was the real problem. We never did know what to call it; we just all got better at noting its presence. It tried to isolate us all from one another—teachers, aides, social workers, doctors, friends. All had ideas for what Matthew needed.

Matthew did, too. Remarkably, the problem hadn't convinced him that his only options were "out" or "revenge," or that a combination would be the ultimate victory. Matthew's reaction to our "helping" actually turned out to be an invitation into relationship. He was relentless with us and gave us chance after chance to see things in new ways and to join him in laughter, including at ourselves. There were so many ideas, positions, and expectations that kept us from joining him there: ideas about help, resistance, and appropriateness; ideas about respect for adults; ideas about his needing to take his upcoming entrance into adulthood seriously. It was he who broke through isolation to let us see absurdity as he saw it, and we discovered how "resistance" had hold of us. Now at times when I feel myself caught in a therapeutic posture—or when I catch myself trying to be clever—I think of Matthew. Sometimes I wince (caught again!); sometimes I shake my head a little in self-reproach. At other times I think of Matthew's dead-on impersonation of me, and I laugh. I am grateful that I can continue to answer to him in my mind.

One of the early dilemmas for us was to reconcile the discrepancies we sometimes felt between the good intentions of school staff members toward most students and some of the attitudes they appeared to hold toward some students. For instance, we met adults with considerable skill and honest commitment to the well-being of students, who somehow seemed separated from their own skills when responding to specific students at certain moments. What was it that was interfering with their talents and redirecting their responsiveness? What was guiding their responses? We also noticed what seemed to be a discrepancy between what teachers wanted and what students wanted. Young people had clear ideas about what and how to learn, and what kind of relationships were important to them. Many of these were consistent with what the adults wanted, yet teachers and students often seemed to be at odds. What was it that got between them? It seemed to us that cultural beliefs about the purposes of education and the most appropriate methods for educating often interfered with the freedom to exercise the intuitive knowledges and wisdom that both adults and young people had about learning. Different cultural beliefs reflected distinct worldviews that supported particular values, attitudes, and practices, and discouraged other values and practices. We found that naming a particular perspective on schooling through a key metaphor made it easier for us to understand the nature and effects of some of these differing cultural beliefs or worldviews. What follows is a list of some such metaphors that form a backdrop against which young people, their families, teachers, other school staff members, and the wider community relate to schools and schooling.

METAPHORS OF SCHOOLING

Most of you, indeed, cannot but have been part and parcel of one of those huge, mechanical, educational machines, or mills, as they might more properly be called. They are, I believe, peculiar to our own time and country, and are so organized as to combine as nearly as possible the principal characteristics of the cotton mill and the railroad with those of the model

state's prison. (Charles Francis Adams, addressing the National Educational Association, 1880; quoted in Bowles & Gintis, 1976, p. 151)

This statement from more than a century ago points to a relationship
that grows more and more disturbing. We might ask in the late 1990s
what the prison system, the factory system, and the education system
have in common and whose interests they serve (Denborough, 1996).
What might it tell us to look at in the history of public education as an
institution? Who would we see exercising power, and what kind of power? Whose culture has been presented as normative, and how has normative status been conferred? What class interests have been represented? What values have been promoted and how? In the hallways, in the
teachers' lounge, in the offices, in the classrooms, in the counselors' offices, and in district meetings where students and policy were discussed,
we[8] noticed some of the discourses of schooling in operation. These discourses overlap with dominant discourses in the wider society: discourses of labor, motivation, psychology, moral worth, adulthood, childhood,
knowledge, and the purpose of knowledge, among others. They had visible effects on all of us—school staffers, contract workers, students, and
families—as well as our relationships with one another and with our
work. The core metaphors[9] in these discourses include the following:

1. *School as factory.* Public schooling is an artifact of the Industrial
Revolution, so it is not surprising that it was constructed according to
beliefs and models of the factory system. According to this metaphor,
students are on an assembly line leading to adulthood, and it is up to
teachers to construct the products. It tells teachers that students are in-
complete and that products can and should be standardized. It also encourages teachers and administrators to measure students and their own
performance according to that standard. Families can be seen as distant,
outside the walls, or as producers of raw materials. The consumers of
the product are society at large and the economy, so accountability is to
those customers. A completed student must be equipped with specific
tasks, tools, and features in order to be "roadworthy." This metaphor
tells students similar things and creates considerable anxiety as they
near the end of the assembly line. By that time they know whether
they're to be deluxe or economy versions, or whether they're headed for
the scrap heap. These ideas can correspond to families' ideas about

---

[8]"We" refers to the three of us and to all those who have worked at BAFTTA since 1990,
as well as those who have worked at Project Respect since 1995.

[9]These metaphors reflect the collected wisdom of those of us who discussed these ideas
over time.

preparing children for the "outside world" and can get caretakers to join in the measurement of teachers based on product. Working conditions can be risky, as in factories. Moreover, possibilities abound for burnout and alienation from the job, especially since teachers are promised professional status; thus, they feel they should have some control over their work, and interpret limits to this control as failure on their parts.

2. *School as surrogate (better) parents.* This metaphor tells teachers, administrators, and policy makers that young people are not getting what they need at home, and that, by default, schools are left with the responsibility of child rearing. This discourse can cite the moral or economic "breakdown of traditional families." This invites parents and caregivers at home to cooperate with school staff members in discounting home and family knowledge and traditions, pathologizing students and families whose home lives don't match those of the evaluators, and privileging professional knowledges and practices. It can construct schools as the site of "moral education" and "character building." It can infiltrate school–caregiver relationships through "parenting classes" and referrals for family therapy. It can alienate families from schools and push for meanings that get students thinking they have to choose between home and school. The pressure on adults in the schools to "save" children can be enormous, adding to a sense of "never-enoughness" for teachers, self-doubt and resentment among parents and caregivers, and confusion among young people.

3. *School as the great equalizer.* In this view, the school's job is to integrate young people into society so that they can assume the places society has waiting for them. This includes ideas about an even playing field, equal opportunities, and personal responsibility for taking advantage of those opportunities. It tells teachers different things, depending on their view of what society is. It can be close to the factory view, with additions and refinements from corporate culture, such as ever newly packaged technologies for managing and motivating people. It tells students that they'd better master certain skills, and, if they can't, it's their fault and their funeral. It can tell them that they are being sorted and trained to fit into slots. It can get teachers to tell them, "This hurts me more than it hurts you," and "You'd better get used to it—that's the way it is." It probably tells different families different things, since the society people are being prepared to fit into is one that discriminates according to skin color, class, ethnicity, sexuality, gender, age, appearance, and so on. It presents an illusion of equality and creates conditions for disillusionment and rage.

4. *School as the last bastion of (Western) civilization.* This is the "barbarians at the gate" discourse. With modern values declining and

them (immigrants, young people, gays, technology, Biblical end times) "taking over", it's up to the schools to preserve what's important. This puts tremendous pressure on school staff members, who get blamed in the mass media, in homes, and on street corners, and can get caught in the belief that it's all up to them. It can tell them and other caregivers that young people are raw and both dangerous and endangered, subject to forces of encroaching evil, and in need of discipline and protection. It encourages vigilance to the first hint of trouble (hence the term "at risk"). It is also akin to the "bad apple" view that justifies expulsion. It can tell young people the same thing, and can also persuade them that adults are out to stifle their self-expression and rob them of identity.

5. *School as bank.* In this view, critiqued by Friere (1970), adults make "deposits" of knowledge in passive students, who can then access it later. This convinces teachers that they hold objective knowledge and convinces students that they don't; the students are seen as empty vessels. This is also known as the "cup-and-jug" metaphor. This can lead to intense frustration when the "cups" do not sit still and receive their allotment of knowledge. It can discourage students and teachers from thinking for themselves, and thus leave the school staff exhausted and students squirming.

6. *School as a safe arena for exploring and experimenting.* This tells teachers that young people can follow their curiosities and interests and can try things out. It can also tell them that they have a responsibility for figuring out how much or what kind of structure to provide. It can put teachers at odds with standardization. Moreover, this view can tell young people that their interests and opinions are valuable, and that adults have differences and struggles and have to negotiate through periods of uncertainty. If caregivers are included in negotiations about safety, it can give them permission to explore and experiment as well. However, the strength of expectations to prepare young people for the economy can leave caregivers shouldering lots of worry and lead them to think they've been abandoned to hold their visions of the harsh, real world alone.

This is not an exhaustive list. It names some threads we found that helped us understand how power relations often had young people feeling "operated upon" by school staff and parents; school staff feeling "operated on," "manipulated," and "taken advantage of" by those above and beneath them in the hierarchy; and parents feeling "outside the loop" as consumers of specialized services provided by professionals. We are not suggesting that we can live outside of metaphors, but that awareness of them may lessen the degree to which they trap us.

We noticed among these schooling metaphors what a powerful impact social and economic conditions in the world of work have on education. School discourses do not arise in a vacuum. It is not surprising, then, that we would start to notice other, broader related discourses in operation as well—pressuring, supporting, infusing certain meanings, shaping relationships in specific ways, and obscuring other possibilities. These grand narratives include patriarchy, with its powerful allies individualism (leading to ideas of individuation and self-actualization), colonialism, militarism, and secularism, which all hook up with white supremacy; capitalism, often masquerading as democracy and accompanied by competition and profit (and colonialism and militarism—all of these discourses overlap and intersect); and morality, focusing on moral worth, heterosexual dominance, and technologies of reproduction. These, along with multiple other justifications of dominance, racism, ageism, and classism, work together to prop up the status quo on spindly but multiple legs. Especially influential on schools are the myths of scarcity (of time, money, qualifications, etc.), technocracy (in which power is accorded to the skilled, and power depends on acquiring those skills), and meritocracy (which assumes an even playing field—those who succeed do so because they deserve to). All these stories are given the status of truth and have very real effects in people's lives. They are the stories that are used to justify injustice. These are the stories most readily available to us as we make meaning of our experience.

　　How do we challenge these metaphors, or at least begin to make visible the negative effects they have on the lives of students, parents, teachers, administrators, counselors . . . in short, all those involved in school as an institution? Certainly we made a start by working one-on-one with students, but also involving others as a community of support. But were there more direct ways we could influence the context? Following are some examples of specific ways we attempted to create contexts of challenge and protest—contexts that would open possibilities for developing other metaphors, more empowering constructions for understanding and performing schooling.

CREATING CONTEXTS WHERE FAILURE IS IMPOSSIBLE[10]

Jorge "Coco" Mendoza,[11] an artist and educator, is one of those adults consistently referred to by students as "a grownup who understands" or one who "knows what kids like." He honors young people's culture and

[10]This is a phrase used by Michael White (1994).

[11]Coco works at Project Respect.

has worked with Latino paraprofessionals at James Lick Middle School[12] to set aside nonacademic space for students to express their culture through visual art. He explained to me how he invites students into the pleasure of artistic expression: "I say to the kids, 'Try a color you don't usually use. Try one you don't even like. Then, if it doesn't work, if you don't like it, you were right. If it does, you can be pleasantly surprised.'"

To me (LB), this expresses the narrative work we do—attending to ways of structuring and pacing questions, what we pay attention to, and what we don't. In the ways we try to structure conversations and activities, people either find they are "right," or they are pleasantly surprised. This is especially poignant in relation to schools, which developed in the same intellectual time and from the same tradition as the Panopticon (described very clearly in White & Epston, 1990), which embodies the practices of evaluation, surveillance, comparison, classification, and isolation—all so pervasive and powerful. In response to these practices, we began to notice and think about counterpractices and counterstructures. This response opened more than the content of our questions to examination and experimentation. In fact, we had to check with ourselves and with the young people we worked with to find out if our way of asking, or our presumption of our right to ask, was in some way exerting and promoting dominance. Not surprisingly, we found that our emphasis on the verbal was cultural (European-American, professional), and that there was more work to do in considering time, space, atmosphere, silences, and cadences. What we show here are some examples of structures that create different sorts of interactions and performances of possibilities than those created in traditional school structures, or even in one-to-one interviews.

Inspired by the work of Durrant (1995), team members in a special education program[13] for students labeled "severely emotionally disturbed" collaborated with students and staff to change the culture from a deficit- and stigma-dominated one to one of pride and community. A first step was to shift the intake process away from the "This is your last chance" message and to create structures of welcome. Students formed a welcoming committee and took charge of introducing themselves in ways that they wanted to be seen. Another step was the reclamation of

---

[12]This is the school in the San Francisco Unified School District where Project Respect is located.

[13]This program, known as the "severely emotionally disturbed—special day class" (SED-SDC), is located at Prospect High School in the Campbell Union High School District (CUHSD), which has contracted with BAFTTA from 1991 to the present to provide therapy services for the students in the program.

individual education plan (IEP) meetings.[14] These meetings all too often become ceremonies for glorification and amplification of deficits (which have traditionally been seen as necessary to justify funding for services); thus, progress may be documented, but not enough progress to call for the end of services. Mithran Cabot, Kaern Kreyling, and Doliene Slater[15] worked to transform these occasions into ceremonies of acknowledgment. Students could invite their friends to the meetings and could be interviewed about preferred developments. Therapeutic letters could be introduced into the record, as could other documentation students considered significant.

Anu Singh and Margy Lim[16] revised school referral forms to involve staff members in an externalizing process from the outset. The forms included such questions as "What percentage of the time does the problem take over?" and "In what areas is its influence strongest?"; they also provided room for descriptions of students when the problem was not in charge. These changes privileged teachers' knowledges of students' successes and were counterpractices to being on the lookout for problems.

Daurice Graves,[17] an artist and teacher, was enthusiastic about what she saw of our narrative work and devised activities that encouraged students to story their experiences visually. In one project the class looked at the functions of parts of a tree, and in their drawings of trees were invited to plot their values, characters in their lives, and preferences on the roots, leaves, or trunks of the trees. Later, students were invited to place the trees on a road map, along with stories of the roads. "There is no wrong way to do this," she told her students, many of whom found that very hard to believe. Seeing what Daurice was doing, a group of English teachers approached us for consultation on using narrative ideas in their lessons.

Osamu Inoue,[18] working at a Silicon Valley high school, began to

---

[14]IEP meetings are required by California state law for any student placed in a special education program in the California school system.

[15]Mithran and Kaern worked as therapists in the CUHSD SED-SDC program from 1995 to the present, Doliene is the classroom teacher, and has worked in that capacity since 1991. She has become one of BAFTTA's and narrative therapy's greatest supporters.

[16]Anu and Margy were two of the first counselors to work at BAFTTA in 1990. They initiated some truly ground-breaking ideas and processes in the schools where they worked.

[17]Daurice is a teacher at Cupertino High School in the Fremont Union High School District, who works closely with the student advocates from BAFTTA involved in her school setting.

[18]Osamu is a Japanese man studying psychology in the United States; he wanted to learn more about how to work within the narrative approach, with the hope of introducing

notice who was referred for counseling and who was not, and so started groups for students who had recently migrated to the United States. These groups grew rapidly by word of mouth from student to student. They reported feeling relieved and gratified to be able to share and name their experiences, and agreed that before the groups, part of their common experience at school had been one of invisibility. Out of this innovation came a request from students for other groups that would address racism's effects on students and on faculty members.

Valerie Minor and Susan Sandler[19] meet regularly with a group of paraprofessionals and teachers who are interested in a "practice–reflection–practice" process. The group examines dominant school culture, with its pressures of time and resource scarcity and its often unacknowledged power differentials, and develops counterpractices. With food, games, art, off-campus meeting space, and a relaxed pace, these meetings provide a bit of what one of us (JZ) calls "cookies and milk time for grownups." This group uses accountability processes to privilege marginalized voices (e.g., at times paraprofessionals and teachers caucus separately, then come back together to listen and respond to each other as a group). This group has been considering the question: "How do we make James Lick Middle School a truly anti-racist community?"

Shad Linscomb and Amy Epstein[20] realized that at a school where most of the teachers are white and most of the students are African-American and Latino, parents of the students labeled "at risk" often experienced schools as hostile and judgmental. They noticed the factors in school culture that created this experience, and, in partnership with parents and students, set up an alternative space and time by inviting parents to a party at the school. The gatherings reflected the great care they took to consider what would actually be welcoming to parents (how the room was set up; who could help attend to children; what would be appropriate kinds of food, music, and games; how or whether to structure the time; what languages would be spoken). Parent turnout was much higher than usually reported at parent meetings at the school, and people had time and room to use their own cultural knowledges to get to know each other and to have fun in ways that were comfortable to them.

As mentioned previously, a group of concerned teachers called the Student Assistance Team had the job of sorting through apparent crises and piles of files of students identified as "at risk." As their responsibility became more and more of a burden, we trained team members to

some of the ideas when he returned to Japan. He worked at BAFTTA from 1995 to 1996.

[19]Both Susan (as noted earlier) and Valerie are from Project Respect at James Lick Middle School.

[20]Both Shad and Amy are counselors with Project Respect.

serve as a reflecting team, and included them more in our work with students as audience to new stories. At times they participated on teams with students, reflecting on their own work and that of other staff members.

Alberto Colorado[21] worked in Spanish with elementary school boys who were referred for aggressive behavior that was getting them in trouble. They externalized the *"diablito"* that kept landing them in the office, and this led to a look at the effects of "temper," at how to show respect in a context where the dominant culture was disrespecting them, and also at ways of being men. Alberto linked this with his community work with a group of adults interested in promoting respectful relationships in a country that was new to them. Both groups are looking to their own cultures for wisdom on ways of standing against violence.

These efforts and many others were created by intern therapists in collaboration with those who provided narrative supervision (i.e., the three of us). The "heart" of narrative work is seeing the problem as located in sociopolitical discourse. We thus see the work of therapy as protesting oppressive practices that are promoted by dominant, subjugating discourses. We also believe that supervision is isomorphic to the therapy process. Our narrative work (and thus narrative supervision) was aimed at privileging local knowledges over global knowledge and at inviting practices that would challenge dominant discourse. This way of thinking and working may be what made room for the amazing proliferation of creative processes that intern therapists were able to construct and in which they participated, even in the short time that they worked in a school context with BAFTTA.

A STUDENT'S COMMENTS ON OUR EFFORTS TO LISTEN

Katerina, aged 12, shared her thoughts in an interview at the end of the school year about her experience with Project Respect. She had been part of a group of Latino students who had objected when it was proposed that Latino students not be allowed to wear any colors that might be associated with gangs. In a dialogue process facilitated by Susan Sandler and Shad Linscomb, the students met in a group and, in a series of meetings, listened to a group of teachers and administrators answer

---

[21]Alberto is a Latino public health worker who took time off from his other job to work with BAFTTA one-half day a week for 1 year. He worked in the Moreland School District. With Jésus Tovar, Pamela Montgomery, Lucero Arréllano, and Raoul Rojas, he has been developing narrative approaches to community work in English, Spanish, and French. They can be reached at P.O. Box 2565, Saratoga, CA 95070.

such questions as "What do we wish students knew about us?" and "What do we most want to know about students?" The young people also caucused; they talked among themselves in an inner circle about their concerns for safety and justice in their lives, and their hopes for their own futures, while the adults formed an outer-circle listening group. "What were the effects of all this?" Katerina was asked. "More trust," she answered. "Grownups heard what we had to say about wanting more things about our culture in the school. Hopefully, next year there will be more about Latinos." Another effect, she said, was that "I feel more trust for the adults involved." How did she know when an adult was trustworthy? "They have to prove it." How? "They can start by trusting kids. We trust grownups who trust kids."

How can we cultivate our trustworthiness? How do we hone our attentiveness to invitations to trust young people? How can we trust ourselves as adults to listen well and to respond respectfully?

ACCOUNTABILITY

These questions make me think of the business of school culture: the moments that come and go; the shorthand stories that can serve as cookie cutters of identity; and the power of reflection in allowing life, intentions, values, and creativity to thrive. The school is an institution—a white, middle-class institution—that is informed by and reproductive of values and injustices of the dominant society. Indeed, the goal of school is to reproduce this society's values. What do we challenge, and how do we stay accountable to young people, to communities of color, to any and all who are marginalized in any form? How do we keep some kind of commitment to justice and to just practices, as well as some kind of awareness of our position in the matrix of power and privilege? (See Waldegrave, 1990).

Our work not only attends to, but is shaped and guided by, voices from the margins. We try to stay aware of power differentials and to make sure they are as visible to those with more power and privilege as they are to those with less. It is incumbent on those of us who are members of dominant groups to take responsibility for the blind spots that come with privilege, to make room for people who have been marginalized to speak, to hear them, to check out whether we have heard, and to learn about our own practices of dominance so that we can establish alternative practices that promote partnership with and self-determination for marginalized groups (Tamasese & Waldegrave, 1993). This is an ongoing process. This needs to be a way of life.

For example, as a white woman of professional status and apparently heterosexual orientation, I (LB) was received differently than some of my colleagues who were "out" about their gay sexuality or had dark skin or spoke in ways that didn't sound like mainstream North American English. It was easier to attune to intentions in white teachers because of my experiences of acceptance in schools as I grew up. I took my welcome for granted among administrators and teachers (most of them white) until my colleagues of color told me of the subtle and not-so-subtle insults and suspicions they faced every day from school staff members. As I started to work in schools, I built relationships first with people who were most like me, and I'm sure I missed a lot of information because of lack of life experience. Listening to young people alerted me to injustices and the role of my people in perpetuating them. This in turn alerted me to further injustices, which helped me hear invitations to partnership and accountability. One of my partners in this journey is John Prowell,[22] an African-American community therapist. John has said: "It is so hard for white people to know what they don't know. They're usually not trained to understand the bind young people of color are in in the schools. As recently as 150 years ago, African-Americans were brutally punished for learning to read and write." I asked him about how white people might come to understand better. John replied: "We can talk to each other. White people can learn the stories of their ancestors, too. What seems to get in the way is when administrators want solutions to problems (thinking racism is a young person's problem) without understanding the problem, the effects of their own racist behavior—not 'name-calling' kind of racist behavior, but 'not-understanding' kind of behavior." This has led me to work harder at understanding, and also makes more obvious the importance of making sure institutions are open to the people who can actually help.

We all came into this work wanting to be helpful. Now we must continually open ourselves to being challenged on what we think we mean by "help." We need to check with the young people we think we are serving and to ask ourselves (and the people who have agreed to consult with us) what is would take to establish the kind of trust that would encourage young people to answer us honestly. How would we need to be standing, speaking, thinking, listening? How do we convey that we don't take for granted our right to ask about people's lives? And if accountability extended outside the therapy office or the school campus, how would we be living? What kinds of relationships would we have with the communities we hope to serve? And do we responsibly receive what they offer? The academic imperialism and entitlement that

[22]John can be reached by fax at (510) 558-1138.

go with our adult privilege might tempt us to take knowledge from young people and to universalize it or build a career on it. How do we make sure that young people are in charge of their own stories? Are we willing to be as "changed and affected by them as they are by us [those of us in dominant positions] every day" (Lewis, 1996)?[23]

THE MATH PROBLEM—COUNTING TRIANGLES

Remember the triangle problem described at the beginning of this chapter, and how hard it can sometimes be to find all the triangles and to count them, especially when they overlap? I (LB) have said that the task of writing about work in the schools is very much like this problem—because there are so many triangles, so many lives and stories that overlap and weave together. I have remarked that in my original experience, it might have helped if there had been someone who could accompany me, and, not assuming she knew how to help, let me teach her what I needed. I have commented that if such a person had made a mark as I outlined the triangles, I could have counted the marks.

In this account, we (LB, VD, JZ) have had lots of people accompany us as we tried to find the triangles and count them. First, we had a vision that something could be done in creating more empowering contexts in working with schools. Then came those who were intrigued by narrative ideas—intern therapists who were interested in learning, and who could look to those who had knowledges about their lives (both students and teachers) and learn from them. Then there were the school district personnel and the administrators who were interested in challenging what they experienced as having negative effects on students and on themselves, and who were willing to keep trying. There were also teachers and administrators at school sites who wanted to participate in this work of protest and wanted to collaborate to be more helpful to students.

We think we have named the central figure here—the interlocking and interrelated discourses that affect the school as institution. We have made visible some of the other figures: working with students one-on-one, helping them create and perform their lives in ways they prefer, and assisting teachers and others in the school community to act as audiences and as communities of support. We have challenged ourselves to continue to notice what has previously been invisible to us—how specifications of adultness, for example, may continue to isolate us from cre-

---

[23]Victor Lewis works at the Center for Diversity and Ethics in Oakland, CA; phone, (510) 204-9567.

ative possibilities; how racism (whiteness for many of us), heterosexual dominance, and professional class ideas continue to limit us. We have worked hard at creating contexts that support and privilege personal knowledges. And we have tried to notice how all these figures overlap, interact, and sometimes mask other meanings. We have missed some figures. That is inevitable. But we no longer feel bad about that. We have taken the position of learners. And our interest is in continuing to privilege that position.

EDITORIAL QUESTIONS

Q: *(CS) I was impressed with how wonderfully open, rich, and vivid your (LB's) own memories of school were. These triggered my own re-membrances of how often well-meaning students and adults seem to miss each other, each seemingly trapped in their own perceptions of the other. I'm also struck by how you all are courageously and successfully bridging these adult and youth worlds, and providing opportunities for both adults and students to listen to each other and to evolve in more mutually satisfying ways!*

It seems to me that you are trying to keep a delicate balance between respecting the life experiences, familiar traditions, and good intentions of administrators, teachers, and other school personnel, while also creating room for a context where "failure is impossible" with students in counseling. You also allow room for students who are marginalized (by race, class, gender, sexual orientation, etc.) to be heard and respected, while recognizing how easy it is for those in more dominant positions to feel threatened and confused by acknowledging these previously silenced students' concerns.

I imagine you have learned a lot from your experiences in these difficult balancing acts with counseling activities and with Project Respect. I am also imagining that some readers who work in schools will be very inspired by what you have accomplished and will want to start something similar, but may feel a little overwhelmed. Some of this may relate to feeling that they don't have much power in the face of long-standing ways of working and thinking more traditionally. Knowing what you know now, what sorts of suggestions might you have for people wanting to build a similar relational ethic for counseling and for school-wide interactions in their own schools, but needing to start from "ground zero"? How did you all begin this process, and how long did it take for change to begin happening? What were the most important building blocks? What might you have done differently with the benefit of hindsight?

A: (LB) It was not my intention to suggest to people how to set up such a program. I wanted to point to some considerations that may not be immediately apparent (that may be obscured by school discourses or mental health discourses). More than anything, I wanted to tell my story of some of the learnings that came from the opportunity to work in schools, and to share some of the questions it raised for us—not to mention to encourage further questioning, collaboration, and reflection.

(JZ and VD) It could be tempting to enter into schools bringing the conventional discourses that relate to joining or entering systems. These would lead to "tried and true" practices and might have some good effects. To the extent, though, that they would stop one from learning about the "alternative knowledge" discourses raised in this chapter and from developing practices related to these discourses, one would be inadvertently participating in supporting oppression and its effects on numerous students and school staff members.

Q: *(CS) You (LB) eloquently describe working narratively with Sid through an approach that externalized the problem as teachers' "tripping" and invited him to consider alternatives to this story. These sorts of things seemed to help empower him and lead to more desired outcomes. Upon reflection, you realized that your externalizing efforts inadvertently precluded you from appreciating his painful experiences of daily racism. You indicated that if you were to do it all over again, you would have asked about the effects of racism and would not have glossed over your racial differences. You also would have seen this as an invitation to open up more conversations with school staff members on racism.*

What I'm curious about is whether you look at these two different directions (helping Sid explore more preferred alternatives and being curious about racism's effects, etc.) as synergistic and mutually compatible or as mutually exclusive? Are you thinking that with hindsight, you might have externalized the effects of "racism" rather than teachers' "tripping" and his resulting reputation? If so, what might this have allowed that would be different from what occurred originally? Can you say some more about what possibilities might have resulted, had you included discussions of racism in your counseling with students?

A: (LB) Well, no, they're not mutually exclusive. Why do you ask? I'm wary about suggesting that externalizing "racism" (or any specific externalization) would be key. That would leave too much room for "therapy by the numbers" and the illusion of neutrality. As always, we try to co-construct in ways that are as close as possible to people's experience. The more blind spots I have, the harder it is to get close to people's experience. There is a history of oppression and violence between my people and the people I'm attempting to serve (Hardy, 1996). The more I learned from people of color, the more I learned that whiteness isn't a neutral thing, and this awareness now informs my conversations.

(VD and JZ) We want to underline the difference that is implicit in this question between work that is strategic/solution-focused or conversational/collaborative-language-based, and the sociopolitical work that is narrative as we know it. (See Dickerson & Zimmerman, 1996.) Not to privilege the sociopolitical context of problems is (again) supportive of oppression and leads to the use of externalization as merely a technique.

ACKNOWLEDGMENTS

As first author, LB made the major contribution to this chapter. The work with students and teachers, the projects created, the description of the work, the metaphors—all have her stamp on them. VD and JZ are grateful for their association and collaboration with her over these past years.

Many interns, student advocates, counselors, and therapists (all the names by which people have been known or called in these school settings) are named here, and many are not named. However, the three of us wish to acknowledge the contribution that all have made who have worked for BAFTTA from 1990 to 1997 and for Project Respect from 1995 to 1997 in the settings described here.

LB wishes to thank Karl Tomm for his questions, suggestions, and encouragement in her process of thinking through these ideas and putting them in written form.

REFERENCES

Bowles, S., & Gintis, H. (1976). *Schooling in capitalist America.* New York: Basic Books.

Brown, L., & Gilligan, C. (1992). *Meeting at the crossroads.* Cambridge, MA: Harvard University Press.

Denborough, D. (1994). The model of hope: Men against sexual assault—Accountability structures. *Dulwich Centre Newsletter,* Nos. 2–3, 44–54.

Denborough, D. (1996). *Beyond the prison: Gathering dreams of freedom.* Adelaide: Dulwich Centre Publications.

Dickerson, V. C., & Zimmerman, J. L. (1996). Myths, misconceptions, and a word or two about politics. *Journal of Systemic Therapies, 15*(1), 79–88.

Durrant, M. (1995). *Residential treatment: A cooperative, competency-based approach.* New York: Norton.

Epstein, E. K. (Ed.). (1996). Socially constructing substance use and abuse [Special issue]. *Journal of Systemic Therapies, 15*(2).

Frank, P. (1996, May). *Diffusing the danger.* Workshop given by VCS Batterer's Intervention Project, Rockland County, New York.

Freedman, J., & Combs, G. (1996). *Narrative therapy: The social construction of preferred realities.* New York: Norton.

Friere, P. (1970). *Pedagogy of the oppressed.* New York: Continuum.

Gilligan, C. (1990). Joining the resistance: Psychology, politics, girls and women. *Michigan Quarterly Review, 29,* 501–536.

Hall, R. (1994). Partnership accountability. *Dulwich Centre Newsletter,* Nos. 2–3, 6–29.

Hardy, K. (1996, November). *The anatomy of oppression.* Workshop sponsored by the Association of Family Therapists of Northern California, Tomales Bay, CA.

Lewis, V. (1996, September). *Beyond the color of fear.* Workshop presented at the Center for Diversity and Ethics, Oakland, CA.

Lobovits, D., Maisel, R., & Freeman, J. (1995). Public practices: An ethic of circulation. In S. Friedman (Ed.), *The reflecting team in action* (pp. 223–257). New York: Guilford Press.

McLean, C. (1994). A conversation about accountability with Michael White. *Dulwich Centre Newsletter,* Nos. 2–3, 68–79.

Nylund, D., & Corsiglia, V. (1996). From deficits to special abilities. In M. Hoyt (Ed.), *Constructive therapies* (Vol. 2, pp. 163–183). New York: Guilford Press.

Tamasese, K., & Waldegrave, C. (1993). Cultural and gender accountability in the "just therapy" approach. *Journal of Feminist Family Therapy, 5*(2), 29–45.

Waldegrave, C. (1990). Just therapy. *Dulwich Centre Newsletter,* No. 1, 6–46.

White, M. (1994, March). *Therapeutic conversations as collaborative inquiry.* Workshop in the Narrative Therapy Series for Bay Area Family Therapy Training Associates, Cupertino, CA.

White, M. (1995). Reflecting teamwork as definitional ceremony. In M. White, *Re-authoring lives: Interviews and essays* (pp. 172–198). Adelaide: Dulwich Centre Publications.

White, M. (1996, October). *Narrative therapy renewed.* Workshop in the Narrative Therapy Series for Bay Area Family Therapy Training Associates, Cupertino, CA.

White, M., & Epston, D. (1990). *Narrative means to therapeutic ends.* New York: Norton.

Zimmerman, J. L., & Dickerson, V. C. (1996). *If problems talked: Narrative therapy in action.* New York: Guilford Press.

Index